Ensuring Quality
C A N C E R *Care*

Maria Hewitt and Joseph V. Simone, *Editors*

National Cancer Policy Board

INSTITUTE OF MEDICINE
and
COMMISSION ON LIFE SCIENCES,
NATIONAL RESEARCH COUNCIL

NATIONAL ACADEMY PRESS
Washington, D.C.

NATIONAL ACADEMY PRESS • 2101 Constitution Avenue, N.W. • Washington, D.C. 20418

NOTICE: The project that is the subject of this report was approved by the Governing Board of the National Research Council, whose members are drawn from the councils of the National Academy of Sciences, the National Academy of Engineering, and the Institute of Medicine. The members of the National Cancer Policy Board, which is responsible for the report, were chosen for their special competences and with regard for appropriate balance.

The Institute of Medicine was chartered in 1970 by the National Academy of Sciences to enlist distinguished members of the appropriate professions in the examination of policy matters pertaining to the health of the public. In this, the Institute acts under both the Academy's 1863 congressional charter responsibility to be an adviser to the federal government and its own initiative in identifying issues of medical care, research, and education. Dr. Kenneth I. Shine is president of the Institute of Medicine.

The National Research Council was organized by the National Academy of Sciences in 1916 to associate the broad community of science and technology with the Academy's purposes of furthering knowledge and advising the federal government. Functioning in accordance with general policies determined by the Academy, the Council has become the principal operating agency of both the National Academy of Sciences and the National Academy of Engineering in providing services to the government, the public, and the scientific and engineering communities. The Council is administered jointly by both academies and the Institute of Medicine. Dr. Bruce M. Alberts and Dr. William A. Wulf are chairman and vice chairman, respectively, of the National Research Council.

This study was supported through funding provided by the National Cancer Institute (Contract No. NO2-CO-71024); the Centers for Disease Control and Prevention; the American Cancer Society; Amgen, Inc.; Abbott Laboratories; and Hoechst Marion Roussel, Inc. The views presented in this report are those of the National Cancer Policy Board and are not necessarily those of the funding organizations.

The full text of this report is available on line at **www.nationalacademies.org/publications/**

For more information about the Institute of Medicine and the National Cancer Policy Board, visit **www4.nationalacademies.org/iom/iomhome.nsf**

Library of Congress Cataloging-in-Publication Data

Ensuring quality cancer care / Maria Hewitt and Joseph V. Simone,
editors ; National Cancer Policy Board, Institute of Medicine and
Commission on Life Sciences, National Research Council.
  p. cm.
 Includes bibliographical references and index.
 ISBN 0-309-06480-5 (pbk.)
 1. Cancer--Treatment--United States. 2.
Cancer--Treatment--Quality control. 3.
Cancer--Patients--Care--United States. I. Hewitt, Maria Elizabeth.
II. Simone, Joseph V. III. National Cancer Policy Board (U.S.)
 RA645.C3 E57 1999
 362.1'96994'00973--dc21

        99-6488
        CIP

Cover: Constellation Cancer, the Crab. "Cancer" comes from the Latin word meaning "crab, malignant tumor."

Printed in the United States of America

NATIONAL CANCER POLICY BOARD

CONSULTANTS

BRUCE E. HILLNER, Medical College of Virginia Campus, Virginia Commonwealth
University
JEANNE S. MANDELBLATT, Georgetown University Medical Center
MARK A. SCHUSTER, University of California at Los Angeles and RAND, Santa Monica
THOMAS J. SMITH, Medical College of Virginia Campus, Virginia Commonwealth
University

INDEPENDENT REPORT REVIEWERS

This report has been reviewed in draft form by individuals chosen for their diverse perspectives and technical expertise, in accordance with procedures approved by the National Research Council's Report Review Committee. The purpose of this independent review is to provide candid and critical comments that will assist the Institute of Medicine in making the published report as sound as possible and to ensure that the report meets institutional standards for objectivity, evidence, and responsiveness to the study charge. The review comments and draft manuscript remain confidential to protect the integrity of the deliberative process. The Board wishes to thank the following individuals for their participation in the review of this report:

LU ANN ADAY, Professor, University of Texas School of Public Health

KATHLEEN ANGEL, Midway, Massachusetts

PAUL CALABRESI, Professor of Medicine and Chairman Emeritus, Brown University School of Medicine

WILLIAM H. DANFORTH, Chairman, Board of Trustees, Washington University

HAROLD P. FREEMAN, Director of Surgery, Harlem Hospital Center, and Professor of Clinical Surgery, Columbia University College of Physicians and Surgeons

PATRICIA A. GANZ, Professor, Schools of Medicine and Public Health, University of California at Los Angeles, and Director, Division of Cancer Prevention and Control Research, Jonsson Comprehensive Cancer Center, University of California at Los Angeles

DONALD R. MATTISON, March of Dimes Birth Defects Foundation, White Plains, New York

RUTH McCORKLE, Professor and Director, Center for Excellence in Chronic Illness Care and Chair, Doctoral Program, Yale University School of Nursing

DAVID P. RALL, Former Director of the National Institute of Environmental Health Sciences, Research Triangle Park, North Carolina

ROSEMARY ROSSO, Greater Baltimore-Washington Breast Cancer Advocacy Group, Washington, D.C.

While the individuals listed above have provided constructive comments and suggestions, it must be emphasized that responsibility for the final content of this report rests entirely with the authoring Board and the Institute of Medicine.

Contents

Summary

We all want to believe that when people get cancer—including ourselves and our relatives—they will get health care of the highest quality. Concerns about a growing lack of public confidence in the nation's system of care prompted the National Cancer Policy Board to undertake a comprehensive review of the evidence on the effectiveness of cancer services and delivery systems, the adequacy of quality assurance mechanisms, and barriers that impede access to cancer care. The National Cancer Policy Board (NCPB) was established in March 1997 at the Institute of Medicine (IOM) and National Research Council to address issues that arise in the prevention, control, diagnosis, treatment, and palliation of cancer. The 20-member board includes consumers, health care providers, and investigators in several disciplines. The NCPB report, *Ensuring Quality Cancer Care*, addresses five questions:

1. What is the state of the cancer care "system"?
2. What is quality cancer care and how is it measured?
3. What cancer care quality problems are evident and what steps can be taken to improve care?
4. How can we improve what we know about the quality of cancer care?
5. What steps can be taken to overcome barriers to access to quality cancer care?

WHAT IS THE STATE OF THE CANCER CARE "SYSTEM"?

The National Cancer Policy Board began its deliberations on quality by trying to describe what an ideal cancer care system would look and feel like from the vantage point of an individual receiving cancer care. The NCPB suggested that, for many, excellence in cancer care would be achieved if individuals had:

- access to comprehensive and coordinated services;
- confidence in the experience and training of their providers;

1

- a feeling that providers respected them, listened to them, and advocated on their behalf;
- an ability to ask questions and voice opinions comfortably, to be full participants in all decisions regarding care;
- a clear understanding of their diagnosis and access to information to aid this understanding;
- awareness of all treatment options and of the risks and benefits associated with each;
- confidence that recommended treatments are appropriate, offering the best chance of a good outcome consistent with personal preferences;
- a prospective plan for treatment and palliation;
- a health care professional responsible (and accountable) for organizing this plan in partnership with each individual; and
- assurances that agreed-upon national standards of quality care are met at their site of care.

The NCPB then described at least some aspects of a cancer care *system* that would support such an ideal state of care. A system of ideal cancer care would

- articulate goals consistent with this vision of quality cancer care;
- implement policies to achieve these goals;
- identify barriers to the practice and receipt of quality care and target interventions to overcome these barriers;
- further efforts to coordinate the currently diverse systems of care;
- ensure appropriate training for cancer care providers;
- have mechanisms in place to facilitate the translation of research to clinical practice;
- monitor and ensure the quality of care; and
- conduct research necessary to further the understanding of effective cancer care.

The NCPB has concluded that for many Americans with cancer, there is a wide gulf between what could be construed as the ideal and the reality of their experience with cancer care.

There is no national cancer care program or system of care in the United States. Like other chronic illnesses, efforts to diagnose and treat cancer are centered on individual physicians, health plans, and cancer care centers. The ad hoc and fragmented cancer care system does not ensure access to care, lacks coordination, and is inefficient in its use of resources. The authority to organize, coordinate, and improve cancer care services rests largely with service providers and insurers. At numerous sites in the federal government, programs and research directly relate to the quality of cancer care, but in no one place are these disparate efforts coordinated or even described. Efforts to improve cancer care in many cases will therefore be local or regional and could feasibly originate in a physician's practice, a hospital, or a managed care plan. Because cancer disproportionately affects the elderly, the Medicare program could be an important vehicle for change. Certainly, issues related to quality cancer care have to be addressed at the national and state levels, in coordination with other quality-of-care efforts.

WHAT IS QUALITY CANCER CARE AND HOW IS IT MEASURED?

Health care can be judged as good to the extent that it increases the likelihood of desired health outcomes and is consistent with current professional knowledge (IOM, 1990). In practical terms, poor quality can mean

- overuse (e.g., unnecessary tests, medication, and procedures, with associated risks and side effects);
- underuse (e.g., not receiving a lifesaving surgical procedure); or
- misuse (e.g., medicines that should not be given together, poor surgical technique).

Quality care means providing patients with appropriate services in a technically competent manner, with good communication, shared decision making, and cultural sensitivity.

The first step in assessing quality of care is establishing which attributes of care are linked to optimal outcomes (e.g., survival, enhanced quality of life). Large, carefully designed clinical trials are usually necessary to establish which specific processes of care or treatments are effective. Early detection of breast cancer through screening mammography, for example, has been shown to reduce mortality significantly for women age 50 and older. Other types of research, notably health services research, also have a role to play in defining high-quality care. Next, observations of current medical practice—for example, through reviews of a sample of medical records—reveal the extent to which effective care is being applied. Measures of quality may assess structural aspects of the health care delivery system (e.g., hospital case volume), processes of care (e.g., use of screening), or outcomes of care (e.g., survival, quality of life). Each of these dimensions of quality could be assessed to provide complementary information.

WHAT PROBLEMS ARE EVIDENT IN THE QUALITY OF CANCER CARE AND WHAT STEPS CAN BE TAKEN TO IMPROVE CARE?

More is known about the quality of care for breast cancer than for any other kind of cancer. Treatment of early breast cancer saves lives, and early detection through screening contributes to early diagnosis, when treatment is most effective. When established quality measures have been used to assess the care women receive, the following quality problems have been identified:

- underuse of mammography to detect cancer early;
- lack of adherence to standards for diagnosis (e.g., inadequate biopsies, poor reporting of pathology studies);
- inadequate patient counseling regarding treatment options; and
- underuse of radiation therapy and adjuvant chemotherapy after surgery.

The consequences of these lapses in care are, in some cases, reduced survival and, in others, compromised quality of life.

Based on the best available evidence, some individuals with cancer do not receive care known to be effective for their condition. The magnitude of the problem is not known, but the National Cancer Policy Board believes it is substantial. The reasons for failure to deliver high-quality care have not been studied adequately, nor has there been much investigation of how appropriate standards vary from patient to patient.

The means for improving the quality of cancer care, which involve changes in the health care system, are the first five of a total of ten recommendations of the National Cancer Policy Board. Implementation of these recommendations may vary by locality and by system of care with, for example, different mechanisms needed in rural versus urban areas, or for particularly high-risk or underserved populations.

Cancer care is optimally delivered in systems of care that:

RECOMMENDATION 1: Ensure that patients undergoing procedures that are technically difficult to perform and have been associated with higher mortality in lower-volume settings receive care at facilities with extensive experience (i.e., high-volume facilities). Examples of such procedures include removal of all or part of the esophagus, surgery for pancreatic cancer, removal of pelvic organs, and complex chemotherapy regimens.

Many aspects of the delivery of health care can potentially affect its quality. There is convincing evidence of a relationship between treatment in higher-volume hospitals and better short-term survival for individuals with several types of cancer for which high-risk surgery is indicated (e.g., pancreatic cancer, non-small-cell lung cancer). Several studies show very large effects, with lower-volume hospitals having postsurgical mortality rates two to three times higher than hospitals that do more such procedures. A dose–response effect is also evident to support the finding that as volume increases, so do good outcomes. The findings cut across cancer types and systems of care, sharing the common element of complicated medical or surgical intervention. Although estimates are imprecise, a relatively large share of high-risk surgery is taking place in lower-volume settings (e.g., from one-quarter to one-half of surgical procedures for pancreatic cancer).

More limited data show a relationship between surgery performed at higher-volume hospitals and better outcomes for men with prostate cancer who undergo radical prostatectomy and for women who undergo breast cancer surgery. A few studies of the management of other types of cancer (i.e., testicular cancer, leukemia) also show a relationship between higher volume and better outcome. This volume–outcome relationship appears to be strong, and consistent with findings from other areas of complex care (e.g., coronary revascularization procedures).

Even in the absence of extensive data for each particular cancer type and stage, evidence strongly indicates that health outcomes are better in high-volume settings for highly technical cancer management.

RECOMMENDATION 2: Use systematically developed guidelines based on the best available evidence for prevention, diagnosis, treatment, and palliative care.

Total quality improvement initiatives, disease management programs, and implementation of clinical practice guidelines all have the potential to improve care within health systems. Information about clinical practice can serve as a powerful tool to change physician and patient behavior and to improve the use of effective treatments. The experience with oncology practice guidelines has been mixed, however, with some examples of success, but other examples of failure to change provider behavior or outcomes. Many guideline efforts have failed because of flaws in the way the guidelines were developed or implemented. Evidence suggests that care can be improved when providers themselves are involved in shaping guidelines and when systems of accountability are in place. Such efforts must be intensified.

RECOMMENDATION 3: Measure and monitor the quality of care using a core set of quality measures.

Once effective care has been identified through the research system, mechanisms to develop and implement measurement systems are needed. Translating research results into quality monitoring measures is a complex process that will require significant research investments. There is now a broad consensus about how to assess some aspects of quality of care for many common cancers (e.g., cancers of the breast, colon, lung, prostate, and cervix), but specific measures of the quality of care for these cancers are still being developed and tested within health delivery systems.

Systematic improvements in health care quality will likely only occur through collaborative efforts of the public and private sectors. As large health care purchasers, both sectors have a stake in improving the quality of care, and both sectors have knowledge and experience concerning quality measurement and reporting. A public–private collaborative approach has recently been recommended by the President's Advisory Commission on Consumer Protection and Quality in the Health Care Industry, and some initial implementation steps are being taken (President's Advisory Commission, 1998).

Cancer care quality measures should span the continuum of cancer care and be developed through a coordinated public–private effort.

To ensure the rapid translation of research into practice, a mechanism is needed to quickly identify the results of research with quality-of-care implications and ensure that it is applied in monitoring quality. In a few areas, evidence suggests that care does not meet national standards for interventions known to improve care. After primary prevention, cancer screening is the most effective method to reduce the burden of cancer, yet screening is underused. It is often health care providers who can be held accountable for the underuse of cancer screening tests. One of the strongest predictors of whether a person will be screened for cancer is whether the physician recommends it, and evidence suggests that physicians order fewer cancer screening tests than they should. Even when screening is accomplished, many individuals fail to receive timely, or any, follow-up of an abnormal screening test. Both screening and follow-up rates can be improved with interventions aimed both at those eligible for screening and at health care providers (e.g., reminder systems). Implementation of accountability systems can greatly increase participation in cancer screening.

Cancer care quality measures should be used to hold providers, including health care systems, health plans, and physicians, accountable for demonstrating that they provide and improve quality of care.

There are many opportunities to exert leverage on the health care system to improve quality. Quality assurance systems are often not apparent to consumers, but have the potential to greatly affect their care:

• large employer groups are holding managed care plans accountable for quality performance goals;

• the Health Care Financing Administration (HCFA, which funds Medicare and the federal component of Medicaid) requires Medicare and Medicaid health plans to produce standard quality reports; and

• state Medicaid programs are beginning to include quality provisions in their contracts with plans and providers.

Six of ten new cancer cases occur among people age 65 and older and, consequently, Medicare is the principal payer for cancer care. There is generally a lack of quality-related data from fee-for-service providers from whom most Medicare beneficiaries receive their care. Information systems are, however, in place that allow the reporting on a regional basis of some quality indicators (e.g., cancer screening rates) relevant to those in fee-for-service systems. For Medicare beneficiaries in managed care plans, accountability systems should incorporate core measures of quality cancer care.

Cancer care quality measures should be applied to care provided through the Medicare and Medicaid programs as a requirement for participation in these programs.

The collection, reporting, and analysis of information about the quality of cancer care will be expensive. Many segments of the health care industry will invest in information systems to maximize efficiency and to stay competitive, however, some may require incentives to provide patient-level data.

Information about quality cancer care is becoming more available to individuals with cancer (or at risk for cancer), but it is not yet easily accessible or understandable to consumers. A number of potential quality indicators can be listed, but most have not been evaluated to assess their ultimate value for consumers. It is unclear, for example, how the following indicators affect an individual's experience of care or health care outcomes:

• a physician's board certification,

• a hospital's approval status, for example, as determined by the American College of Surgeons' Commission on Cancer, and

• a health plan's accreditation status and quality scores from the National Committee for Quality Assurance.

By the time a diagnosis of cancer is made and individuals have a clear reason to seek quality care, it is often too late to switch health plans. Also, even if they wanted to, most people do not have access to alternative plans. Individuals may use available quality indicators to choose doctors and hospitals within their plans, and perhaps to choose alternative courses of treatment, but evidence suggests that individual consumers can exert only a modest "market" pressure for quality improvement through access to better information about the quality of cancer care. Large purchasers, such as employers are likely to exert more leverage and to have designated staff to assess alternative plans.

Cancer care quality measures should be disseminated widely and communicated to purchasers, providers, consumer organizations, individuals with cancer, policy makers, and health services researchers, in a form that is relevant and useful for health care decision-making.

Quality measures enable consumers and purchasers to judge the quality of a system of care by its performance relative to evidence-based standards.

RECOMMENDATION 4: Ensure the following elements of quality care for each individual with cancer:

- **that recommendations about initial cancer management, which are critical in determining long-term outcome, are made by experienced professionals;**
- **an agreed-upon care plan that outlines goals of care;**
- **access to the full complement of resources necessary to implement the care plan;**
- **access to high-quality clinical trials;**
- **policies to ensure full disclosure of information about appropriate treatment options;**
- **a mechanism to coordinate services; and**
- **psychosocial support services and compassionate care.**

Some elements of care simply make sense—that is, they have strong face validity and can reasonably be assumed to improve care unless and until evidence accumulates to the contrary. This recommendation amounts to a statement of the ideal, based on principles of cancer care articulated by cancer survivors. Details of how to interpret and apply the principles will vary according to health plan, cancer type, stage of disease, and preferences of the individual needing care.

RECOMMENDATION 5: Ensure quality of care at the end of life, in particular, the management of cancer-related pain and timely referral to palliative and hospice care.

Cancer is the second leading cause of death in the United States. A strong body of evidence suggests that the experience of dying for many with cancer can be greatly improved with better palliative care (IOM, 1997). Many individuals with cancer suffer pain needlessly and have their treatment preferences ignored. Practice guidelines are available to assist health care providers in this area, but they have not been adopted widely. Financial barriers limit effective care for people at the end of life. Additional studies are needed to identify nonfinancial barriers to appropriate end-of-life care.

HOW CAN WE IMPROVE WHAT WE KNOW ABOUT THE QUALITY OF CANCER CARE?

For many aspects of cancer care, it is not yet possible to assess quality because the first step in quality assessment has not been taken—the conduct of clinical trials. Consequently, for many types of cancer, answers to the following basic questions are not yet available:

• How frequently should patients be evaluated following their primary cancer therapy, what tests should be included in the follow-up regimen, and who should provide follow-up care?
• What is the most effective way to manage recurrent cancers, or cancers first identified at late stages?

> **RECOMMENDATION 6: Federal and private research sponsors such as the National Cancer Institute, the Agency for Health Care Policy and Research, and various health plans should invest in clinical trials to address questions about cancer care management.**

For some questions regarding cancer management, a health services research component could possibly be integrated into a clinical trial designed to assess the efficacy of a new treatment. For other questions, innovative units of randomization could be used, for example, randomizing providers (instead of patients) to test different clinical management strategies. Such trials have been used to assess educational and service delivery topics (e.g., colorectal screening performed by nurse clinicians, counseling patients to quit smoking).

> **RECOMMENDATION 7: A cancer data system is needed that can provide quality benchmarks for use by systems of care (such as hospitals, provider groups, and managed care systems).**

Toward that end, in 1999, the National Cancer Policy Board will hold workshops to:

• identify how best to meet the data needs for cancer in light of quality monitoring goals;
• identify financial and other resources needed to improve the cancer data system to achieve quality-related goals; and
• develop strategies to improve data available on the quality of cancer care.

The second step of quality assessment involves surveillance—making sure that evidence regarding what works is applied in practice. Ideally, quality assessment studies would include recently diagnosed individuals with cancer in care settings representative of contemporary practice across the country, using information sources with sufficient detail to allow appropriate comparisons. The available evidence on the quality of cancer care is far from this ideal.

Two national databases are available with which to assess the quality of cancer care, but each has limitations.

1. The Surveillance, Epidemiology, and End Results (SEER) cancer registry, maintained by the National Cancer Institute (NCI), when linked to Medicare and other insurance administrative files, has been valuable in assessing the quality of care for the elderly and other insured populations. It is also useful in identifying a sample of cases for in-depth studies of quality-related issues. The SEER registry, however, covers only 14 percent of the U.S. population in certain geographic locations, so it may not adequately represent the diversity of systems of care. Finding ways to capture measures of process of care, treatment information, and intermediate outcomes—and to improving the timeliness of reporting—would enhance the registry's use in quality assessment.

2. The National Cancer Data Base (NCDB), a joint project of the American College of Surgeons' Commission on Cancer and the American Cancer Society, now holds information on more than half of all newly diagnosed cases of cancer nationwide and includes many of the demographic, clinical, and health system data elements necessary to assess quality of care. A limitation of the NCDB is the absence of complete information on outpatient care. The NCDB has not yet been widely used to assess quality of care, but it has great potential for doing so.

Existing data systems must be enhanced so that questions about quality of care can be answered comprehensively, on a national scale, without delays of many years between data collection and analysis. An effective system would capture information about:

- individuals with cancer (e.g., age, race and ethnicity, socioeconomic status, insurance or health plan coverage);
- their condition (e.g., stage, grade, histological pattern, comorbid conditions);
- their treatment, including significant outpatient treatments (e.g., adjuvant therapy, radiation therapy);
- their providers (e.g., specialty training);
- site of care delivery (e.g., community hospital, cancer center);
- type of care delivery system (e.g., managed care, fee for service); and
- outcomes (e.g., satisfaction, relapse, complications, quality of life, survival time, death).

It may be costly and difficult to obtain all of the desired data elements for all individuals with available sources, so sampling techniques could be used to make the task manageable for targeted studies. Alternatively, it may be feasible to link some databases (e.g., those describing structural aspects of care such as hospital characteristics) to other existing databases. It is unlikely that one single database can meet all of the various objectives of such systems, for example, cancer surveillance, research, and quality monitoring. Data systems need to be monitored to assure accuracy, and should be automated to improve the timeliness of quality data. Data gathered into national databases, in particular, should be made available quickly for analysis by investigators and evaluators.

RECOMMENDATION 8: Public and private sponsors of cancer care research should support national studies of recently diagnosed individuals with

cancer, using information sources with sufficient detail to assess patterns of cancer care and factors associated with the receipt of good care. Research sponsors should also support training for cancer care providers interested in health services research.

Grants to support the analysis of data that focus on pressing health policy questions, especially about how the organization and financing of cancer care affect the processes and outcomes of care, should be a high priority. Methodologic research is also needed to improve the quality of cancer-related health services research, for example, to develop tools for "case-mix" adjustments to reduce the potential for bias inherent in observational cancer research.

An annual report that provides a description of the status of cancer-related quality-of-care research, and summarizes relevant published literature in the area would serve as a valuable resource for health services researchers and those involved in quality assessment. Such a report would also help organizations set priorities for research, ensure that their research portfolios address important quality-of-care questions, and ensure that their research programs are complementary and coordinated.

WHAT STEPS CAN BE TAKEN TO OVERCOME BARRIERS OF ACCESS TO QUALITY CANCER CARE?

RECOMMENDATION 9: Services for the un- and underinsured should be enhanced to ensure entry to, and equitable treatment within, the cancer care system.

Cancer is among the most expensive conditions to treat, and individuals with cancer and their families invariably bear some of the financial burden. Most individuals diagnosed with cancer are elderly and have Medicare coverage, but an estimated 7 percent of individuals facing a new diagnosis of cancer lack any health insurance at all. For these individuals, cancer can be catastrophic to their finances as well as their health. The problem that affects far more individuals, however, is underinsurance—health plans and insurance coverage offer some, but often incomplete, protection against the high costs of cancer care. High deductibles, copayments or coinsurance, and coverage caps can all contribute to high out-of-pocket expenditures. Medicare, for example, was estimated to cover only 83 percent of typical total charges for lung cancer and 65 percent of charges for breast cancer in 1986. Some individuals have additional protection through other insurers (e.g., Medigap policies or Medicaid), but despite this, the financial burden of cancer can be substantial even among those covered by a health plan. Limits on prescription drug coverage, an expensive and widely used benefit (e.g., outpatient pain medications), are a particular problem for many with cancer because the drugs are often expensive. A limited number of free services or financial assistance programs are available to people with cancer, but they do not substitute for adequate insurance coverage for cancer treatment.

RECOMMENDATION 10: Studies are needed to find out why specific segments of the population (e.g., members of certain racial or ethnic groups, older patients) do not receive appropriate cancer care. These studies should

measure provider and individual knowledge, attitudes, and beliefs, as well as other potential barriers to access to care.

While access problems persist throughout cancer care, overcoming barriers to screening and early detection is a priority because after primary prevention, the greatest improvements in outcomes will be realized by identifying cancers early, when treatments are most effective. Moreover, initial planning is extremely important for many types of cancer, because failure on the first treatment severely limits subsequent treatment options due to the nature of cancer progression. Evidence suggests that much of the disparity in mortality by race could be reduced by improving access to primary care and cancer screening.

A number of public and private programs have enhanced access to care. The Centers for Disease Control and Prevention's National Breast and Cervical Cancer Early Detection Program provides screening for women unable to afford care. A few states have launched special programs to pay for cancer care for the poor and uninsured (e.g., the Maryland program for women with breast cancer). Many pharmaceutical companies have patient assistance programs to help defray the costs of expensive chemotherapy drugs. These programs and services cannot substitute for adequate insurance coverage for cancer treatment, but they can ease the financial burden for those eligible to receive them.

Although having health insurance coverage improves access, it does not guarantee good care. Several factors other than insurance status and cost can prevent people from "getting to the door" of a health care provider. These include fear of a diagnosis of cancer, distrust of health care providers, language, geography, and difficulties in getting through appointment systems. Incomplete understanding of cancer risk or certain beliefs, such as the belief that one is not at risk or that nothing can be done to change one's fate, may also prevent people from seeking care. Once "in the door," other barriers to access may surface when attempting to navigate the system: for example, getting from a primary care provider to a specialist. Within the system, providers may have difficulty communicating with patients or have insufficient staff to coordinate care and provide all the services patients need. The cancer care system is complex, and different barriers may impede access to care at different phases.

Individuals who have low educational attainment or are members of certain racial or ethnic minority groups face higher barriers to receiving cancer care and tend to have less favorable outcomes than other groups.* Limited access to primary care and cancer screening contributes to having cancer diagnosed at latter stages when prognosis is worse. Differences in treatment by race have been well documented; however, it appears that the effect may actually be more closely related to social class than to race.

Those of advanced age also appear to be vulnerable in the cancer care system. Older people are less likely than younger people to receive effective cancer treatments, despite evidence that the elderly can tolerate and benefit from them. Some undertreatment is explained by provider attitudes toward treating the elderly, who are perceived as less willing or able to tolerate aggressive treatment. Some undertreatment may also be due to patient preferences and unwillingness to experience the side effects of certain treatments.

---

*Research in this area sponsored by the National Institutes of Health is addressed in the 1999 IOM report, *The Unequal Burden of Cancer: An Assessment of NIH Research and Programs for Ethnic Minorities and the Medically Underserved* (IOM, 1999).

REFERENCES

IOM (Institute of Medicine). 1990. *Medicare: A Strategy for Quality Assurance*, KN Lohr, ed. Washington, D.C.: National Academy Press.

IOM. 1997. *Approaching Death: Improving Care at the End of Life*. MJ Field, CK Cassel, eds. Washington, D.C.: National Academy Press.

IOM. 1999. *The Unequal Burden of Cancer: An Assessment of NIH Research and Programs for Ethnic Minorities and the Medically Underserved*. MA Haynes, BD Smedley, eds. Washington, D.C.: National Academy Press.

President's Advisory Commission on Consumer Protection and Quality in the Health Care Industry. 1998. *Quality First: Better Health Care for All Americans*. Washington, D.C.

1

Introduction

We all want to believe that when people get cancer—including ourselves and our relatives—they will get health care of the highest quality. This report is about how closely we currently approach this ideal in the United States. Concerns about a growing lack of public confidence in the nation's system of care prompted the National Cancer Policy Board to undertake a comprehensive review of the evidence on the effectiveness of cancer services and delivery systems, the adequacy of quality assurance mechanisms, and barriers that impede access to cancer care. This report is the result of that review; it summarizes the state of knowledge about quality cancer care and makes recommendations about how to improve it.

The stakes are high. In 1999, more than 8 million Americans, or 3 percent of the population, will require some form of care because of a diagnosis of cancer: 1.2 million of these individuals will be newly diagnosed this year and initiate treatment; some, diagnosed in previous years, will continue treatment; others, who have been successfully treated and no longer have evidence of cancer, will require follow-up care; and over 500,000 people will die from cancer. Even larger numbers of adults in the United States will have been screened for cancer (ACS, 1999; Ries et al., 1997).

As exciting new scientific advances are making the news, there are concerns that what is already known to be effective for individuals with cancer is not reaching those who can benefit. This concern is not new; it was prominent among the reasons for the 1971 National Cancer Act (P.L. 92-218) and was expressed again as recently as 1994 in a report of the National Cancer Advisory Board (NCAB, 1994), *Cancer at a Crossroads*. At the same time, there is both uncertainty about the relative effectiveness of many interventions that are being used and a growing recognition that research efforts need to be expanded to identify standards of care (IOM, 1994). Complicating the picture is the rapid evolution of new health care delivery systems, whose impact on cancer care outcomes remains unclear.

Major shifts in the organization and financing of health care in the United States have precipitated a crisis in confidence. A growing number of Americans are uninsured, even more are underinsured, and many who are covered in health plans are worried that the system for delivering health care is more focused on cost than on quality. They wonder whether they will be referred appropriately to someone expert in cancer treatment and whether health professionals will be their advocates or the guardians of expenditures. The general concerns about health care are magnified among those with cancer because of the fearsome nature of the disease, the complexity of cancer management, the frequent reliance upon new and experimental interventions, and the high costs associated with cancer care.

The experience of each individual with cancer is unique, affected by the type of cancer (there are more than 100) and the extent to which it has progressed. Each individual's experience is also influenced by socioeconomic status, insurance coverage, geographic location, and culturally based attitudes and beliefs. Finding the best cancer care and navigating through the complex care system can be difficult. Care spans screening, early detection, treatment, follow-up, palliative care, and sometimes end-of-life care. Numerous health professionals in hospitals, clinics, and private offices may all be involved. For certain individuals with cancer the best treatment option might only be available far from home at a specialized cancer center.

Primary care physicians may guide patients through the initial stages of the diagnostic process. In some cases, entry into the cancer care system may be the result of public health screening rather than primary care. Once a diagnosis is made, charting a course for treatment may involve second or multiple opinions from cancer specialists, who might recommend different treatment options. Clinicians have agreed upon standard ways to treat some types of cancer, but for others, no evidence-based consensus exists. While adjusting to having cancer and the fear that it engenders, individuals frequently need to learn quickly about unfamiliar treatments and make difficult treatment choices.

Some evidence suggests that quality falls short for many individuals with cancer. Various cancer control and treatment strategies of known effectiveness, such as regular screening for cervical cancer and mammography in women over 50, are underutilized (NCHS, 1997). In certain regions, radical or modified mastectomies are still performed for breast cancer, despite evidence that less invasive procedures are at least as effective in many situations (Fisher et al., 1985; Sarrazin et al., 1984; Veronesi et al., 1981). In some circumstances, most notably care in the latter phases of advanced cancer, providers fail to elicit, understand, and heed patient preferences (SUPPORT, 1995).

ROLE OF THE NATIONAL CANCER POLICY BOARD

The National Cancer Policy Board (NCPB) was established in March 1997 at the Institute of Medicine (IOM) and National Research Council to address issues that arise in the prevention, control, diagnosis, treatment, and palliation of cancer. The 20-member board includes health care consumers, providers, and investigators in several disciplines (see membership roster). In its first report, *Taking Action to Reduce Tobacco Use*, the NCPB addressed the foremost known cause of cancer in the nation (NCPB, 1998).

This second NCPB report, *Ensuring Quality Cancer Care,*

• describes important elements of the current cancer care "system," from early detection to end-of-life care, in the context of the rapidly changing health care environment;

- identifies major barriers that impede access to quality cancer care;
- defines quality cancer care and describes its measurement;
- provides examples of problems that limit early detection, accurate diagnosis, optimal treatment, and responsive supportive care;
- reviews and critiques systems of accountability that are in place to help ensure the receipt of quality cancer care;
- assesses whether ongoing cancer-related health services research is addressing outstanding questions about the quality of cancer care; and
- presents recommendations to enhance cancer care for consideration by Congress, public and private health care purchasers, health plans, individual consumers, health care providers, and researchers.

The NCPB convened a public forum on March 31, 1997 and also listened to presentations by federal agency representatives at its quarterly meetings. Staff and Board members participated in a series of President's Cancer Panel meetings on quality issues in cancer care (PCP, 1998a–c). In addition, five background papers on cancer care quality issues were commissioned to support this report:[*]

- two reviews of the health services literature related to quality cancer care (Hillner and Smith, 1998; Schuster et al., 1998);
- a case study of model cancer care programs (Smith et al., 1998);
- an analysis of the state of clinical practice guidelines for cancer care (Smith et al., 1998); and
- a review of the literature on barriers to access to cancer care (Mandelblatt et al., 1998).

Primary cancer prevention (i.e., preventing people from getting cancer in the first place), recognized as key to effectively curbing cancer, was viewed by the NCPB as outside the scope of this report. The Board believes strongly in the value of prevention, as witnessed by its first report on tobacco control, but prevention merits its own specific attention and fits better into other activities the Board anticipates undertaking in the future than into this report, which focuses on the system of medical care.

FRAMEWORK OF THE REPORT

Chapter 2 describes the trajectory of cancer management, from early detection and treatment to end-of-life care, and the existing cancer care infrastructure. The chapter concludes with a summary of the effects on cancer care of recent changes in the organization, financing, and delivery of health care.

Chapter 3 discusses barriers to access to cancer care. A new diagnosis of cancer in the absence of comprehensive health insurance coverage provides a case illustration of the difficulties of achieving access to care and the potentially devastating financial consequences of cancer.

---

[*]These papers are available on the NCPB website (www.nas.edu/cancerbd).

Even in the absence of financial barriers, individuals may not receive quality care because of where they live, language or cultural barriers, and late adoption on the part of health care providers of effective interventions.

Chapter 4 defines quality cancer care, describes the ways in which it can be measured, and documents important gaps in the quality of care for individuals with breast or prostate cancer, two cancers for which there have been quality assessments.

Chapter 5 summarizes evidence on the ways in which three aspects of the health care delivery system can affect the quality of cancer care: (1) the volume of services provided either by institutions or by individual providers; (2) specialization in cancer care either by institutions or by individual providers; and (3) managed care.

Chapter 6 reviews and critiques the means of monitoring quality and accountability that are in place.

Chapter 7 surveys ongoing health services research that addresses cancer-related quality issues sponsored by selected federal agencies and private organizations.

Chapter 8 summarizes the key findings and presents the Board's recommendations for action by Congress, health care purchasers, health plans, health care providers, individual consumers, and health services researchers.

REFERENCES

American Cancer Society. 1999. *Cancer Facts and Figures—1999*. Atlanta, GA.

Chassin MR, Gavin RW. 1998. The urgent need to improve health care quality. Institute of Medicine National Roundtable on Health Care Quality. *Journal of the American Medical Association* 280(11):1000–1005.

Fisher B, Bauer M, Margolese R, et al. 1985. Five-year results of a randomized clinical trial comparing total mastectomy and segmental mastectomy with or without radiation in the treatment of breast cancer. *New England Journal of Medicine* 312:665–673.

Hillner BE, Smith TJ. 1998. The quality of cancer care: Does the literature support the rhetoric? National Cancer Policy Board commissioned paper.

IOM (Institute of Medicine). 1990. *Medicare: A Strategy for Quality Assurance*, KN Lohr, ed. Washington, D.C.: National Academy Press.

IOM. 1994. *America's Health in Transition: Protecting and Improving Quality*. A Statement of the Council of the Institute of Medicine. Washington, D.C.: National Academy Press.

Mandelblatt J, Yabroff KR, Kerner J. 1998. Access to quality cancer care: Evaluating and ensuring equitable services, quality of life and survival. National Cancer Policy Board commissioned paper.

National Cancer Advisory Board. 1994. *Cancer at a Crossroads: A Report to Congress for the Nation*. Bethesda, MD: National Cancer Institute.

National Cancer Policy Board. 1998. *Taking Action to Reduce Tobacco Use*. Washington, D.C.: National Academy Press.

National Center for Health Statistics. 1997. *Healthy People 2000 Review*. Hyattsville, MD: U.S. Department of Health and Human Services, Public Health Service.

President's Cancer Panel. 1998a. Meeting on Quality of Care/Quality of Life. Los Angeles, California, April 23.

President's Cancer Panel. 1998b. Meeting on Quality of Care/Quality of Life. New Haven, Connecticut, June 2.

President's Cancer Panel. 1998c. Meeting on Quality of Care/Quality of Life. Buffalo, New York. October 6.

Ries LAG, Kosary CL, Hankey BF, et al., eds. 1997. *SEER Cancer Statistics Review, 1973–1994.* NIH Pub. No. 97-2789. Bethesda, MD: National Cancer Institute, National Institutes of Health.

Sarrazin D, Le M, Rouesse J, et al. 1984. Conservative treatment versus mastectomy in breast cancer tumors with macroscopic diameter of 20 millimeters or less: The experience of the Institut Gustave-Roussy. *Cancer* 53:1209–1213.

Schuster MA, Reifel JL, McGuigan K. 1998. Assessment of the quality of cancer care: A review for the National Cancer Policy Board of the Institute of Medicine. National Cancer Policy Board commissioned paper.

Smith TJ, Hillner BE. 1998. Ensuring quality cancer care: Clinical practice guidelines, critical pathways, and care maps. National Cancer Policy Board commissioned paper.

Smith TJ, Desch CE, Hillner BE. 1998. Ensuring quality cancer care: Models of excellence. National Cancer Policy Board commissioned paper.

SUPPORT Principal Investigators. 1995. A controlled trial to improve care for seriously ill hospitalized patients. The study to understand prognoses and preferences for outcomes and risks of treatments (SUPPORT). *Journal of the American Medical Association* 274(20):1591–1598.

Veronesi U, Saccozzi R, Del Vecchio M, et al. 1981. Comparing radical mastectomy with quandrantectomy, axillary dissection, and radiotherapy in patients with small cancers of the breast. *New England Journal of Medicine* 305:6–11.

2

The Cancer Care "System"

There is no national cancer care program or system of care in the United States. Like other chronic illnesses, efforts to diagnose and treat cancer are centered on individual physicians, health plans, and cancer care centers. The authority to organize, coordinate, and improve cancer care services rests largely with service providers and insurers, although employers and other payers are increasingly holding providers accountable for quality, and consumers are calling for action by state and federal legislatures. Nevertheless, there is a federal research and programmatic infrastructure that greatly affects the quality of cancer care obtained within the U.S. health care system. This chapter describes:

- elements of the federal cancer care effort;
- elements of cancer care: who gets care, what services are provided, who provides care, where it is provided, and at what cost; and
- aspects of health care organization and financing that affect cancer care.

ELEMENTS OF THE FEDERAL CANCER CARE EFFORT

Although there is no national cancer care system, substantial public investments in research, training, prevention, and information dissemination have been made in an attempt to improve cancer care in the United States. The federal infrastructure is larger and more complex than that for other medical conditions. Since the "War on Cancer" was launched in 1971, a large share of federal medical research funding has been invested at the National Cancer Institute (NCI) to understand the underlying mechanisms of cancer, to evaluate progress against cancer through surveillance, to test promising diagnostic and treatment modalities, and to make information on how to prevent, treat, and live with cancer available to health care providers and to the public. At the Centers for Disease Control and Prevention, ongoing efforts to reduce the burden of cancer include providing cancer screening to low-income populations and monitoring the achievement of cancer-related public health goals (see Chapter 6). Elsewhere in the federal government, the Agency for Health Care Policy and Research disseminates information about clinical practice guidelines to health providers and supports health services research aimed at understanding the links between the organization and delivery of health care and the resulting health outcomes (see Chapter 7). The federal Health Care Financing Administration (HCFA), as the nation's largest payer for health care, has established quality assurance programs targeting cancer care and is developing tools to more effectively monitor the quality of cancer care delivered to Medicare beneficiaries (see Chapter 6).

Although there are numerous sites within the federal government whose programs and research directly relate to the quality of cancer care, there is no system in place to coordinate these efforts. This has not always been the case. Although the effort failed, an attempt was made during the 1970s to coordinate federal and private cancer research programs through the National Cancer Program.

The 1971 War on Cancer Act (P.L. 92-218) created a National Cancer Program, headed by the director of the NCI to coordinate both federal and private cancer research programs (McGeary, 1997). The National Cancer Program concept saw NCI as primarily a research agency that was also involved in translating research into applications to improve prevention, diagnosis, treatment, and rehabilitation efforts. The National Cancer Program was not supposed to become the cancer care system, but it was supposed to interact enough with the system through planning and coordination to improve the delivery of patient care. These broader coordination and planning goals that should have extended the reach of the National Cancer Program beyond NCI to other federal and private parties could not be met, and when the 1971 act was recodified in 1978, the scope of the program was redefined to include only NCI (McGeary, 1997).

Cancer care is often provided as part of research initiatives; consequently, the current National Cancer Program intersects with the health care delivery system. The majority of children with cancer, for example, fall within an NCI-sponsored system of care because they are participants in NCI-sponsored research protocols (Simone and Lyons, in press). Furthermore, a system of NCI-funded cancer centers extends research opportunities to community hospitals throughout the country. Nevertheless, most cancer care services are provided by hospitals and centers falling outside the purview of the National Cancer Program, and there is no national effort to coordinate the disparate federal efforts related to the quality of cancer care.

The lack of national coordination in cancer-fighting efforts in the public, private, and voluntary sectors is a problem that hinders progress against cancer, according to the findings of the NCI-appointed National Cancer Advisory Board (NCAB) in their review of the National Cancer Program in the early 1990s (NCAB, 1994). In its final report, the NCAB recommended that the National Cancer Program should extend "beyond research to its application to the people and include all non-research, non-governmental, and community constituents whose actions impact the cancer problems" (NCAB, 1994). To date, the legislative authority to have the National Cancer Program coordinate federal and nonfederal cancer programs has not been reinstated (McGeary, 1997).

ELEMENTS OF CANCER CARE

Individuals Receiving Cancer Care

In 1999, more than 8 million Americans, or 3 percent of the population, will require some form of care because of a diagnosis of cancer: 1.2 million of these individuals will be newly diagnosed this year and initiate treatment; some, diagnosed in previous years, will continue treatment; others, who have been successfully treated and no longer have evidence of cancer, will require follow-up; and over 500,000 people will die from cancer (ACS, 1999; Ries et al., 1997). Even larger numbers of adults in the United States will have been screened for cancer.

Cancer is characterized by abnormal cell growth, but it is really more than 100 different diseases, each with a unique profile of population at risk, symptoms, effective treatments, and prognosis. Some cancers are extremely rare, but relatively few cancer sites account for more than half (54 percent) of all new cases of cancer: prostate; breast; lung and bronchus; and colon and rectum (Table 2.1) (ACS, 1999).

Cancer most often strikes after middle age. Six of ten new cancer cases occur among those age 65 and older (Ries et al., 1997). With the aging of the "baby-boom" cohort, the number of new cancers diagnosed annually in the United States among the elderly is projected to more than double by the year 2030 (Polednak, 1994). Roughly four of ten new cases of cancer occur among working-age adults who often must meet the demands of supporting and raising a family while undergoing treatment. In terms of potential years of life lost, lost productivity, and lost earnings, cancer that strikes at younger ages has graver consequences than cancers that affect the elderly. Cancer among children is rare (e.g., 14.2 cases per 100,000 infants and children up to age 14 in 1993–1994) (NCI, 1998a); however, with the success of treating cancer in childhood, estimates are that 1 in 1,000 people reaching adulthood is a cured survivor of childhood cancer (NCI, 1997).

Cancer disproportionately affects the African-American community. Cancer incidence rates are higher for several sites, and once cancer is diagnosed, survival is poorer (Figures 2.1 and 2.2). Limitations in access to health care explain some, but not all, of these differences (see Chapter 3).

Slightly more men than women are diagnosed with cancer each year, but as women succumb to the effects of increased rates of smoking over the past two decades, they are becoming more equally represented among those with cancer (ACS, 1999).

TABLE 2.1 Estimated Number and Distribution of New Cancer Cases, United States, 1999

	Estimated No.	Distribution (%)
All Sites	1,221,800	100.0
Prostate	179,300	14.7
Female breast	175,000	14.3
Lung and bronchus	171,600	14.0
Colon and rectum	129,400	10.6
All other sites	566,500	46.4

SOURCE: ACS, 1999.

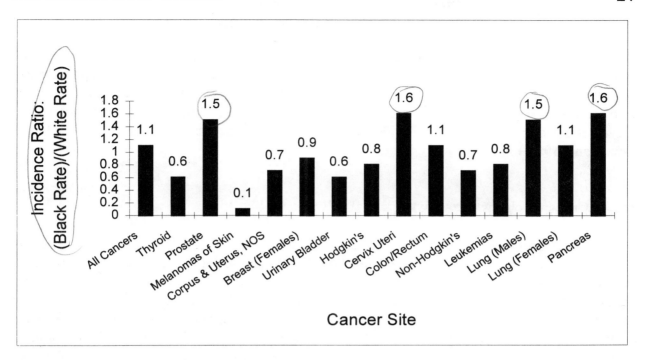

FIGURE 2.1 Cancer incidence rates, ratio of black rate to white rate, all ages, SEER Program, 1990–1994.

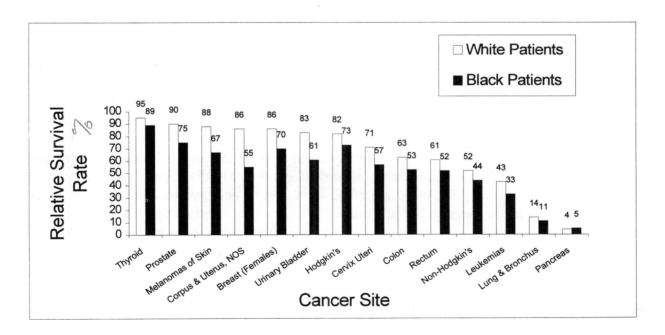

FIGURE 2.2 Five-year relative survival rates (percent), males and females, SEER Program, 1986–1993.

Trajectory of Cancer Care

The continuum of cancer care spans prevention, early detection and screening, diagnosis and treatment of new cancer cases, care of survivors, palliative care, and finally, support for terminally ill patients and their families (Mandelblatt et al., 1998). In this section, phases of cancer care are described beginning with early detection and screening. Primary prevention (efforts to prevent the occurrence cancer) is outside the scope of this report. (Much of this section is adapted from Ganz, 1996.)

Early Detection and Screening

The goals of early detection and screening are to identify cancers before they invade nearby tissue or spread to new sites. Visual examination of the colon using a colonoscope, for example, can find polyps that can be removed before they turn into invasive tumors. Other common screening and early detection methods are mammography, testing for bleeding in the digestive tract, Pap smears of the cervix, blood tests for prostate-specific proteins, and examination of the skin surface. Early detection of cancer is also influenced by attention to symptoms of cancer (e.g., blood in stool, lump in breast) and prompt follow-up. Once cancer is detected by screening or because of symptoms, the diagnostic evaluation phase of cancer management begins.

Diagnostic Evaluation

When a cancer screening test is positive or symptoms lead to its detection, further examinations are conducted to confirm the diagnosis and make it more precise. Pathologists attempt to identify the type of cell causing the cancer and may try to identify prognostic factors from a biopsy or tumor removed surgically to judge whether the cancer is fast growing or slow growing. Breast cancer tissue, for example, is usually examined for the presence of hormone receptors. If the receptors are present, therapy with hormone-blocking drugs may be prescribed to prevent a recurrence. Results of diagnostic and prognostic tests may be reviewed by a team of specialists as a decision is made on the first approach to treatment. Most newly diagnosed cancer patients go through a series of staging tests, including blood tests, x-rays, and various types of scans, to determine the extent of the disease. Initial planning is unusually important for many types of cancer, because choice of the first treatment severely limits subsequent treatment options due to the nature of cancer progression.

Primary and Adjuvant Treatment

Traditionally, most cancers have been treated with surgery, radiation, chemotherapy, or some combination of the three. Surgery has the longest history and is the mainstay of primary treatment for solid tumors (i.e., most cancers other than leukemias and lymphomas). For cancers that have not yet metastasized to distant sites, surgery is often curative, particularly for tumors that are completely localized.

Radiation is the primary treatment for some cancers (e.g., Hodgkin's disease and other lymphomas), but more often, it is used in conjunction with surgery. As an adjuvant to surgery, it is used to destroy remaining cancer cells in and around the site of the primary cancer. It is particularly important, for instance, as an adjunct to lumpectomy for women with early-stage breast cancer and has been demonstrated definitively in randomized trials to reduce the likelihood of a local recurrence. In some cases, radiation is used to shrink the size of a tumor before surgery or in late stages of disease to offer symptom relief by shrinking growths that interfere with eating, breathing, or other functions.

Chemotherapy (including hormone therapy) may be used alone to treat some cancers (e.g., some lymphomas and leukemias), but it is more often used in combination with radiation and surgery. If cancer is found at diagnosis to have spread from its original site (i.e., metastasized), the only potentially curative treatment option is chemotherapy, which can reach cancerous cells around the body. In most cases, patients begin an extended course of chemotherapy, which may last months, after surgery. Like radiation, it may also be used as "neoadjuvant therapy," given before a tumor is surgically removed, with the intent of shrinking the tumor.

With most forms of cancer, higher doses of chemotherapy and radiation are more effective, but they also cause more damage to healthy tissue. The bone marrow (from which most elements of the blood are continuously formed) is particularly sensitive to chemotherapeutic agents and radiation, and doses high enough to control cancer can easily wipe out the bone marrow, killing the patient as well. Over the past decade, oncologists have increasingly used a controversial strategy that employs high-dose chemotherapy and/or radiation treatment in conjunction with autologous bone marrow transplantation, in which patients have some bone marrow removed and stored before they are treated. After treatment, the stored bone marrow cells are reinfused into the patient to repopulate the bone marrow and begin producing blood cells. Bone marrow transplantation using marrow from healthy donors ("allogeneic transplantation") is established as a primary treatment for some leukemias and lymphomas—diseases in which the cancer has arisen in the blood elements themselves—but autologous transplantation still remains of unknown value for the treatment of solid tumors.

Other types of treatment use the body's own immune system to resist disease or invasions. Agents known as biologic response modifiers, which are derived from or modeled on the body's own natural products (e.g., interferon, the interleukins, tumor necrosis factor) are being used in cancer treatment, generally in combination with other treatments.

For most cancers, the majority of physicians and researchers have agreed on one or more "standard treatment approaches"—usually based on research findings, a consensus of expert opinion, or both. Doctors may have different opinions about how to treat some cancers because definitive evidence on what treatment works best (if there are any effective treatments) is not available.

In a few cases, treatments that appear to be of equal effectiveness, but have different implications for quality of life, are available (e.g., watchful waiting versus surgery for some prostate cancers). In these situations, patient preferences often determine the choice of treatment. *Patient-centered care* is care that incorporates respect for patients' values and preferences, provides information in clear and understandable terms, promotes autonomy in decision making, and attends to the need for physical comfort and emotional support.

Much of cancer treatment involves managing cancer symptoms, including pain and the side effects of cancer treatment. The latter may include fatigue; problems related to nutrition and eating (e.g., loss of appetite, nausea and vomiting); hair loss; neurotoxicity (e.g., damage to nerve cells, causing numbness or tingling in hands and feet); loss of concentration; psychological distress; sexual problems; and infertility. Some effects of cancer treatment are short-lived (e.g., hair loss, nausea), but others are permanent (e.g., increased susceptibility to infection after removal of the spleen, infertility after certain chemotherapy drugs). Likewise, some treatment side effects are immediate (e.g., hair loss), whereas others may arise only after a substantial delay (e.g., congestive heart failure many years after anthracycline chemotherapy, leukemia secondary to alkylating agents or radiation therapy). Information about the long-term side effects of treatment on important organs, such as the heart and lungs, is becoming more available.

Cancer patients in the United States have long been interested in treatments not traditionally offered as part of mainstream medicine. The incorporation of some alternative or complementary approaches as adjuncts to conventional treatments is a direct result of patients' desires for better cancer treatment, both curative and palliative, and generally for treatment that leaves them with a better quality of life than they might otherwise expect (Box 2.1).

BOX 2.1 Alternative or Complementary Cancer Treatments

Certain approaches to pain relief and coping (e.g., guided imagery, acupuncture, therapeutic touch) are increasingly being offered in mainstream cancer centers alongside conventional treatment. Other alternative approaches such as combinations of unknown drugs and chemicals given with the promise of cure fall squarely outside what mainstream medicine accepts, and patients may go to clinics inside and outside the United States to obtain them.

Among the more popular alternative or complementary approaches are the following:

- dietary, ranging from low-fat "conventional" or vegetarian diets to a strict "macrobiotic" diet (which supporters believe to be curative);
- spiritual approaches based on Western and Eastern religions, as well as Native American belief systems;
- mind–body techniques such as hypnosis, relaxation, meditation, yoga, and guided Imagery;
- physical approaches such as massage and therapeutic touch; and
- Chinese medicine of various types.

Patients may use mind–body approaches, in particular, throughout the course of cancer treatment (and survivorship)—for example, to alleviate the side effects of chemotherapy, to improve their psychological state, and to increase their energy levels. Some of these techniques have been studied and have been shown objectively to benefit patients, although this cannot be said for each approach or claim of benefit.

At present, there is little evidence available for judging which, if any, alternative treatments are actually beneficial, particularly in terms of improved survival and, in some cases, safety. It is reasonable to assume, however, that patient interest will continue to maintain a focus on these treatments and that the government will continue its modest efforts to foster reliable evaluations of them.

Posttreatment Surveillance and Follow-Up Care

The follow-up care phase of treatment is the time after completion of the initial course of therapy. Life-long follow-up is necessary to identify problems following cancer treatment, such as new cancers or recurrence of the same cancer.

Treatment of Recurrent Cancer

Cancer may recur in the same part of the body in which it was found originally (a local recurrence), or it may reappear in a more distant part of the body (a metastasis). The type of treatment that is selected for a recurring cancer depends on the specific type of cancer, how large it is, how it behaves biologically, and what previous therapy was given. Recurrent cancers can be cured, but the chance of cure is usually far lower than it is for the initial treatment of cancer. Advanced and incurable cancer may exist at the time of diagnosis, or it may occur after many years of treatment and follow-up care. In either case, the usual goal of care for the patient with advanced cancer resistant to anti-cancer therapy is symptom relief. Some patients may also want to participate in clinical trials of new experimental treatments.

Palliative Care

Much can be done to relieve symptoms, ease distress, provide comfort, and in other ways improve the quality of life of someone with cancer. This care may be referred to as palliative care, supportive care, or comfort care. Palliative care is important at any stage of cancer care management. For a person with cancer, maintenance of quality of life requires, at a minimum, relief from pain and other distressing symptoms; relief from anxiety and depression, including the fear of pain; and a sense of security that assistance will be readily available if needed. Hospice care is an approach to care during the final stages of life.

End-of-Life Care

One-half of cancer patients die of the disease, making death and end-of-life care important issues that must be addressed (American Society of Clinical Oncology, 1998). Poor symptom control, fear, and a lack of acceptance of death before dying, can be minimized by ensuring that appropriate medical and social support services are available (Foley, 1998). End-of-life care is in itself a diverse set of services and may involve the following (Lynn, 1997):

- management of physical or emotional symptoms and limitations of function;
- provision of pain relief and palliation to improve or maintain the quality of remaining life;
- counseling on the potential harm or benefit of aggressive life-extending treatments;
- respite, social support, and other services to relieve caregiver burden;
- advance care planning (e.g., living wills); and
- bereavement support.

End-of-life care extends beyond physical treatments to include supportive psychological, spiritual, and emotional care, and the goals of care shift from the quantity of life to the quality of life and symptom relief.

Providers of Cancer Care

It is common for cancer patients to see a number of specialist providers during the course of cancer care. *Interdisciplinary care* refers to the reliance on health care and other providers with a range of backgrounds and expertise. An interdisciplinary cancer care team might include an oncology nurse, pathologist, radiation oncologist, medical oncologist, surgeon, nutritionist, social worker, occupational therapist, pastoral counselor, hospice volunteer, and pain management team made up of physicians, nurses, and pharmacists. Individuals being cared for in a cancer center may have the most direct access to the full range of cancer care providers. In other settings—for example, rural areas—a community-based primary care provider may become the local member of a geographically dispersed team and, through communication, serve as a link between these providers and patients.

A wide range of physicians can be involved in cancer care, from pathologists, radiologists, surgeons, and medical oncologists, to specialists in pain management. It is difficult to obtain a precise count, but there are roughly 10,000 cancer physician specialists according to information from medical boards, the American Medical Association's (AMA's) annual survey of physicians, and the American Society of Clinical Oncology (ASCO).

Specialty medical boards are private, voluntary, nonprofit organizations founded to conduct examinations and issue certificates of qualifications. As of 1997, four medical specialty boards had certified nearly 10,000 cancer specialists:

1. The American Board of Internal Medicine had certified 6,550 medical oncologists.
2. The American Board of Radiology had certified 1,468 radiation oncologists.
3. The American Board of Pediatrics had certified 1,348 pediatric hematology oncologists.
4. The American Board of Obstetrics and Gynecology had certified 568 gynecologic oncologists.

Many practicing "oncologists" are not board certified as such. For example, among physicians identifying themselves as radiation oncologists on the AMA survey, as many as one-quarter were not certified by the American Board on Radiology (AMA, 1997). The reasons experienced oncologists might not be board certified include age (board certification is relatively recent) and primary involvement in research activities rather than patient care. Board certification is used as a quality indicator for physicians, but subspecialty certification is not always available for cancer specialists (e.g., there is no board certification for surgical oncology).

According to the AMA, in 1996 there were an estimated 6,731 self-identified medical oncology specialists representing 1 percent of the U.S. physician workforce. Nearly all of these oncologists (87 percent) were involved in patient care, and of these, more than three-quarters (77 percent) were in office-based practices. An estimated 8 percent of oncologists were primarily clinical researchers (AMA, 1998).

As of 1997, about 9,000 U.S.-based physicians belonged to the American Society of Clinical Oncology, the largest professional society dedicated to clinical oncology issues (Linda Mock, American Society of Clinical Oncology, personal communication to Maria Hewitt, March 1998).

Ambulatory Cancer Care Providers

National data on ambulatory medical care is available from two large surveys conducted by the National Center for Health Statistics, the National Ambulatory Medical Care Survey (NAMCS), and the National Hospital Ambulatory Medical Care Survey (NHAMCS) (Schappert, 1997). Only nonfederally employed physicians are included in the NAMCS sample and certain specialties are excluded—anesthesiologists, pathologists, and radiologists. Clinics specializing in radiology were excluded from the NHAMCS. Radiologists are important providers of cancer care and their omission limits the interpretation of cancer-specific analyses. Nevertheless, data from these surveys are presented to obtain some insights into the characteristics of adult ambulatory cancer care provided in physician office-based practices and hospital outpatient departments (care provided in hospital emergency rooms was excluded from the following analyses).

Each year, an estimated 19 million adults (age 25 and older) visit physicians' offices and hospital outpatient departments for cancer care.[1] These visits represent 3 percent of adult ambulatory care visits. The five physician specialties (excluding radiologists) providing most adult office-based ambulatory cancer care are the following (Table 2.2):

1. oncologists,
2. primary care providers,
3. dermatologists,
4. urologists, and
5. general surgeons.

The predominant physician provider (excluding radiologists) of adult ambulatory cancer care varies by type of cancer (see Table 2.2):

- Urologists are the main providers of ambulatory care for adults with prostate cancer (72 percent of visits).
- Dermatologists are the main providers of ambulatory care for adults with skin cancer (nonmelanoma) (67 percent of visits).
- Oncologists see roughly one-half of adults with cancer of the lung or larynx (46 percent of visits), female breast (45 percent visits), and colorectal cancer (51 percent of visits), and nearly two-thirds of adults seeking care for lymphoma or leukemia (73 percent of visits).

---

[1]This annual estimate represents the 3-year average (1994–1996) for visits for which the primary reason for the visit was care for malignant neoplasms, International Classification of Diseases (ICD-9) codes 140 to 208. The diagnosis represents the physician's best judgment at the time of the visit and could have been tentative, provisional, or definitive. Excluded from this estimate are cancer-related visits made by individuals without a diagnosis of cancer (e.g., for cancer screening tests).

TABLE 2.2 Distribution of Adult (age 25 and older) Ambulatory Cancer Care Visits, by Type of Cancer, Site of Visit, and Physician Specialty, 1994–1996[a]

	Type of Cancer[b]							
	All	Larynx, Lung	Female Breast	Prostate	Colon, Rectum	Lymphoma, Leukemias	Skin (non-melanoma)	Other Type
Sample Size	5,609	455	1,122	698	606	705	713	1,310
Site of Visit								
Physician office-based visits	100.0	100.0	100.0	100.0	100.0	100.0	100.0	100.0
	88.6	83.5	88.4	94.0	87.9	86.5	94.5	84.8
Hospital outpatient department visits	11.4	16.5	11.6	6.0	12.1	13.5	5.5	15.2
Physician Office-Based Visits[c]								
All physicians	100.0	100.0	100.0	100.0	100.0	100.0	100.0	100.0
Oncology	33.8	45.5	45.1	9.9	51.0	72.9	0.3	27.3
Primary care	15.4	23.0	12.8	14.3	24.1	16.0	10.5	14.7
General surgery	10.4	3.0	29.9	0.7	16.3	1.5	5.9	8.0
Specialty surgery	5.1	4.4	6.6	0.2	1.8	0.8	12.7	5.4
Dermatology	14.3	0.0	0.0	0.0	0.0	1.6	67.3	14.4
Urology	12.3	0.0	0.0	71.5	0.1	0.0	0.0	13.4
Other specialty	8.8	24.0	5.5	3.5	6.7	7.3	3.3	16.9
Hospital Outpatient Department Visits[d]								
Total	100.0	100.0	100.0	100.0	100.0	100.0	100.0	100.0
General medical	81.0	73.1	87.0	66.6	91.3	96.0	82.2	69.8
Surgery	18.0	26.8	13.0	33.4	8.7	3.7	17.8	26.7
Other	1.0	0.1	0.0	0.0	0.0	0.3	0.0	3.5

aPercentages are adjusted using sampling weights to produce national estimates.

bAccording to the Ninth Edition of the International Classification of Diseases (ICD-9): larynx, lung = 161, 162; female breast = 174; prostate = 185; colon, rectum = 153, 154; lymphomas, leukemias = 200–208; skin = 173; other = all other malignancies. Visit was considered cancer related if the principal diagnosis was coded as a malignant neoplasm (ICD-9 140 to 208).

cOncology includes medical oncology and gynecological oncology; primary care includes family practice, internal medicine, and general practice; specialty surgery includes the following surgical specialties: colorectal, head and neck, neurosurgery, orthopedic, plastic, thoracic, cardiovascular, abdominal, and vascular. Other specialty includes hematology, gastroenterology, pulmonary disease, and others. Radiologists are not included in the NAMCS sample.

dRadiology clinics are not included in the NHAMCS sample.

SOURCE: USDHHS, 1999a, b.

Social Workers?

Nurses and social workers are also essential providers of cancer care. More than 17,000 nurses are certified by the Oncology Nursing Society as oncology nurses (ONS, 1998). These nurses have extensive experience with the management of cancer, including the administration of chemotherapy, monitoring of pain and nausea, and patient counseling and education. An estimated 1,000 social workers with special training in oncology provide psychosocial services to people with cancer and their families (Susan Hedlund, Association of Oncology Social Workers, personal communication to Maria Hewitt, September 1998).

Cancer care often involves numerous practitioners across a variety of settings, physicians' offices, outpatient diagnostic centers, hospitals, nursing homes, patients' homes, and hospices, making communication and coordination of care difficult. *Comprehensive and coordinated care management* refers to the ability to fully access necessary services and to have components of care efficiently planned and integrated. Clear and ongoing communication among care providers and among providers, patients, and family members is a prerequisite to coordinated care. Too often, adults newly diagnosed or suspected of having cancer see one doctor and then others sequentially, without having an overall plan of care devised at the outset by, or in consultation with an interdisciplinary team. This can have deleterious consequences because the first treatment offers the best chance for cure and because every treatment used may limit subsequent treatment options (Moore, 1985).

Sites of Cancer Care

Although the locus of cancer care in the past has been the hospital, an increasing number of cancer care services, from diagnostic imaging to the administration of chemotherapy, are being shifted from the hospital to outpatient settings. According to the NAMCS and the NHAMCS, most cancer-related adult ambulatory care is provided in physicians' offices (89 percent), with the balance (11 percent) provided in hospital outpatient departments (Table 2.3).[2] Relatively few types of cancer account for more than three-quarters (79 percent) of all adult ambulatory visits—female breast; skin (nonmelanoma); lymphomas and leukemias; prostate; colon and rectum; and lung and respiratory cancers (Table 2.3). Management of cancer-related symptoms and the need for follow-up care and pre- or postoperative checks are among the most common reasons for adults' making cancer-related ambulatory care visits (Table 2.3). Chemotherapy is administered during about one in five adult ambulatory care visits (22 percent). As would be expected given the age of onset of most cancers, more than one-half (56 percent) of adult ambulatory care visits are made by the elderly, and Medicare is the principal source of payment for adult ambulatory care visits (Table 2.3).

In 1997, nearly 1,000 hospital-based cancer care programs discharged 276 or more patients with a primary diagnosis of cancer (Comarow, 1997; Ehrlich, 1997). These hospitals range from relatively small, community-based hospitals to large referral centers that treat cancer patients exclusively. Available evidence suggests that cancer patients are concentrated in a few U.S. hospitals. Only one in three of the 5,080 general hospitals in the United States has a cancer program approved by the American College of Surgeons' Commission on Cancer (ACoS-COC)

---

[2]These estimates exclude ambulatory care visits to radiologists and to hospital radiology clinics. These providers are excluded from the NAMCS and the NHAMCS.

(1,500 programs), but these hospitals, most of them community hospitals, provide care for 80 percent of newly diagnosed patients (Carol Cook, Administrative Coordinator, American College of Surgeons, personal communication to Maria Hewitt, February 1999; American Hospital Association, 1999).[3]

TABLE 2.3 Characteristics of Adult (age 25 and older) Cancer-Related Ambulatory Cancer Care Visits, 1994–1996

Characteristic	Cancer Care Visits[a]	
	Sample Size	Distribution (%)[b]
Type of cancer[c]		
Lung, other respiratory	455	7.3
Female breast	1,122	18.4
Prostate	698	12.7
Colon, rectum	606	11.0
Lymphomas, leukemias	705	14.0
Skin (nonmelanoma)	713	15.7
All others	1,310	20.9
Age		
25–44	649	9.8
45–64	1,970	33.9
65–74	1,604	29.2
75+	1,386	27.1
Site of visits		
Physician office	3,075	88.6
Hospital outpatient department	2,534	11.4
Reason for visit[d]		
Symptoms	1,297	26.4
Exam, tests, medication	735	12.3
Chemotherapy, other therapy	680	11.6
Follow-up, pre- or post-op check	1,158	19.2
Cancer, no specific reason provided	1,474	25.8
Other	265	4.8
Oncolytic therapy administered[e]		
Yes	1.090	21.9
No	4,519	78.1
Result of referral[f]		
Yes	1,740	28.0
No	3,869	72.0

Continued

---

[3]See Chapter 6 for a description of the ACoS-COC survey process.

TABLE 2.3 *Continued*

Characteristic	Cancer Care Visits[a]	
	Sample Size	Distribution (%)[b]
Insurance		
Medicare	2,671	49.2
Medicaid	299	2.4
Non-Medicare, private commercial	1,316	23.9
Non-Medicare, HMO, other prepaid	653	14.6
Self-pay or no charge	295	4.6
Other insurance	92	1.0
Unknown	283	4.2

[a] Visit was considered cancer related if the principal diagnosis was coded as a malignant neoplasm (ICD-9 140 to 208). Radiologists and radiology clinics are not included in the survey samples and ambulatory visits to these providers are not represented.

[b] Percentages are adjusted using sampling weights to produce national estimates.

[c] In the Ninth Edition of the International Classification of Diseases (ICD-9): larynx, lung = 161, 162; female breast = 174; prostate = 185; colon, rectum = 153, 154; lymphomas, leukemias = 200–208; other = all other malignancies.

[d] Reason for visit is the most important patient complaint, symptom, or other reason given by the patient for the visit.

[e] Oncolytic therapy ordered, supplied, or administered during the visit including antineoplastics; hormonal or biological response modifiers; antimetabolites; antibiotics, alkaloids, or enzymes; or DNA-damaging drugs (National Drug Code Directory Drug Classes).

[f] Was patient referred for this visit by another physician?

SOURCE: USDHHS, 1999a, b.

Each year, individuals with cancer incur 1.4 million hospitalizations (5 percent of all hospital discharges) (Graves and Gillum, 1997). In 1994, relatively few types of cancer accounted for the majority (52 percent) of hospitalizations—lung and other respiratory cancers, lymphomas and leukemias, and cancers of the colon and rectum, female breast, and prostate (Table 2.4). Most individuals hospitalized with a principal diagnosis of cancer are elderly (55 percent), and Medicare is the payer for most hospital care (Table 2.4). A greater share of cancer-related hospitalizations occurs in larger than in smaller hospitals (i.e., 45 percent of cancer-related hospitalization are in hospitals with 300 beds or more, and 37 percent are in hospitals with fewer than 200 beds) (Table 2.4).

With the advent of earlier hospital discharges, there has been a growing demand for services provided in the home. About 6 percent of the 2 million individuals estimated to be receiving home health care services each year have cancer (Jones and Strahan, 1997). Most individuals who die as a result of cancer spend the end of their lives in hospitals, but individuals with cancer are more likely than those with other conditions to use hospice care. The majority of individuals residing in hospice care facilities have cancer (Jones and Strahan, 1997).

TABLE 2.4 Characteristics of Hospital Discharges with Primary Diagnosis of Cancer, 1994

Characteristic	Sample Size	Estimate No. of Cancer-Related Hospital Discharges Nationally (se)[a]	Percent Distribution (se)[a]
All cancer discharges	11,021	1,408,600 (66,300)	100.0
Type of cancer[b]			
Lung, other respiratory	1,415	194,000 (14,800)	13.8 (0.8)
Female breast	1,092	137,300 (11,900)	9.7 (0.7)
Prostate	838	110,000 (10,400)	7.8 (0.6)
Colon, rectum	1,172	142,900 (12,200)	10.1 (0.7)
Lymphomas, leukemias	1,116	152,000 (12,700)	10.8 (0.7)
All others	5,388	672,300 (35,800)	47.8 (1.2)
Age			
0–24	455	53,600 (10,100)	3.8 (0.2)
25–44	1,029	129,900 (8,100)	9.2 (0.4)
45–64	3,434	444,900 (27,300)	31.6 (0.5)
≥65	6,103	780,100 (48,900)	55.4 (0.6)
Sex			
Male	5,227	664,100 (44,800)	47.1 (0.6)
Female	5,794	744,600 (31,100)	52.9 (0.8)
Race			
White	7,382	1,012,600 (62,700)	71.9 (1.1)
Black	1,059	127,100 (11,500)	9.0 (0.4)
Other	642	54,600 (10,400)	3.9 (0.2)
Not stated	1,938	214,300 (29,000)	15.2 (0.6)
Hospital size (No. of Beds)			
6–99	896	190,800 (14,600)	13.5 (0.8)
100–199	1,822	329,800 (21,100)	23.4 (1.0)
200–299	2,627	254,200 (17,600)	18.0 (0.9)
300–499	3,521	384,100 (23,500)	27.3 (1.1)
≥500	2,155	249,600 (17,400)	17.7 (0.9)

Continued

TABLE 2.4 *Continued*

Characteristic	Sample Size	Estimated No. of Cancer-Related Hospital Discharges Nationally (se)[a]	Percent Distribution (se)[a]
Principal expected source of payment			
Medicare	5,352	733,500 (64,300)	52.1 (0.8)
Medicaid	683	82,900 (11,400)	5.9 (0.7)
Other government	117	20,100 (5,500)	1.4 (0.3)
Blue Cross	1,097	119,500 (28,131)	8.5 (1.9)
Other private or commercial	2,965	354,600 (49,100)	25.2 (3.0)
Self-pay or no charge	298	36,700 (8,800)	2.6 (0.6)
Other	352	38,200 (6,372)	2.7 (0.3)
Not stated	157	23,100 (5,700)	1.6 (0.2)

[a] Numbers and percentages are adjusted using sampling weights to produce national estimates. Variance estimates were calculated using the Taylor series approximation technique taking into account the complex design the survey (StataCorp, 1997).

[b] According to the Ninth Edition of the International Classification of Diseases, (ICD-9): lung, larynx = 161, 162; female breast = 174; prostate = 185; colon, rectum = 153, 154; lymphomas, leukemias 200–208; other = all other malignancies. Table includes discharges for which the first listed diagnosis was cancer.

SOURCE: USDHHS, 1999c.

The Intersection of Cancer Care and Research

The majority of children with cancer (an estimated 70 percent), but only about 2 percent of adults, receive their care through a research protocol, most often sponsored by the National Cancer Institute (NCI, 1998a). There are 35 NCI-designated "comprehensive cancer centers" with extensive research portfolios covering basic science, epidemiology, medicine, and public health. Another 23 NCI-designated "basic" and "clinical" cancer centers have research programs with a narrower focus (Figure 2.3). In addition to conducting research, NCI-designated cancer centers also provide community outreach activities and public education (NCI, 1999).

NCI's Cooperative Group Program conducts and promotes multi-institutional clinical trials. Twelve cooperative groups involve 1,700 institutions and 6,000 investigators throughout the United States, Canada, Europe, and Australia. Each year, approximately 20,000 new patients participate in cooperative group clinical trails (NCI, 1999).

The Community Clinical Oncology Program (CCOP) links community cancer specialists and primary care physicians with clinical cooperative groups and cancer centers to conduct clinical trials. There are currently 48 CCOP offices in 30 states, with 330 participating hospitals at which some 2,300 physicians enter individuals into NCI-approved clinical trials. An additional seven minority-based CCOPs enhance the participation of minority populations in clinical trials. Altogether, more than 4,000 patients are entered into NCI-sponsored cancer treatment clinical trials each year through CCOPs and an additional 4,000 participants are entered into cancer prevention and control clinical trials (NCI, 1999).

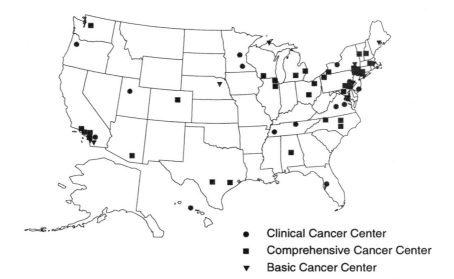

FIGURE 2-3 National Cancer Institute-designated cancer centers.

FINANCIAL COSTS OF CANCER CARE

The financial costs of cancer care are substantial, both in societal terms and to individuals paying for care. This section describes estimates of national cancer care expenditures and, with the limited data that are available, the distribution of costs by cancer site or phase of care. Chapter 3 discusses financial costs from a patient perspective and reviews potential financial barriers to access to care related to the absence of insurance coverage or to inadequate insurance coverage for care.

In 1998, the "direct" health care cost of delivering cancer care (e.g., hospital and outpatient care, nursing home care, home health care, doctors and other providers, drugs) was estimated to be roughly $50 billion, representing about 5 percent of U.S. health care expenditures (Martin Brown, Head, Health Services and Economics Section, Applied Research Branch, Cancer Surveillance Research Program, National Cancer Institute, personal communication, October 19, 1998; Schuette et al., 1995). Most "direct" cancer care expenditures cover hospital care (65 percent) and physicians' services (24 percent) (Brown and Fintor, 1995). The economic burden of cancer is substantially higher if "indirect" costs are considered, for example, those associated with lost earnings and reduced work productivity (Brown and Fintor, 1995).

Direct medical costs for cancer exceed those for most other chronic illnesses. In one study of chronic health care direct costs in a large staff-model health maintenance organization (HMO), the annual costs for cancer exceeded by far the annual costs associated with other chronic diseases such as heart disease, diabetes, depression, and multiple sclerosis. A person diagnosed with heart disease accounted for 40 percent more in annual costs than someone without such a diagnosis, after controlling for age, sex, and presence of other chronic conditions. For cancer, there was more than a ninefold increase in annual cost (Fishman et al., 1997). Factors contributing to the high costs associated with cancer care include the specialized facilities and personnel used to deliver therapy, the inherent toxicity and other risks associated with anticancer treatments, the complexity of the disease and variability in patient response, and the advent of new technologies (e.g., radiotherapeutic equipment, new drugs, diagnostic tests) (Bailes, 1995; Lazar and Desch, 1998).

Cancer is a diverse set of conditions, so it is not surprising that the cost of cancer care varies by the type of cancer. In one analysis within a large staff-model HMO, the costs of initial, continuing, and terminal care were found to vary for three cancers: colon, prostate, and breast. The costs associated with each treatment phase varied by stage at diagnosis, patient age, and the presence or absence of other diseases, and the patterns of variation differed for each type of cancer. The total costs of initial care, for example, increased with stage at diagnosis for colon and breast cancer, but not for prostate cancer (Taplin et al., 1995).

The variation in cost by type of cancer and stage of illness is also seen in a study of Medicare payments. Among the Medicare population, average payments varied among cancer sites, especially in the initial care phase, where payments were highest for lung and colorectal cancers and lowest for female breast cancer (Table 2.5).

Efforts to promote cancer screening among the elderly will likely increase Medicare costs. Persons diagnosed at earlier stages incur higher total Medicare payments between diagnosis and death than those diagnosed at later stages, reflecting their longer survival. Total Medicare payments from diagnosis to death were lowest for those with lung cancer, mainly because of short survival times (Table 2.6).

IMPACT OF A CHANGING HEALTH CARE SYSTEM ON CANCER CARE

Cancer is a common chronic illness whose management is costly, technology dependent, and interdisciplinary and extends from prevention to end-of-life care. It thus illustrates the challenges posed by the increasingly complex and dynamic American health care system. This section describes how one dominant force of change, the rise in managed health care, has affected essential aspects of health care delivery that are important to individuals with cancer. Another trend, the tendency for employers to assume financial risk and to self-fund or insure their own health plans, is also described because it has limited the applicability of cancer-related, state-mandated health benefits and consumer protections.

TABLE 2.5 Average Medicare Payments by Site and Phase of Cancer (1990 dollars per person-year)

	Lung	Female Breast	Prostate	Colon or Rectum	Bladder
Less than 1 year survival	$19,199	$16,475	$18,698	$22,473	$21,529
Survived 1 year or more					
Initial	17,518	8,913	10,235	17,505	10,717
Continuing care	4,305	3,138	3,788	3,625	4,656
Pre-final	9,985	7,633	8,542	9,056	10,036
Final	13,2!7	11,129	12,061	12,028	13,633

SOURCE: Riley et al., 1995.

TABLE 2.6 Medicare Payments, Average Age at Diagnosis, and Average Years of Survival by Site of Cancer

	Lung	Female Breast	Prostate	Colon or Rectum	Bladder
Total payments from diagnosis to death[a]	$29,184	$50,448	$48,684	$51,865	$57,629
Average payments per year[a]	$17,371	$5,333	$7,005	$8,016	$7,927
Average age at diagnosis	73.6	74.9	75.3	76.2	75.6
Average years of survival	1.68	9.46	6.95	6.47	7.27

[a] 1990 dollars per person-year.

SOURCE: Riley et al., 1995.

Managed Care

Although the majority of Americans insured through employment-based plans, 73 percent in 1995, are enrolled in some type of managed care plan (President's Advisory Commission, 1998), less than one-half of newly diagnosed cancer patients are in such a system. This decreased exposure to managed care occurs because 60 percent of individuals newly diagnosed with cancer are elderly and covered by Medicare, and 87 percent of Medicare beneficiaries have opted for traditional fee-for-service (FFS) care (HCFA, 1998).

Managed care can be defined as *an entity that assumes both the clinical and the financial responsibility for the provision of health care for a defined population* (Donaldson, 1998). It is, however, difficult to distinguish one type of managed care organization from another (Box 2.2).

With the shift to managed care, health insurance products have adopted features that directly influence how care is delivered—what services are offered, who provides them, and how they are organized (President's Advisory Commission, 1998). The relationship between managed care and quality is not clear, and evidence can suggest that managed care is as good as, worse than, or better than fee-for-service care—depending on which research one turns to (Miller and Luft, 1997). Managed care presents "both a problem and an opportunity for cancer care" according to the President's Cancer Panel (President's Cancer Panel, 1997). On one hand, managed care organizations (MCOs) may restrict patients' access to oncology specialists, limit the use of new therapeutic agents (e.g., closed drug formularies, off-label use of drugs), or deny coverage of care offered as part of a clinical trial. Furthermore, physicians within MCOs may be at financial risk and so may not fully assume the role of patient advocate. On the other hand, proponents of managed care applaud the success of MCOs in curbing health care spending and suggest that managed health care promotes preventive services, standardizes "appropriate" care by adopting clinical practice guidelines, and often provides comprehensive disease management for those with chronic illnesses such as cancer. For Medicare beneficiaries, more extensive coverage of outpatient drugs and other ancillary services by HMOs than FFS plans is also viewed as particularly beneficial for cancer patients. The limited evidence regarding the way in which managed care has affected the quality of cancer care is reviewed in Chapter 5.

BOX 2.2 Defining Managed Care

Although managed care has a long history in the United States, adoption of the federal Health Maintenance Organization Act in 1973 (as well as the term "health maintenance organization") marked the beginning of an era of accelerating growth for the managed care industry. In the 1970s and 1980s, HMOs typically were one of four distinct types:

1. staff-model HMOs hired and supervised salaried physicians;
2. group-model HMOs contracted with a single group of physicians without directly hiring them;
3. independent practice association (IPA) models contracted with individual physicians or small groups in private practice and often arose when groups of physicians affiliated for the purpose of securing contracts;
4. network HMOs contracted with two or more groups and were largely centrally organized as a means of securing discounted contracts with providers.

Currently, this typology fails to describe accurately new forms of managed care. Many new systems now have components of both IPAs and groups, and share many of the same physician groups and intermediary organizations (e.g., IPAs). Most managed care organizations now have multiple options or "products" from which consumers can choose. Thus, the evolution of health care organizations has surpassed the current taxonomy, and even experienced observers of the health care system cannot adequately distinguish different health plans from one another.

SOURCE: Landon et al., 1998.

A key concern of individuals with cancer is how they access cancer care specialists. In managed care systems, access to oncology specialists is often through a "gatekeeper," a primary care provider who authorizes referrals to specialists. In recent years, nearly one-third of primary care physicians report an increase in the severity and complexity of patient conditions they care for without referring to a specialist (St. Peter et al., 1997). Oncologists have expressed concerns that delays in referrals from primary care providers in managed care settings can negatively affect the outcome of therapy (Mortensen, 1997). While there are public concerns about access to specialists within managed care, there is little information on how managed care has affected oncology referral patterns. Furthermore, it is not entirely clear what the respective roles of primary care physicians and specialists should be in the provision of some aspects of care (e.g., follow-up care). The limited available evidence on the effect of provider specialization on quality is reviewed in Chapter 5.

Access to treatments and procedures has also changed in recent years. Utilization review has become a standard feature of both conventional and managed care. In a 1995 national survey, physicians said that on average, 59 percent of their patients were reviewed for length of stay, 45 percent for site of care, and 39 percent for the appropriateness of treatment. Although utilization review is common, denials of recommended procedures or referrals to specialists are relatively rare. Physicians reported that only 1 percent of recommended surgical procedures and 3 percent of referrals to specialists were ultimately denied (Remler et al., 1997).

Most Medicare HMO enrollees report having few problems accessing care—in a 1996 survey, 6 percent said that they did not get a desired referral to a specialist. People with chronic illnesses, disabilities, or functional impairments were, however, more likely to report problems of access (Gold et al., 1997). Medicare beneficiaries enrolled in HMOs are generally satisfied with their plans, and those whose cancer is diagnosed after they enroll are no more likely than others to disenroll and opt for fee-for-service care (Riley et al., 1996).

When patients (or their physicians) disagree with a plan's coverage decision, a resolution procedure is available, but the timeliness and processes (e.g., option of external review) may vary greatly from plan to plan. Licensed health plans are subject to numerous state and federal laws, and many also comply with standards of private accrediting bodies (e.g., National Committee for Quality Assurance, Joint Commission on Accreditation of Healthcare Organizations) (see Box 2.3) (President's Advisory Commission, 1998).

BOX 2.3 Selected Federal and State Regulations Regarding Resolution of Complaints or Appeals*

Medicare

Under the Medicare fee-for-service system, fiscal intermediaries and carriers must provide a two-step internal review and notification of their final decision before a beneficiary is entitled to seek reconsideration from the Social Security Administration (SSA) and the Health Care Financing Administration (HCFA). HMOs that participate in Medicare are required to provide meaningful internal procedures for resolving complaints about the quality of care, untimely provision of care, or improper demeanor of health care personnel. HMO decisions to deny coverage for certain treatments, referral outside a plan, or reimbursement for emergency or out-of-area care are subject to an external review and administrative appeal. HCFA has contracted with a private organization, the Center for Health Dispute Resolution, to perform these reconsiderations. After external review, a Medicare beneficiary dissatisfied with the results of the review has a right to SSA review.

Medicaid

The federal Medicaid statute requires state agencies to provide beneficiaries with a fair hearing and an administrative appeal when their eligibility or requests for services are denied or not acted upon within reasonable time. These determinations can be challenged in state court under state administrative procedure acts or in federal court. In addition, HMOs that contract to serve Medicaid beneficiaries must establish an internal complaint procedure that will resolve disputes promptly. These internal procedures are subject to review and approval by the state.

*A "complaint" is any expression of dissatisfaction to a health plan, provider, or facility by a consumer made orally or in writing, for example, concerning waiting times, the demeanor of health care personnel, respect paid to consumers, or provision of services. An "appeal" is a consumer's request for a health plan, facility, provider, or other body to change an initial decision.

Continued

BOX 2.3 *Continued*

ERISA Plans

All employers offering health benefits to their employees through managed care organizations or traditional indemnity insurers must comply with requirements of the Employee Retirement Income Security Act (ERISA). ERISA requires private employer-provided health benefit plans to disclose certain information to plan participants, to report information to the federal government, and to pay benefits that are promised under the plans. ERISA regulations generally require employer health plans to approve or deny claims within 90 days and to approve or deny an appeal of claims denials within 60 days. Although ERISA health plans are required to establish and disclose complaint and appeals procedures to participants, and to notify participants of claims denials, the plans are not required to provide a particular complaint procedure.

State-Licensed Insurance Products

Some state insurance regulations require health insurers doing business in the state to provide certain complaint procedures to enrollees. In addition, all 50 states have laws licensing or governing HMOs doing business in the state, which are separate from their laws regulating indemnity insurance products. Many states' laws are based on the model HMO law drafted by the National Association of Insurance Commissioners, which requires HMOs to establish complaint procedures approved by the state's insurance commissioner.

An estimated 30 states have some specified complaint procedures that HMOs must follow, and at least seven states now require an expedited appeal for denials of urgently needed care.

SOURCE: President's Advisory Commission, 1998.

Changes in the way physicians are paid have altered the financial incentives of clinical practice. Whereas providers under fee-for-service generally have financial incentives to provide more care, managed care plans have attempted to shift the incentive system toward the use of performance indicators. Common measures used by half or more HMOs with such physician incentive systems include utilization and cost, quality of care (e.g., adherence to practice guidelines), patient complaints, and the results of consumer surveys. Usually, these performance-based bonuses or "withholds" represent a small share of a physician's total income. Managed care organizations still tend to pay individual specialists on a fee-for-service basis, but elements of risk are being introduced. Some plans are capitating (i.e., paying a flat fee per patient covered) or competitively bidding for specific specialty services such as mental health, radiology, podiatry, and cardiology (InterStudy, 1997). Some managed care organizations offer cancer care as a "carve-out" through a network of cancer care providers (e.g., Value Oncology Services) (Bell, 1997). In these arrangements, an employer removes coverage for cancer care from the regular health benefits plans and arranges for coverage through a contract with a separate set of specialized providers.

Cancer care is often resource intensive, and some managed care companies are hiring disease management specialists to track costs and manage patient care (Bennett, 1997; Piro and Doctor, 1998). Disease management systems can reduce costs and improve care if they coordinate care and reduce unnecessary visits or redundant diagnostic tests or if they manage pain and other symptoms better, thereby reducing the use of emergency rooms. Disease management can contribute to greater patient satisfaction if coordination of care and provider communication improve.

Several versions of a patient's Bill of Rights were considered during the 105th Congress, but no federal legislation was passed (Medical Payment Advisory Commission, 1998). A range of protections that are particularly relevant to people with cancer in managed care plans were considered, including guaranteed access to health care specialists, continuity of care if a health provider is dropped in the middle of treatment, reimbursement for care while participating in clinical trials, and access to a meaningful internal and external appeals process for consumers to resolve their differences with their health plans and health care providers.

Self-Funded Health Insurance Plans

Nearly one-half of insured workers in 1995 were employed by organizations that self-fund their health insurance plans (Jensen, 1997). Many states have mandated the coverage of certain health benefits and consumer protections, but self-funded plans are regulated under the federal Employee Retirement Income Security Act of 1974 (ERISA) and are not subject to these mandates. Several state laws affect cancer care (Box 2.4). Rhode Island, Georgia, and Maryland, for example, require insurers to pay for new investigational cancer therapies provided as part of a qualified clinical trial, and at least 17 states prohibit insurers from excluding coverage for the off-label use of prescription drugs to treat cancer (e.g., use of a drug approved by the U.S. Food and Drug Administration [FDA] for one type cancer or other condition to treat another type of cancer for which the drug has not yet been FDA approved) (NCI, 1998b). States can affect the care provided under ERISA plans by mandating what providers licensed in the state must do (e.g., requiring physicians to give patients with breast cancer information about treatment options) (Murphy et al., 1997).

KEY FINDINGS

A single national system or program to ensure access to comprehensive, coordinated care for cancer does not exist. This situation is not unique to cancer, and in fact, pluralism, dynamism, and diversity are hallmarks of the U.S. health care industry (President's Advisory Commission, 1998). The ad hoc and fragmented nature of the existing "system," however, is especially problematic for individuals with cancer because of the complex nature of cancer care.

The trajectory of cancer care services—from early detection to treatment, follow-up, and palliative care—can span decades, occur in a variety of settings, involve numerous providers from different medical disciplines, and incorporate an ever-changing set of treatment modalities. The course of care through this trajectory varies widely by type of cancer (of which there are more than 100) and stage of disease. In addition to being highly complex, cancer is one of the most expensive conditions to treat, consuming about one out of every twenty health care dollars spent in the United States.

BOX 2.4 State Laws Mandating Cancer Care Benefit Coverage

Screening

- At least 15 states have enacted laws requiring coverage for prostate cancer screening, applying primarily to people over age 50 or over 40 for high-risk individuals. Most state laws require coverage of the prostate specific antigen (PSA) test, and slightly more than half of the laws require coverage of digital rectal examination. The laws apply mostly to private insurers and specialized managed care providers (Alaska, Colorado, Delaware, Georgia, Illinois, Louisiana, Maine, Maryland, Minnesota, New Jersey, North Carolina, North Dakota, South Carolina, Texas, Virginia).
- Twenty-two states have enacted laws requiring coverage for cervical cancer screening. In most cases, the law calls for coverage of an examination annually or as recommended by a physician. The laws apply primarily to private insurers and specialized managed care providers, with only a few states mandating this of public employee health plans and Medicaid or state medical assistance programs (Alaska, California, Delaware, District of Columbia, Georgia, Illinois, Kansas, Louisiana, Maine, Massachusetts, Minnesota, Nevada, New Jersey, New Mexico, New York, North Carolina, Ohio, Oregon, Rhode Island, South Carolina, Virginia, West Virginia).
- All 50 states have enacted laws requiring third-party payers to offer or provide coverage for mammograms. For most states there is required coverage for annual exams for women over 50.

Treatment

- At least 16 states have enacted laws requiring physicians to distribute information to patients about breast cancer treatment (California, Florida, Georgia, Illinois, Kansas, Kentucky, Massachusetts, Maryland, Maine, Michigan, Minnesota, Montana, New Jersey, New York, Pennsylvania, Texas). For most states, this includes information about the specific treatment (e.g., surgery, radiation) and information about reconstructive surgery and mammography.
- Several states have also enacted regulations requiring third-party payers to provide a specified amount of inpatient care following a mastectomy, lumpectomy, or lymph node dissection. For mastectomy the minimum length of stay ranges from 24 hours (Virginia) to 72 hours (New Jersey) following modified radical mastectomy. Most other states that have such laws require coverage for a 48-hour stay or as directed by the physician (Arkansas, Connecticut, Florida, Illinois, Kentucky, Maine, Montana, New Mexico, New York, North Carolina, Oklahoma, Pennsylvania, Rhode Island, South Carolina, Texas).
- A number of states have laws requiring third-party payers, particularly private insurers and private managed care providers, to cover reconstructive surgery and/or prosthetic devices following mastectomy (Arizona, Arkansas, California, Connecticut, Florida, Illinois, Indiana, Kentucky, Louisiana, Maine, Maryland, Michigan, Missouri, Montana, Nevada, New Hampshire, New Jersey, New York, North Carolina, Oklahoma, Pennsylvania, Rhode Island, South Carolina, Tennessee, Texas, Virginia, Washington, West Virginia).

Continued

BOX 2.4 *Continued*

Clinical Trial Reimbursement

• Three states (Georgia, Maryland, and Rhode Island) have laws requiring insurance reimbursement for cancer treatment provided as part of a clinical trial, but not all studies are applicable.

Protections for the Indigent

• The Maryland legislature has passed a law requiring screening and treatment for needy women without access to care.

SOURCE: NCI, 1998b.

Over the past few decades, managed care has grown to become the dominant organizing and financing mechanism for U.S. health care, changing dramatically the way in which health care services are delivered. Individuals with cancer are less likely to be covered by managed care plans because they are elderly and tend to have Medicare's traditional fee-for-service coverage. Nevertheless, many aspects of cancer care—for example, access to specialists, coverage for drugs and ancillary services, and use of practice guidelines—differ in managed care compared to fee-for-service care. In response to market forces, managed care organizations have consolidated, diversified, and become quite heterogeneous, making it difficult to generalize about their impact on cancer care. States, in some instances, have tried to counter the effects of managed care by mandating certain benefits or consumer protections. These mandates, however, do not apply to many Americans whose health plans are self-funded by an employer and therefore exempt from state regulation.

REFERENCES

American Cancer Society. 1999. *Cancer Facts and Figures—1999.* Atlanta, GA: American Cancer Society.

American Hospital Association, 1999. *Hospital Statistics: 1999 Edition.* Chicago: American Hospital Association.

American Medical Association. 1997. *Physician Characteristics and Distribution in the U.S. 1996–1997 Edition.* Chicago: American Medical Association.

American Medical Association. 1998. *Physician Characteristics and Distribution in the U.S. 1997–1998 Edition.* Chicago: American Medical Association.

American Society of Clinical Oncology. 1998. Cancer care during the last phase of life. *Journal of Clinical Oncology* 16(5):1986–1996.

Bailes JS. 1995. The economics of cancer care. *Cancer* 76(10 Suppl.):1886–1887.

Bell N. 1997. Approaches to cancer management vary widely. *Faulkner & Gray's Medicine and Health Perspectives* 51(27):3.

Bennett C, Buchner D, Ullman M. 1997. Approaches to prostate cancer by managed care organizations. *Urology* 50(1):79–86.

Brown ML, Fintor L. 1995. Economic burden of cancer. In Greenwald P, Kramer BS, Weed DL, eds. *Cancer Prevention and Control*. New York: M. Dekker.

Comarow A. 1997. 1997 annual guide to America's best hospitals: Inside the rankings. *U.S. News & World Report*, July 28.

Donaldson MS. 1998. Accountability for quality in managed care. *Journal of Quality Improvement* 24(12):711–725.

Ehrlich, RH, Hill CA, Winfrey KL 1997. The 1997 index of hospital quality. Chicago: National Opinion Research Center, University of Chicago.

Fishman P, Von Korff M, Lozano P, et al. 1997. Chronic care costs in managed care. *Health Affairs* 16(3):39–47.

Foley K. 1998. Presentation on "Policy issues for physicians and caregivers," at President's Cancer Panel Quality of Cancer Care/Quality of Life Conference, New Haven, CT.

Ganz P. 1996. Understanding cancer, its treatment, and the side effects of treatment. Chapter one in Hoffman B, ed. *A Cancer Survivor's Almanac: Charting Your Journey*. National Coalition for Cancer Survivorship.

Gold M, Nelson L, Brown R, et al. 1997. Disabled Medicare beneficiaries in HMOs. *Health Affairs* 16(5):149–162.

Graves EJ, Gillum BS. 1997. National hospital discharge survey: Annual summary, 1994. *Vital and Health Statistics. Series 13: Data from the National Health Survey* (128):i–v;1–50.

Health Care Financing Administration. 1998. http://www.hcfa.gov.

InterStudy. 1997. *The InterStudy Competitive Edge: Part II, HMO Industry Report*. No. 7.2. Excelsior, MN.

Jensen GA, Morrisey MA, Gaffnet S, Liston DK. 1997. The new dominance of managed care: Insurance trends in the 1990s. *Health Affairs* 16(1):125–136.

Jones A, Strahan G. 1997. The National Home and Hospice Care Survey: 1994 summary. National Center for Health Statistics. *Vital Health Statistics. Series 13: Data from the National Health Survey* 13(126):i–v; 1–125.

Landon B, Wilson I, Cleary P. 1998. A conceptual model of the effects of health care organizations on the quality of medical care. *Journal of the American Medical Association* 279(17):1377–1382.

Lazar GS, Desch CE. 1998. Performance measurement in cancer care: Uses and challenges. *Cancer* 82(10 Suppl):2016–2021.

Lynn J. 1997. Measuring quality of care at the end of life: A statement of principles. *Journal of the American Geriatrics Society* 45(4):526–527.

Mandelblatt J, Yabroff KR, Kerner J. 1998. Access to quality cancer care: Evaluating and ensuring equitable services, quality of life and survival. National Cancer Policy Board commissioned paper.

McGeary M. 1997. The National Cancer Program: Enduring Issues. Washington, D.C.: National Academy of Sciences, National Cancer Policy Board.

Medical Payment Advisory Commission. 1998. *Report to the Congress: Context for a Changing Medicare Program*.

Miller R, Luft H. 1997. Does managed care lead to better or worse quality of care? *Health Affairs* 16(5): 7–25.

Moore C. 1985. Multidisciplinary pretreatment cancer planning. *Journal of Surgical Oncology* 28:79–86.

Mortensen L, Leader S, Mallick R, et al. 1997. The impact of managed care on oncology practice. *Oncology Issues* 22–27.

Murphy GP, Morris LB, Lange D. 1997. *Informed Decisions: The Complete Book of Cancer Diagnosis, Treatment, and Recovery*. New York: Penguin Group.

National Cancer Advisory Board. 1994. *Cancer at a Crossroads: A Report to Congress for the Nation*.

National Cancer Institute. 1997. *Cancer Research: Because Lives Depend on It*. Bethesda, MD: National Institutes of Health.

National Cancer Institute. 1998a. *The Nation's Investment in Cancer Research: A Budget Proposal for Fiscal Year 1999*. Bethesda, MD: National Institutes of Health.

National Cancer Institute. 1998b. *State Cancer Legislative Database Program. 1990–98*. Bethesda, MD: National Institutes of Health.

National Cancer Institute. 1999. *The Nation's Investment in Cancer Research: A Budget Proposal for Fiscal Year 2000*. Bethesda, MD: National Institutes of Health.

Oncology Nursing Society. 1998. http://www.ons.org.

Piro L, Doctor J. 1998. Managed oncology care: The disease management model. *Cancer* 82(Suppl. 10):2068–2075.

Polednak AP. 1994. Projected numbers of cancer diagnosed in the U.S. elderly population, 1990 through 2030. *American Journal of Public Health* 84(8):1313–1316.

President's Advisory Commission on Consumer Protection and Quality in the Health Care Industry. 1998. *Quality first: Better health care for all Americans*. Washington, D.C.

President's Cancer Panel. 1997. *Fighting the War on Cancer in an Evolving Health Care System*. Bethesda, MD: National Cancer Program, National Cancer Institute.

Remler D, Donelan K, Blendon R, et al. 1997. What do managed care plans do to affect care? Results from a survey of physicians. *Inquiry* 34 (Fall):196–204.

Ries LAG, Kosary CL, Hankey BF, et al., eds. 1997. *SEER Cancer Statistics Review, 1973–1994*. NIH Pub. No. 97-2789. Bethesda, MD: National Cancer Institute, National Institutes of Health.

Riley, GF, Feuer EJ, Lubitz JD. 1996. Disenrollment of Medicare cancer patients from health maintenance organizations. *Medical Care* 34(8):826–836.

Riley GF, Potosky AL, Lubitz JD, et al. 1995. Medicare payments from diagnosis to death for elderly cancer patients by stage at diagnosis. *Medical Care* 33(8):828–841.

Schappert SM. 1997. Ambulatory care visits to physician offices, hospital outpatient departments, and emergency departments: United States, 1995. *Vital and Health Statistics. Series 13: Data from the National Health Survey* (129):1–38.

Schuette HL, Tucker TC, Brown ML, et al. 1995. The costs of cancer care in the United States: Implications for action. *Oncology* 9(11 Suppl.):19–22.

Simone J, Lyons J. In press. Superior cancer survival in children compared to adults: A superior system of cancer care? Salt Lake City: Huntsman Cancer Institute, University of Utah.

StataCorp, 1997, Stata Statistical Software: Release 5.0, College Station, TX: Stata Corporation.

St. Peter R, Reed MC, Blumenthal D, Kemper P. 1997. The scope of care provided by primary care physicians: Physician assessments of change and appropriateness. Paper presented at the Association for Health Services Research Annual Meeting, Chicago.

Taplin SH, Barlow W, Urban N, et al. 1995. Stage, age, comorbidity, and direct costs of colon, prostate, and breast cancer care. *Journal of the National Cancer Institute* 87(6):417–426.

U.S. Department of Health and Human Services, National Center for Health Statistics. 1999a. *National Ambulatory Medical Care Survey, 1994–1996, special tabulations*. Washington, D.C.

U.S. Department of Health and Human Services, National Center for Health Statistics. 1999b. *National Hospital Ambulatory Medical Care Survey, 1994–1996, special tabulations*. Washington, D.C.

U.S. Department of Health and Human Services, National Center for Health Statistics. 1999c. *National Hospital Discharge Survey, 1994, special tabulations*. Washington, D.C.

3

Ensuring Access to Cancer Care

The link between poor access to care and poor health outcomes is well established (Hoffman, 1998; IOM, 1994), but the reasons for inadequate access are not well understood. Some of the connections are intuitive and obvious: women without health insurance have breast cancer detected at later stages and have poorer survival rates than women with insurance (Ayanian et al., 1993). One in seven Americans lacks health insurance, which creates a general barrier to getting medical care of any kind. Some other barriers to receiving appropriate medical care are less obvious. Nonfinancial barriers that may prevent people from "getting to the door" of a health care provider include geography, language, fear and distrust of health care providers, and difficulties getting through appointment or "gatekeeper" systems. Once "in the door," other barriers to access may surface when attempting to navigate the system: for example, getting from a primary care provider to a specialist. Within the system, providers may lack current information on treatment, have difficulty communicating with patients, or have insufficient staff to coordinate care and provide all the services patients need. The cancer care system is complex; consequently, various barriers that serve to limit access may surface during each phase of care.

Access, as defined by the Institute of Medicine (IOM, 1994), **is the timely use of personal health services to achieve the best possible health outcomes.** This definition of access incorporates both the use of health services and the quality of such services to assess the degree of access that has been achieved. The test of equity of access involves first determining whether there are systematic differences in use and outcomes among groups in U.S. society and, if there are, the reasons for these differences (IOM, 1994).

This report brings together the best evidence from the published literature about the barriers to health care for cancer patients and the roots of these barriers. The body of available literature clearly documents differences in access to particular phases of care for particular cancers, at specific points in time and place. In no case, however, does it provide an overall picture of access to cancer care across society in the late 1990s, and in some cases conflicting evidence is presented on the same topic. Some discrepancies may be due to different research methods, but many of them probably reflect the actual situation—that access has varied across time and place and that the variation has multidimensional causes and effects. Nonetheless, the material presented here is a useful guide to general patterns of differential access and to some of the interventions that have been successful in improving access.

EVIDENCE OF ACCESS PROBLEMS

Individuals who are poor, have low educational attainment, or are members of racial or ethnic minority groups tend to have poorer cancer outcomes than members of other groups. This is supported by findings from the literature relating to different aspects of cancer care:

- Survival from cancer is associated with social class (characterized by income and education): lower social classes tend to have poorer survival (Gordon et al., 1992; Greenwald et al., 1996; Kogevinas and Porta, 1997; Savage et al., 1984).
- Overall cancer mortality is higher in the lower social classes, even after risk factors such as smoking are taken into account (Lantz et al., 1998).
- Death rates among African-American hospital patients with colorectal cancer are higher than rates for white patients, even when differences in patient characteristics, insurance status, clinical factors, and providers are accounted for (Ball and Elixhauser, 1996; Cooper et al., 1996).
- Hispanic cancer patients have lower colorectal survival rates than non-Hispanics (Goodwin et al., 1996).
- Five-year survival rates for Native American compared to white, non-Hispanic individuals, ascertained in 1978–1981, were substantially lower for colorectal cancer (37 versus 51 percent), lung and bronchial cancer (5 versus 12 percent), and female breast cancer (53 versus 75 percent) (Miller 1996).
- Individuals with cancer who are elderly, women, and members of racial/ethnic minority groups are more likely to have poor pain relief than others (Bernabei et al., 1998; Cleeland et al., 1994, 1997).

Why Do These Differences Exist?

Some of the factors that have been investigated as possibly affecting access to optimal cancer care are

- health insurance coverage and type of coverage;
- cost, including health insurance and out-of-pocket costs;
- attributes of the health care delivery system (e.g., geographic distribution of cancer care facilities, lack of service coordination);
- attributes of individuals (e.g., lack of knowledge or misperceptions about cancer prevention and treatment, linguistic or cultural attributes); and
- attributes of health care providers (e.g., lack of knowledge about cancer prevention and treatment, communication styles).

These factors and others may come into play in different ways at one or more of the steps along the path from cancer detection and treatment to care at the end of life, and all can potentially contribute to differences in outcomes. In this chapter, the role of financial barriers in the context of cancer care is reviewed, in particular, problems related to health insurance coverage and out-of-pocket costs. Then the literature exploring the sources of the mortality differentials among sociodemographic groups is summarized by the following phases of care (For a more in-depth review of this literature and a conceptual framework regarding issues of access to cancer care, see the NCPB commissioned paper by Mandelblatt and colleagues [Mandelblatt et al., 1998, available on line at: www.nas.edu/cancerbd], upon which this review is based):

- Phase 1: Early detection,
- Phase 2: Evaluation of abnormal screening results,
- Phase 3: Cancer treatment,
- Phase 4: Posttreatment surveillance and recurrence care, and
- Phase 5: End-of-life care.

Financial Barriers to Access to Cancer Care

Health Insurance and Type of Coverage

Individuals with cancer are very likely to be insured, because the large majority is over age 65 and covered by Medicare. Nevertheless, of the 1.3 million new cases of cancer diagnosed in 1997, an estimated 86,000 individuals, or 7 percent, would be expected to be uninsured (estimate based on age-specific cancer incidence rates and the age distribution of the uninsured). Nationally, 16 percent of the population was uninsured in 1997 (U.S. Bureau of the Census, 1998). In addition, many individuals with health insurance experience lapses in coverage (an estimated 12 million in 1992).

The diagnosis of cancer can, in itself, lead to a loss of health insurance coverage or to higher insurance premiums. In 1992, 7 percent of cancer survivors who were insured prior to their diagnosis reported that their health insurance changed following their cancer diagnosis (e.g., 5 percent said that their insurance costs increased) (Hewitt, 1998). Congress tried to remedy this problem in 1996, enacting the Health Insurance Portability and Accountability Act (Kennedy–Kassebaum Act) to improve the portability and continuity of health insurance coverage in private insurance markets and among employer-sponsored group health plans. The act limits the ability of insurers to deny or discontinue coverage because of preexisting conditions such as cancer. The increased cost of premiums for portable insurance products and difficulties in implementing the law, however, have limited the value of these new protections for consumers (U.S. General Accounting Office, 1997).

If individuals are uninsured, medical expenses related to cancer may force them to "spend down" to become eligible for Medicaid—that is, to deplete their assets until they meet eligibility criteria. Alternatively, individuals who are disabled by cancer for a period of two years may become eligible for Medicaid coverage through the Supplemental Security Income (SSI) program. Some hospitals are obligated to provide some charity care to the uninsured (i.e., under the Hill-

Burton Act of 1946); some state and federal programs provide free cancer screening and sometimes treatment for the uninsured (e.g., the Centers for Disease Control and Prevention [CDC] National Breast and Cervical Cancer Early Detection Program; the Maryland state program that pays for treatment for uninsured women with breast cancer); at least 50 pharmaceutical companies have patient assistance programs to help defray the costs of expensive chemotherapy drugs for those who are poor and uninsured (or underinsured);[1] and some charitable organizations provide free services or financial assistance to individuals with cancer. These programs and services cannot substitute for adequate insurance coverage for cancer treatment, but they can ease the financial burden for those who receive them.

• The American Cancer Society has a volunteer-based program called Road to Recovery that provides transportation for cancer patients to and from medical appointments and treatments (Anne Marie Oria, Texas American Cancer Society, personal communication to Elizabeth Kidd, October 1998).
• Cancer Care, a nonprofit, voluntary agency serving primarily the New York City area provides, on a limited basis, financial assistance for treatment-related expenses (e.g., transportation, child care, home care, pain medication) (Sherry Fremont, personal communication to Elizabeth Kidd, October 1998).
• St. Jude Children's Research Hospital provides free medical care, transportation, and other supportive services for children with cancer and other conditions (Jerry Chipman, personal communication to Elizabeth Kidd, September 1998).
• The Organ Transplant Fund provides health care support services, financial assistance, and advocacy programs to transplant candidates and their families (Organ Transplant Fund, 1998).

At least 27 states sell comprehensive health insurance to state residents with serious medical conditions who cannot find a company to insure them or who cannot afford the high cost of coverage. The insurance provided through these so-called state risk pools (also known as Guaranteed Access Programs) generally costs more than regular insurance, and in some states, there are waiting periods for coverage of preexisting conditions and lifetime caps on benefits (e.g., sometimes as low as $250,000) (Matt Hayes, Patient Advocate Foundation, personal communication to Elizabeth Kidd, September 1998).

---

[1]Bristol-Myers Squibb Company, for example, provides financial assistance to pay for the near 25 chemotherapy drugs that it makes. One of its products, Vepesid, (etoposide, oral), could cost an uninsured (or underinsured) cancer patient more than $1,000 per month. This program approved more than 5,000 applications from January through September 1998 (individuals must reapply for assistance every six months) (Betsey Grasser, personal communication to Elizabeth Kidd, October 1998). The Bristol-Myers Squibb program and those of other pharmaceutical companies have stringent eligibility requirements based on income and insurance status.

Cost, Including Health Insurance and Out-of-Pocket Costs

Health insurance coverage may not adequately protect individuals from the high costs associated with cancer treatment. Some policies have high deductibles (e.g., catastrophic policies typically contain a deductible of $15,000 or more), and copayments or coinsurance over the course of cancer treatment can be substantial (HIAA, 1998). Furthermore, many insurers, including Medicare, do not cover all of the drugs and treatments used by cancer patients (see discussion of prescription drug coverage below).

Relatively few studies specific to cancer exist regarding the magnitude of the financial burden associated with out-of-pocket costs, but available evidence suggests that it is substantial. In a study conducted in 1986, Medicare was found to cover an estimated 83 percent of typical total charges for lung cancer and 65 percent of typical charges for breast cancer (Sofaer et al., 1990). For these two cancers, investigators assessed the extent to which supplemental Medigap plans reduced out-of-pocket costs and found that plans varied widely in the financial protection offered. Out-of-pocket expenses ranged from less than $100 under some health maintenance organization (HMO) plans to nearly $4,000 under some private Medigap plans (1986 dollars) (Sofaer et al., 1990). Unlike the great majority of employer-provided insurance plans, Medicare does not cap beneficiaries' total payments for cost sharing (AARP, 1997). Medicare HMOs typically have lower cost sharing than the traditional Medicare program and may offer additional benefits, such as outpatient prescription drug coverage (AARP, 1997).

Prescription Drug Coverage. Insurance policies often lack comprehensive coverage for prescription drugs, a benefit needed by most individuals with cancer. Medicare, for example, does not cover the costs of most outpatient prescription drugs, which can include pain medications and other drugs to treat the effects of cancer and its treatment. Many Medicare beneficiaries are subject to these costs because only one-third of them have insurance policies that cover prescription drugs (e.g., Medicaid, employer-provided, or privately purchased policies) (Gluck, 1999). Most chemotherapy is administered in outpatient settings and is covered by Medicare. Even when insurance does offer prescription drug coverage, out-of-pocket expenses can be high because of limits to coverage.[2] An estimated 7 percent of the elderly with chronic illnesses spend at least 10 percent of their household income on prescription drugs (Rogowski et al., 1997).

REVIEW OF THE LITERATURE, BY PHASE OF CARE

Phase 1: Early Detection

Early detection tests for breast, cervical, and colorectal cancers are effective in reducing mortality. For women age 50 to 69, for example, mammography screening reduces the death rate from breast cancer by about one-third (USDHHS, 1991). Although effective, these tests are underutilized, for example,

---

[2]Available Medigap policies, for example, vary in their coverage of outpatient prescriptions. For some plans, the patient pays 50 percent per prescription. Others have an annual deductible (e.g., $250) and then cover up to $1,250 or $3,000 of the cost of prescription drugs.

- 56 percent of women age 50 and older in 1994 had had a mammogram to detect breast cancer within the past 2 years,
- 77 percent of women age 18 and older in 1994 had had a Pap smear to detect cervical cancer within the past 3 years,
- 30 percent of people age 50 and older in 1992 had had a fecal occult blood test (FOBT) to detect colorectal cancer within the past 2 years, and
- 33 percent of people age 50 and older in 1992 had ever had a proctosigmoidoscopy to detect colorectal cancer (NCHS, 1997).

For those cancers for which effective screening tests exist, diagnosis at advanced stages among those eligible for screening suggests that tests are underused. Overall, 6 percent of breast cancers, 8 percent of cervical cancers, and 21 percent of colorectal cancers are diagnosed late (i.e., advanced) (Ries et al., 1997), but late stage at diagnosis is more common among some sociodemographic groups than others:

- People living in areas with high rates of poverty and unemployment are more likely to have their colorectal cancer diagnosed at a late stage than those living in other areas (Mandelblatt et al., 1996).
- Women living in poorer neighborhoods are more likely than women living in wealthier areas to have invasive, rather than localized, cervical cancer at diagnosis (Breen and Figueroa, 1996).
- African-American and other minority group members diagnosed with cancer are more likely to be diagnosed at advanced stages of disease than are whites (Farley and Flannery, 1989; Mandelblatt et al., 1991, 1996; Wells et al., 1992). For cervical cancer, this racial gap has increased over time despite greater use of Pap tests among African-American, compared to white women (Mitchell and McCormack, 1997).
- African-American and Hispanic women are more likely to have breast cancer diagnosed at late stages than white women, when setting of care, income, and education are controlled for (Mandelblatt et al., 1991).
- Women are more likely than men to have late-stage colorectal cancer at diagnosis (Mandelblatt et al., 1996).

Financial Barriers to Cancer Screening

Lack of health insurance is clearly linked to lower rates of cancer screening (Ayanian, 1993; Hedegaard et al., 1996; Katz and Hofer, 1994; Mickey et al., 1997) and to diagnosis at more advanced stages of disease (Figure 3.1). However, even in countries where health care coverage is universal, screening rates are not uniformly high. In Canada, for example, individuals with high compared to low household incomes are more likely to be screened for cancer (Katz and Hofer, 1994). Conversely, despite not having health insurance, 40 to 50 percent of uninsured women in the United States report that they have been screened for cervical and breast cancer (Hoffman, 1998).

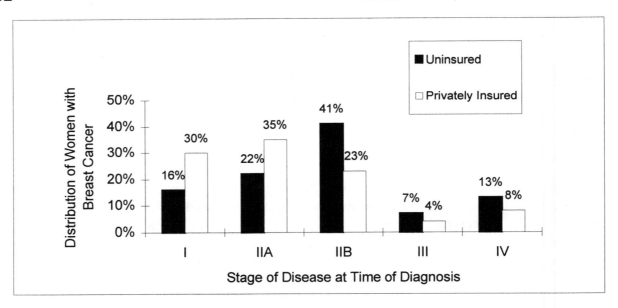

FIGURE 3.1 Distribution of women with breast cancer by disease stage at time of diagnosis. SOURCE: Hoffman, 1998.

Insurance policies vary in the extent of coverage they offer for cancer screening. People covered by plans with no or low levels of cost sharing are more likely to be screened for cancer than those in plans with higher out-of-pocket costs (Lurie et al., 1987). Among Medicare beneficiaries, those with private supplemental insurance are more likely to be screened for cancer than beneficiaries with Medicare supplemented by Medicaid or with Medicare alone (Blustein, 1995; Potosky et al., 1998). Cancer screening tests were a covered benefit for Medicare beneficiaries, but until 1998 a copayment was required for these tests.

Health Care Delivery and Cancer Screening

The way health care is delivered also affects the use of cancer screening tests. Individuals covered by managed care plans have higher rates of cancer screening than those covered by fee-for-service plans (Burack and Gimotty, 1997; Potosky et al., 1998). This is true also of Medicare beneficiaries in HMOs, whose cancer screening rates are the highest of the elderly population (Potosky et al., 1998).

Even for those with insurance, screening tests may be inaccessible because there are no facilities within a reasonable distance. Perhaps for this reason, residents of rural areas use cancer screening tests less often than their urban counterparts (Hayward et al., 1988b; Katz and Hofer, 1994). Some specific findings include the following:

• Women living in areas with no or few mammogram facilities are less likely to have mammograms than those living in areas with more facilities (Mandelblatt, 1995).

• Women living in areas with primary care shortages are less likely to have regular mammograms than women living elsewhere (Phillips et al, 1998).

Role of Patient Beliefs, Knowledge, and Racial or Socioeconomic Characteristics in Screening

A lack of awareness of the benefits of cancer screening can pose as significant a barrier as lack of insurance or distance from screening facilities. Many individuals know little about cancer, and do not know that it can be successfully treated or when and why screening tests are useful (Grady et al., 1992; Myers et al., 1991). Low level of education (which usually occurs in conjunction with low household income) is associated with lower cancer screening (and re-screening) use (Lannin et al., 1998; Mickey, 1997; Rutledge et al., 1988).

Concerns about inconvenience, discomfort, trouble, embarrassment, fear of radiation, and pain involved in screening are among the reasons people forgo cancer screening tests (Davis et al., 1996; Glanz et al., 1996; Myers et al., 1991; Stein et al., 1990). Other attitudes—fatalism, a feeling that one's health cannot be affected by traditional medicine, and religious or cultural beliefs—may also preclude cancer screening (Kagawa-Singer, 1997; Lannin et al., 1998; Mo, 1992).

In one breast cancer study, culturally based attitudes and beliefs were more predictive of advanced stage at diagnosis (suggesting low screening rates) than were social class and race (Lannin et al., 1998). In this study, African-American women had three times the odds of white women (i.e., an "odds ratio" of 3) of being diagnosed with late-stage disease (Stages III and IV). When social class was taken into account in the analysis, the odds ratio decreased to 1.8. When measures of cultural beliefs (e.g., the devil can cause you to get cancer, air causes cancer) were also controlled for in the analysis, African-American women no longer had increased odds of late-stage disease.

Use of mammography appears to account for much of the variation of stage at diagnosis of breast cancer that can be attributed to race (Breen and Figueroa, 1996; Mandelblatt et al., 1995). Studies have found the following:

• There were no differences in stage at diagnosis among women who were regular mammography users according to comparisons of mammography histories of elderly African-American and white women. However, among women who had not participated in screening mammography, the odds of being diagnosed with late-stage breast cancer were 2.5 times greater for African-American than for white women (McCarthy et al., 1998).

• Women who receive medical care through the Department of Defense, and who should therefore all have the same access to care, demonstrate no difference in stage among Caucasian, African-American, and Hispanic women diagnosed with breast cancer (Zaloznik, 1995, 1997).

• Among elderly women, African-Americans as compared to whites use mammography less often. More frequent use of mammography is associated with more visits to a primary care physician in both groups, but the deficit for African-American women persists at each income level, even after primary care use is considered. Primary care visits are less likely to "boost" mammography use for African-American women than for white women (Burns et al., 1996).

Some evidence suggests that certain racial and ethnic groups that appear to have adequate access to care are not getting appropriate screening services. In one study, women living in Appalachia and Hispanic women living in urban Texas had relatively low cancer screening rates despite having access to care (NCI, 1995b). Hispanics and some Asian groups (e.g., Chinese, Vietnamese) tend to have lower screening rates than whites or African Americans, which may be attributable, at least in part, to language and cultural barriers on the part of patients and providers (Hiatt and Pasik, 1996). Studies have found that

- physicians discussed mammography less often with Hispanic than with non-Hispanic patients (Fox and Stein, 1991),
- African-American women enrolled in managed care plans were less likely than white women to have had a doctor advise them to get a mammogram. Nevertheless, African-American and white women had similar self-report mammography use (Glanz et al., 1996); and
- African-American patients were less likely to report receiving advice about cancer screening or receiving screening tests than white patients seeing the same physicians (Gemson et al., 1988).

The older people are, the less likely they are to be screened for breast and cervical cancers (Fox et al., 1994; Hedegaard et al., 1996; NCHS, 1997; NCI, 1995). The elderly may hold beliefs that inhibit testing, but they are likely to comply with physicians' recommendations to be screened (Fox et al., 1994; Mandelblatt et al., 1991). Some physicians may also mistakenly believe that routine cancer screening is unimportant in elderly patients (Weisman et al., 1989).

Many people who are screened for cancer once do not have the tests repeated at recommended intervals. Rates of adherence to regular or "interval" screening are significantly lower than for the initial screening procedure (Burack and Gimotty, 1997; De Waard et al., 1984). Adherence to lifetime cancer screening is measured as the number of cancer screens received per number recommended. For example, if five screens were recommended for a 55-year-old woman and she had received only four of the five, she would be considered 80 percent adherent. The effect of age on adherence to interval screening appears to vary by cancer type, with higher screening rates observed for the elderly with colorectal cancer (Brown et al., 1990; Mandelblatt et al., 1996), but lower rates for cervical cancer (De Waard et al., 1984; Fink et al., 1972; Mandelblatt et al., 1998). One study indicates that adherence to lifetime breast cancer screening is higher among women who are younger, are members of a higher social class, and have access to care, especially membership in an HMO (the study compared women of similar age, race, education, and income) (Philips et al., 1998).

Role of the Physician in Cancer Screening Access

With or without insurance, lacking a regular source of care also leads to lower rates of cancer screening (Bindman et al., 1996; Fox et al., 1994; Gordon et al., 1998; Zapka, 1994; Zapka et al., 1992). In one study, women who did not have a regular doctor were 3.5 times more likely to be diagnosed with late-stage breast cancer than women who had seen their regular doctor within the past year (Lannin et al., 1998). In a study of multiethnic black and Hispanic women in New York, breast and cervical cancer screening rates increased when women had a usual source of care and when they had a regular clinician at their usual source (O'Malley et al., 1997). One of the strongest predictors of whether a person will be screened for cancer is whether the physician recommends testing (Fox and Stein, 1991; Grady et al., 1992; Mickey et al., 1997; Zapka et al., 1991). Overall, physicians order fewer cancer screening tests than are recommended in preventive health care guidelines (Fox et al., 1988; Schwartz et al., 1991). Some researchers have looked into the reasons physicians may not recommend screening tests and have found the following:

- Physicians are generally aware of guidelines, but they may not perceive screening tests to be beneficial in the absence of symptoms (Schapira et al., 1993).
- Screening recommendations change, and some providers may not keep up with current standards, whereas others may be confused by conflicting guidelines.
- Many individuals seek health care only when they have an acute illness and providers may miss opportunities to provide screening if they focus only on the presenting illness.
- A lack of reimbursement for counseling about screening, time pressures, and health system infrastructure limitations (e.g., a lack of tracking or reminder systems) may also contribute to providers' underuse of cancer screening tests.

Screening practices also vary by physician specialty. Obstetrician–gynecologists are more likely than family practitioners to order cancer screening tests for women. Internists generally recommend screening at lower rates than other primary care providers, and subspecialists providing primary care tend to screen at the same, or lower rates than primary care providers (Albanes et al., 1988; Bassett, 1985; Bergner et al., 1990; Mann et al., 1987; Schwartz et al., 1991; Weinberger et al., 1991; Weisman et al., 1989; Zapka et al., 1992). Some studies suggest that women cared for by female physicians are more likely to be screened for cancer than women cared for by male physicians (Lurie et al., 1997).

The manner in which screening is presented by health care providers can affect whether a person actually has the test. A higher level of enthusiasm for the recommendation can influence the likelihood of screening (Mickey et al., 1997). Women who say that they participated in the initial decision to be screened for breast cancer were also more likely to adhere to the recommended follow-up mammography regimen than those who felt the doctor had made the decision for them (Phillips et al., 1998).

Interventions to Improve Screening Rates

A number of interventions have been demonstrated to increase cancer screening rates. Telephone and mailed reminders from providers, multimedia educational interventions, financial incentives, and peer counseling can all increase women's use of mammography (Clementz et al., 1990; Davis et al., 1997; Irwig et al., 1990; Janz et al., 1997; Kendall, 1993; Kiefe et al., 1994; King et al., 1994; Landis et al., 1992; Lantz et al., 1995; Mickey et al., 1997; Mohler, 1995; Taplin et al., 1994). Among women already screened for cancer, reminders to return for screening increase interval testing (Mayer et al., 1994; Schapira et al., 1992). Providing general information about cancer screening alone to those who are eligible, however, has not been effective in increasing test use (Champion, 1994b; Nattinger et al., 1989; Skinner et al., 1994).

Interventions aimed at providers can also improve screening use. Physician reminder systems, chart audit with feedback, and physician education about appropriate screening practices contribute to higher screening test use (Becker et al., 1989; Burack et al., 1997; Chambers et al., 1989; Cheney and Ramsdell, 1987; Cowan et al., 1992; Landis et al., 1992; McPhee et al., 1989, 1991; Nattinger et al., 1989; Ornstein et al., 1991; Tierney et al., 1986; Yarnall et al., 1993). However, in one study, written feedback and financial incentives were ineffective in improving physician compliance to cancer screening guidelines in primary care sites serving women age 50 and older cared for in a Medicaid HMO (Hillman et al., 1998).

Phase 2: Evaluation of Abnormal Screening Results

Follow-Up of Abnormal Results

Screening tests alone do not provide a diagnosis of cancer; this can be made only with further testing. In fact, most people with abnormal results from a single cancer screening test will not be found to have cancer, so definitive testing is essential if the benefits of screening are to be realized (Mandelblatt et al., 1997). Nonetheless, many individuals fail to receive timely, or any, follow-up of an abnormal screening test, with large variations in the rates of nonresolution across settings and populations. Different studies have reported that 20–99 percent of women who have abnormal mammograms receive *appropriate* diagnostic follow-up (Kerlikewske, 1996; Manelblatt et al., 1993b), and 20–74 percent of women with abnormal Pap smears receive *appropriate* follow-up (Lacey et al., 1993; Marcus et al., 1992; Mandelblatt et al., 1997; Michielutte et al., 1985).

In one study of the reasons for delays between the time of the initial medical consultation and the establishment of a diagnosis among women with breast cancer, providers and the health care systems were found to be responsible for 45 percent of cases with significant delays. Delays were attributed to difficulties in scheduling or physician inaction. In about 25 percent of the cases, the delay was attributed to patients, and the most common reason for inaction provided by women was that the problem was not perceived as important. In another 17 percent of cases, both the patient and system were determined to be responsible. For the balance of cases, no reason for the delay was ascertained (Caplan et al., 1996). Several patient characteristics are associated with inadequate follow-up of abnormal cancer screening results: rural residence (Fox et al., 1997), relatively less education (Michielutte et al., 1985), low income (McCarthy et al., 1996a), and being a member of a racial or ethnic minority group (Chang et al., 1996; Kerlikowske, 1996; Mandelblatt et al., 1996; Rojas et al., 1996), but these factors are not all independent predictors of follow-up. Some of the observed racial differences may, in part, be attributable to socioeconomic status, age, marital status, and history of previous mammogram. For instance, when these factors were controlled for in an analysis of the effect of race on screening follow-up, the effect of race diminished substantially (McCarthy et al., 1996a). It is unclear whether certain patients fail to heed advice about follow-up; whether personal characteristics predict the likelihood that a physician will make follow-up recommendations; whether certain institutions lack tracking systems; or whether certain patients have difficulties navigating the system.

Studies have shown that out-of-pocket costs and the type of health care delivery system may influence follow-up rates. Women in HMOs who made copayments waited an average of 1.25 months longer between initial suspicion of cancer and obtaining a definitive diagnosis than women without copayments (Greenwald, 1987). In another study, colorectal cancer patients treated in HMOs had delays in diagnosis or treatment relative to patients in fee-for-service settings (Francis et al., 1984).

Some inadequate follow-up may be traced to poor provider–patient communication. In one study, more than half of the women with abnormal mammograms who had not sought follow-up care indicated that they thought their mammograms were normal (McCarthy et al., 1996b).

Among those who are informed of an abnormal screening test, some may not seek follow-up care for a variety of reasons:

- concern about cost,
- fear of learning that something is wrong,
- anxiety about painful diagnostic procedures (Rojas et al., 1996), or
- concern that they are too old for treatment (Mandelblatt, 1993a).

Interventions to Improve Follow-Up Rates

Several techniques have been tested to improve follow-up rates. Findings from key studies include the following:

- Telephone reminders are more effective than letters in increasing the follow-up of screening tests among women with abnormal Pap smears (Lerman et al., 1992; Marcus et al., 1992; Miller et al., 1997; Paskett, 1990).
- Computerized tracking systems can improve follow-up of abnormal screening results, but their success depends on adequate system staffing and support (Monticciolo and Sickles, 1990; Mandelblatt et al., 1998).
- A comprehensive review of interventions to increase colorectal cancer screening adherence found that the most intensive strategies delivered to eligible persons rarely increased adherence to FOBT above 50 percent. These intensive strategies included the use of a letter signed by one's own physician and including FOBT kits in the mailout to intensive follow-up with instructional telephone calls (Vernon, 1997).
- A review of the literature on strategies to increase adherence to breast and cervical cancer screening among underserved women determined that management systems directed to both patients and providers were consistently effective for most underserved women. Community-based outreach and integration of preventive services at the primary health care site are effective strategies for both African-American and Hispanic women. Use of mass media has been successful when targeted toward Hispanic women, but not when targeted toward African-American women. Mobile units and integration of preventive services at primary health care sites are effective strategies for elderly women (Vellozzi et al., 1996).

• One hospital serving a low-income population instituted a "patient navigator" system that was successful in improving follow-up of abnormal screening or cancer diagnostic tests. Patient navigators were employed to ensure that individuals with abnormal tests were brought into care. Navigators made intensive efforts to contact women, including home visits, and facilitated follow-up appointments once women had been contacted (e.g., arranged child care, transportation) (Freeman et al., 1995).

Access to Definitive Cancer Staging

After a cancer diagnosis, additional tests are used to further classify and stage the disease. These staging tests provide critical information for selecting among treatment options and also provide prognostic information (e.g., likelihood of survival). Cancer patients who have a complete set of staging tests have better survival compared to those who do not (although the reason for this is not obvious) (Lee-Feldstein et al., 1994; Mandelblatt et al., 1998).

There is significant variation in oncologists' and surgeons' use of tests for diagnosis and staging for cancer (Plawker et al., 1997), and standard diagnostic workup and staging are not performed consistently in all population groups. There is evidence suggesting that appropriate staging is completed more frequently for

• younger women with breast cancer (Hillner et al., 1996; Kosary et al., 1995; Lash and Silliman, 1998; Silliman et al., 1989);
• men compared to women (e.g., for colorectal cancers, lung cancers) (Kosary et al., 1995);
• Medicare beneficiaries in HMOs compared to those in fee-for-service (e.g., for breast, cervical, colon, and prostate cancers) (Riley et al., 1994);
• whites compared to African Americans (e.g., for bladder, breast, colorectal, lung or bronchus, uterine, cervical, renal, and prostate cancers) (Ball and Elixhauser, 1996; Harris et al., 1997; Kosary, 1995; Liff et al., 1991); and
• urban compared to rural residents (Liff et al., 1991).

Phase 3: Cancer Treatment

Physicians use information from the diagnostic workup and staging process to formulate treatment recommendations. The treatment that patients actually receive depends on a number of factors, however, including the availability of health care resources, insurance coverage, physicians' awareness of treatment options, and patients' treatment preferences. These variations often show up as differences in the geographic distribution of cancer treatments (Ballard-Barbash et al., 1996; Farrow et al., 1992, 1996; Harlan et al., 1995; Nattinger et al., 1992; Samet et al., 1990). For example, use of breast conserving therapy ranged from 48 percent in Minnesota to 74 percent in Massachusetts (Guadagnoli et al., 1998). Rates of use of systemic chemotherapy also show wide geographic variation (Osteen and Karnell, 1994).

The availability of health care resources explains some geographic variation in cancer treatment:

• Women with breast cancer were more likely to get breast conserving surgery (BCS) than other types of surgery if they resided in counties with a cancer center or in a large city (Samet et al., 1994).

• Women were more likely to receive BCS when they were treated in hospitals with a high volume of breast cancer cases, a medical school affiliation, radiation facilities, and geriatric services (Nattinger et al., 1992).

• In two studies, women with early breast cancer, who were cared for in teaching hospitals, were more likely to receive BCS than those seen in nonteaching settings (Lee-Feldstein et al., 1994; Studnicki et al., 1993).

Having health insurance and the type of coverage one has are also associated with differential treatment patterns:

• Among individuals with non-small-cell lung cancer, patients without private insurance receive surgery less often than those with it (Greenberg et al., 1988).

• Rates of bone marrow transplantation for leukemia or lymphoma have been from one-third to one-half lower among self-pay and Medicaid patients than among privately insured patients (Mitchell et al., 1997).

Physicians may not recommend expensive chemotherapy for uninsured or underinsured patients for financial reasons or because they believe that such groups are less likely to comply with the treatment regimen (Begg and Carbone, 1983).

In one study, one-third or more patients undergoing treatment for cancer in Texas reported out-of-pocket costs exceeding $100 per visit for chemotherapy or radiotherapy. Hispanics were more likely than whites or blacks to have out-of-pocket costs higher than $200 per visit, probably because they were uninsured or underinsured (Guidry et al., 1998).

These same investigators found that black and Hispanic cancer patients being treated in Texas with chemotherapy or radiotherapy consistently reported that barriers such as distance, access to an automobile, and availability of someone to drive them to the treatment center were major problems (Guidry et al., 1997).

The major barriers influencing whether or not patients with cancer seek or continue treatment identified in a recent review of the literature include (Guidry et al., 1996):

• communication problems between patients and providers,
• lack of information about side effects,
• cost of treatment,
• difficulties in obtaining and maintaining insurance coverage, and
• absence of social support networks.

Access barriers generally were found to be greater for older women, members of minority groups, and patients of lower socioeconomic status.

Variation in Cancer Treatment by Age

In many cases (though not all), older people are less likely to get effective cancer treatments than are younger people, despite evidence that the elderly can tolerate and benefit from them (Begg and Carbone, 1983). The underuse of aggressive treatment among older people is often assumed to be related to the presence of coexisting conditions, but even among those without potentially complicating conditions, treatment differences exist by age (Newschaffer et al., 1996). Physicians may underuse some cancer treatment for elderly patients because they do not know that the elderly can tolerate aggressive therapy, they make mistaken assumptions about patient preferences, or they underestimate life expectancy. Some evidence suggests that the elderly are as likely as younger patients to prefer aggressive, lifesaving treatment (McQuellon et al., 1995; Yellen et al., 1994). Several research studies have documented the underuse of cancer treatments among older patients:

- Older patients with localized or regional non-small-cell lung cancer were less likely than younger patients to receive any therapy, and among those who did receive therapy, older patients were more likely to receive radiotherapy than the more aggressive surgical treatment (Smith et al., 1995).
- The elderly are less likely to receive bone marrow transplantation for leukemia or lymphoma (Mitchell et al., 1997).
- Among women with breast cancer, older women are less likely to receive BCS instead of mastectomy (Chu et al., 1987; Farrow et al., 1992; Mor et al., 1985; Newschaffer et al., 1996; Satariano, 1992), and among those getting BCS, older women have lower rates of adjuvant radiotherapy (Greenfield et al., 1987).
- Use of adjuvant chemotherapy declines with age among women with localized breast cancer (Hillner et al., 1996).
- Physicians deviate from recommended chemotherapy regimens more frequently when treating older patients with cancer (Schleifer et al., 1991).
- In New Mexico between 1984 and 1986, 43 percent of women age 85 and older, 84 percent of women age 75–84, and 92 percent of women age 65–74 received definitive treatment for localized breast cancer (defined as lumpectomy or excisional biopsy followed by radiation therapy or mastectomy). Age remained significant when access to transportation, physical activity levels, income, social support, ability to perform activities of daily living, mental status, and the presence of other medical illnesses were taken into account (Goodwin et al., 1993).
- In a comparable population of women in Virginia in 1985–1989, 66 percent of women age 65–69 and 7 percent of women age 85 and older received the appropriate radiation therapy after BCS. In addition, 44 percent of patients with positive lymph nodes received any adjuvant therapy, and 33 percent received hormone therapy (even though adjuvant therapy is recommended for all patients with node-positive disease) (Hillner et al., 1996).
- Based on Surveillance, Epidemiology, and End Results Program (SEER) data, 76 percent of women age 65–69, 68 percent age 70–74, 56 percent age 75–79, and 24 percent age 80 years or older received radiation therapy after breast conserving surgery for Stage I or II cancer. Controlling for differences in comorbidity narrowed, but did not eliminate, the difference associated with age (Ballard-Barbash et al., 1996).

Similar differences in treatment by age have been reported from other studies (Farrow et al., 1992; Greenfield et al., 1987; Lazovich et al., 1991).

Not all the evidence points to underuse of treatment in older people, however. One of the more thorough studies, of postmenopausal women with early breast cancer treated in 1993 in Minnesota, found that most (92 percent) women with node-positive breast cancer received some form of adjuvant therapy (Guadagnoli et al., 1997). The likelihood of treatment with adjuvant therapy did decline slightly with age, but the decline was not statistically significant. The use of adjuvant therapy was less frequent in women with node-negative breast cancer and did decline with age, but the age-associated differences were not significant after adjusting for various demographic and disease-associated factors.

Variations in Cancer Treatment by Race, Social Characteristics, and Gender

Differences in treatment by race have been well documented: African-American patients are less likely than white patients to undergo surgical resection for colorectal cancer (Cooper et al., 1996), to receive bone marrow transplantation for leukemia or lymphoma (Mitchell et al., 1997), to receive radical prostatectomy and radiation for localized prostate cancer (Harlan et al., 1995), or to have breast conserving surgery (BCS) for breast cancer or receive radiation therapy following BCS (Farrow et al., 1992; Muss et al., 1992; Nattinger et al., 1992). However, it appears that these effects may actually be more closely related to social class than to race.

In one study, elderly residents of areas characterized by low compared to high educational attainment were more likely to have received no treatment for non-small-cell lung cancer and, when treated, to receive radiation instead of surgical therapy, despite having similar clinical profiles (Smith et al., 1995). In another study, low educational attainment and a high percentage of the population with poverty-level incomes were associated with lower rates of BCS for women with breast cancer (Samet et al., 1994).

There are few large differences in survival among cancer patients by gender and studies of patterns of treatment by gender for bladder or colorectal cancer, leukemia, and lymphoma do not suggest any differences in care for men and women (Harris et al., 1997; Mitchell et al., 1997).

Physician-Associated Variation in Cancer Treatment

Physicians' treatment recommendations are influenced by a number of factors, including physician age (Liberati et al., 1987), gender (GIVIO, 1988), specialty (Deber and Thompson, 1987), and belief in efficacy of care (Liberati et al., 1987). The content of physician communication also varies according to patient characteristics, including age, income, education, race or ethnicity, and expected prognosis (Waitzkin, 1985).

Variations in the use of breast conserving surgery (BCS) instead of mastectomy for patients with early breast cancer may, in part, be explained by physician specialty, training, and experience. When asked about treatment preferences, medical oncologists were more likely than surgeons to prefer BCS (Deber and Thompson, 1987), surgeons were more likely than primary care physicians to prefer BCS, and among surgeons, those with postgraduate specialty training in surgical oncology were more likely than surgeons with general board certification to recommend BCS to elderly patients (Mandelblatt et al., 1998).

Delays in adoption or lack of compliance with practice guidelines can limit access to recommended cancer care. In 1985, for example, a consensus statement of expert opinion was published accepting the use of BCS and radiation therapy in selected patients with early-stage breast cancer (Harris, et al., 1985). By 1990, the rates of BCS among women 65 to 79 in the Medicare program ranged from only 8 to 26 percent across regions of the United States and rates of BCS use had not increased appreciably nationally (i.e., from 14 percent in 1986 to 15 percent in 1990) (Nattinger et al., 1996). Physicians have also not adhered to recommended chemotherapy regimens. In one study, more than half of patients had their chemotherapy modified by their physicians in ways that were considered inappropriate (Schleifer et al., 1991).

The quality of physician–patient communication can affect clinical outcomes (Greenfield et al., 1988; Kaplan et al., 1989), adjustment to cancer (Roberts et al., 1994), patient quality of life, and satisfaction with care (Greenfield et al., 1988; Kaplan et al., 1989). Evidence of communication gaps is therefore worrisome. Patients and their physicians report the content of their interactions differently (Mackillop et al., 1988; Mosconi et al., 1991; Siminoff et al., 1989), assess the role of the patient in the decision-making process differently (Strull et al., 1984), and have different expectations of treatment benefits (Mackillop et al., 1988; Mosconi et al., 1991; Siminoff et al., 1989). In one study, relatively few women with breast cancer (15 to 27 percent) who had had a mastectomy reported that their physicians discussed BCS as a treatment option (Guadagnoli et al., 1998). Physicians who believe that patients should participate in treatment decisions are more likely to recommend BCS (Liberati et al.,1991).

Cancer Treatment in Clinical Trials

Clinical trials are the mechanism through which new technologies, pharmaceuticals, or therapeutic strategies are evaluated against current standards of care. For patients with cancer, clinical trials can provide access to the best available and most promising new treatments.

There are striking variations in age-specific rates of participation in cancer clinical trials: more than 70 percent of children with cancer participate, but fewer than two percent of individuals age 50 and older with cancer participate in cooperative group clinical trials sponsored by the National Cancer Institute (Tejeda et al., 1996). Pediatric cancers are relatively rare and care within the context of a clinical trial has become standard practice (Simone and Lyons, in press). The elderly have historically been excluded from cancer clinical trials because of concerns about treatment complications or side effects, comorbid conditions, and interactions with current medications (although this has been changing).

Studies conducted to identify inequalities in access to clinical trials among racial or ethnic groups suggest that African Americans are represented in treatment trials, but underrepresented in screening and chemoprevention trials, in proportion to their age-specific rates of cancer (Bleyer et al., 1997a, b; Chlebowshi et al., 1993; Tejeda et al., 1996; Thompson et al., 1995). Negative attitudes toward medicine and research may inhibit African-American participation in clinical trials (Mouton et al., 1997; Robinson, 1996). The National Institutes of Health (NIH) Revitalization Act of 1993 specified that women, minorities, and other subpopulations must be included in all government-sponsored Phase III clinical trials (which are usually large, randomized trials), or justification for their exclusion must be documented (NIH, 1994).

Physicians underrefer patients to clinical trials because of concerns about patient age, frailty, inadequate health insurance coverage, ability to travel to the clinical trial center, and other aspects of participation that might be considered a burden to the patient (Foley and Moertel, 1991). Physicians also report being concerned about the amount of time associated with participation in a trial (patient and physician), being uncomfortable with discussions of the uncertainty of trial treatment, and being concerned about changes in the physician's role as a result of trial participation (Farrar, 1991; Kaluzny et al., 1993; Taylor et al., 1984).

Access to clinical trials can be limited by insurance policies. Most insurers do not cover the cost of participation in clinical trials as a matter of policy (e.g., Medicare, most state Medicaid programs, most managed care organizations).

Phase 4: Posttreatment Surveillance and Recurrence Care

Patients are monitored for recurrent cancer and psychosocial distress for the first several years following their primary and adjuvant treatment when the probability of recurrence and adjustment difficulties is greatest (Schiffer et al., 1997). For most cancers, however, little evidence exists from which to develop guidelines for "appropriate" follow-up procedures, so variations in treatment cannot necessarily be interpreted as better or worse care. Not surprisingly, there is relatively little research on access to care during this phase of disease management, although there are indications that the intensity of follow-up care does vary, at least for some cancers (e.g., lung and colorectal cancers) (Johnson et al., 1996a, b; Virgo et al., 1995). Some of this variation is explained by physician experience and training (Johnson et al., 1996c). One study of the effect of race on the follow-up care of men with prostate cancer in the U.S. military health care system suggests that when health care is uniformly available, follow-up care is similar for whites and African Americans (Moul et al., 1996).

Phase 5: End-of-Life Care

Care at the end of life for patients dying from cancer may include heroic attempts at cure, pain management, treatment for psychological problems, or combinations of these. Caregivers may be the same as those involved in earlier phases of treatment but are likely to include others, among them, hospice caregivers from various disciplines. For most patients, palliation eventually becomes the focus of care. Barriers to the best end-of-life care may stem from financial constraints, and from provider and patient attitudes and knowledge.

Financial Factors

The uninsured and inadequately insured may not be able to afford important components of end-of-life care (e.g., pain medication, nutritional supplements, outpatient nursing services)

(Underwood, 1995). Even among the well insured, the costs of end-of-life care can contribute to financial hardship. In one study, more than half of the families involved in the care of a seriously ill family member reported at least one severe burden ranging from loss of family savings, or loss of income, to changes in future educational plans or employment status (Covinsky et al., 1994). One commonly cited financial burden relates to Medicare reimbursement policy. Medicare will reimburse for pain management at an inpatient facility, but not for outpatient oral analgesics. This is a major barrier to adequate pain management for terminal cancer patients who choose to die at home.

An additional barrier to end-of-life care is the absence of a primary care provider. The poor and uninsured may be less likely to have a regular clinician with whom they are comfortable discussing end-of-life care issues.

Patient Factors

Patients dying of cancer often suffer avoidable pain and distress (Cleeland et al., 1994; Passik et al., 1998). Certain patient attitudes or beliefs can act as barriers to good end-of-life care. Stoicism can lead to underreporting of pain, nausea, or depression; concerns about becoming addicted to pain medication or a belief in the inevitability of pain with cancer can contribute to the underuse of pain medication (Ward et al., 1993). Some patients are reluctant to communicate symptoms to their providers for fear of diverting attention from the pursuit of a cure (Ward et al., 1993). Some evidence suggests that these attitudinal barriers may be more prevalent among certain sociodemographic groups (e.g., those with low educational attainment) and certain racial or ethnic minority groups (Cleeland et al., 1997; Rimer et al., 1987; Ward et al., 1993).

Provider Factors

Aside from financial barriers, most impediments to adequate end-of-life care are associated with health care providers. For example, although there are effective pharmacological strategies to manage pain, providers consistently undertreat pain (Levin et al., 1998; Levy, 1996; McCaffery and Ferrell, 1995). In one study, 42 percent of patients with recurrent or metastatic cancer were inadequately managed for their pain (Cleeland et al., 1994). The elderly, women, and members of racial or ethnic minority groups are more likely than others to have poor pain relief (Bernabei et al., 1998; Cleeland et al., 1994, 1997). Physicians report concerns about management of side effects, patient tolerance of analgesia, and regulatory scrutiny when prescribing narcotics as barriers to effective pain management (Van Roenn et al., 1993). Simple measures, such as attaching a patient-completed pain assessment sheet to the front of the medical chart, can increase effective pain management (Trowbridge et al., 1997).

Physicians also do not adequately identify signs of depression among patients with cancer. In one study, only 13 percent of patients with evidence of moderate to severe depression were identified by their physicians (Passik et al., 1998). Providers may not have clear guidance on how to manage terminal cancer care. Guidelines are available to assist in the management of cancer-associated pain (e.g., from the Agency for Health Care Policy and Research), but there are no standards of care for other common symptoms of cancer such as anxiety, anorexia, or the wasting often associated with cancer.

Communication among various members of the end-of-life care team and with patients may be less than optimal. In one study of terminally ill patients, communication between physicians and patients was poor—only 41 percent of patients in the study reported talking to their physician about prognosis or about their wishes regarding resuscitation (SUPPORT, 1995; Lo, 1995). Physicians infrequently discuss advance directives, and when these are discussed, there is considerable disagreement on the outcome of such discussions. Patients' requests for end-of-life care (e.g., withholding of CPR) are frequently not documented in the medical chart (Haidet et al., 1998; SUPPORT, 1995).

A recent study reports that the vast majority of people with terminal cancer overestimate their chances of surviving their illness (Smith et al., 1998; Weeks et al., 1998). Those who thought they were going to live for six months were more than two times as likely to choose aggressive anticancer therapy instead of palliative or hospice care, which is designed to relieve symptoms. The overoptimistic patients did indeed live longer than those who had more realistic expectations. Patients who overestimated their survival and received aggressive therapy, however, had exactly the same median survival as those who received palliative care and were more likely to have a hospital readmission, undergo attempted resuscitation, or die while receiving ventilatory support. Some patients choose aggressive chemotherapy, even when there is little chance of benefit (Slevin et al., 1990). To achieve the goals of supporting patient values and minimizing the prospect of utilizing therapies that will not increase survival, physicians must make sure that patients understand their prognosis by initiating a dialogue, asking what patients want to know, providing estimates of survival duration, explaining the poor efficacy and debilitating side effects of therapy common at this stage, and discussing all treatment options, including palliative care alone (Smith et al., 1998).

About half of cancer patient deaths involve hospice care. "Hospice" is a philosophy of care that emphasizes the coordinated delivery of many services for terminally ill patients and their families including: nursing care; physician services; homemakers and home health aides; physical, occupational, and speech therapy; and psychological counseling and social services. Medicare provides a hospice benefit that has criteria for patient admissions and use of therapies. Eligibility for hospice services under Medicare requires an expected survival of less than six months, but most hospice patients live for less than two months following their admission. Physicians appear to delay referring patients for hospice care, in part because it is difficult to predict accurately the expected survival of the terminally ill. Delays in referral may also be due to a physician's lack of knowledge of hospice services, poor communication with the palliative care team, or reluctance to engage in uncomfortable discussions or feelings about end-of-life care (Christakis and Escarce, 1996). Hospice benefits for non-Medicare patients are variable and Medicaid coverage of hospice care varies from state to state.

The National Cancer Policy Board sought additional information about barriers to effective end-of-life care for cancer patients by commissioning interviews with 19 expert physicians, nurses, social workers, and health services researchers. The findings are summarized in the paper, *Issues in End of Life Care for People with Cancer: Interviews with Selected Providers and Researchers* (Gelband et al., 1999). This approach was taken to complement the 1997 report, *Approaching Death: Improving Care at the End of Life,* completed by IOM's Committee on Care at the End of Life (IOM, 1997). The 1997 report is a thorough review of end-of-life issues, ending with a series of recommendations that were accepted by the NCPB for cancer patients (Box 3.1). For more detail and context, the reader is referred to the complete IOM report.

A recent review examined outcome measures that have been used, or proposed for use in the clinical audit of palliative care of patients with advanced cancer. Identified measures met some, but not all of the objectives of measurement in palliative care, and fulfilled some, but not all of the criteria established for validity, reliability, responsiveness, and appropriateness (Hearn et al., 1997).

KEY FINDINGS

A persistent, vexing problem for many Americans is lack of health insurance or insufficient coverage to help defray the expense of a costly illness such as cancer. Although most individuals diagnosed with cancer are elderly and have Medicare coverage, an estimated 7 percent of those facing a new diagnosis of cancer lack health insurance. Health insurance offers some, but often incomplete, protection against the high costs of cancer care. High deductibles, copayments or coinsurance, and limits on coverage can all contribute to high out-of-pocket costs. Medicare was, for example, estimated to cover only 83 percent of typical total charges for lung cancer and 65 percent of typical charges for breast cancer in 1986. Some individuals have additional protection through other insurers (e.g., Medigap policies, Medicaid), but even then, the financial burden of cancer can be substantial. A particular problem for many with cancer involves limitations on prescription drug coverage, an expensive and widely used benefit.

Individuals who are poor, have low educational attainment, or are members of racial or ethnic minority groups tend to have less favorable outcomes with cancer than other groups. Limited access to primary care or cancer screening contributes to having cancer diagnosed at later stages when the prognosis is worse. Having health insurance coverage improves access, but does not guarantee that cancer screening tests are used. Other factors that can impede access to screening are culturally based attitudes and beliefs, not having services available in the local community, and health care providers not able to speak the language of the people they serve.

It is often health care providers who can be held accountable for the underuse of cancer screening tests. One of the strongest predictors of whether a person will be screened for cancer is whether the physician recommends testing, and evidence suggests that physicians order fewer screening tests than they should. The use of screening tests is improved in managed care plans, compared to fee-for-service plans.

Even when screening is used, many individuals fail to receive timely, or any, follow-up of abnormal screening results. Both screening and follow-up rates can be improved with interventions aimed at those eligible for screening (e.g., telephone and mailed reminders from providers, educational interventions) and health care providers (e.g., reminder systems).

Differences in treatment by race have been well documented. However, it appears that the effect may actually be related more closely to social class than to race. Another group that appears to be vulnerable in the cancer care system is the elderly. Older people are often less likely to get effective cancer treatments than are younger people, despite evidence that the elderly can tolerate and benefit from them. Some undertreatment is explained by provider attitudes toward treating the elderly, who are perceived as less willing or able to tolerate aggressive treatment.

There is evidence of widespread quality problems in end-of-life care, especially in the area of pain management. The elderly, women, and members of racial or ethnic minority groups are more likely than others to have poor pain relief, which appears to be due to a combination of factors: poor palliative care practices on the part of providers, attitudes of patients (e.g., stoicism), and miscommunication between patients and health care providers.

BOX 3.1 "Recommendations and Future Directions" from
Approaching Death: Improving Care at the End of Life

1. People with advanced, potentially fatal illnesses and those close to them should be able to expect and receive reliable, skillful, and supportive care.

2. Physicians, nurses, social workers, and other health professionals must commit themselves to improving care for dying patients and to using existing knowledge effectively to prevent and relieve pain and other symptoms.

3. Because many deficiencies in care reflect system problems, policymakers, consumer groups, and purchasers of health care should work with health care providers and researchers to:

   a. strengthen methods for measuring the quality of life and other outcomes of care for dying patients and those close to them;

   b. develop better tools and strategies for improving the quality of care and holding health care organizations accountable for care at the end of life;

   c. revise mechanisms for financing care so that they encourage rather than impede good end-of-life care and sustain rather than frustrate coordinated systems of excellent care; and

   d. reform drug prescription laws, burdensome regulations, and state medical board policies and practices that impede effective use of opioids to relieve pain and suffering.

4. Educators and other health professionals should initiate changes in undergraduate, graduate, and continuing education to ensure that practitioners have the relevant attitudes, knowledge, and skills to care for dying patients.

5. Palliative care should become, if not a medical specialty, at least a defined area of expertise, education, and research.

6. The nation's research establishment should define and implement priorities for strengthening the knowledge base for end-of-life care.

7. A continuing public discussion is essential to develop a better understanding of the modern experience of dying, the options available to dying patients and families, and the obligations of communities to those approaching death.

SOURCE: IOM, 1997.

REFERENCES

Albanes D, Weinberg GB, Boss L, Taylor PR. 1988. A survey of physicians' breast cancer early detection practices. *Preventive Medicine* 17(5):643–652.

American Association of Retired Persons Public Policy Insitute and the Lewin Group. 1997. *Out-of-Pocket Health Spending by Medicare Beneficiaries Age 65 and Older: 1997 Projections.*

Ayanian JZ, Kohler BA, Abe T, Epstein AM. 1993. The relation between health insurance coverage and clinical outcomes among women with breast cancer. *New England Journal of Medicine* 329:326–331.

Ball JK, Elixhauser A. 1996. Treatment differences between blacks and whites with colorectal cancer. *Medical Care* 34:970–984.

Ballard-Barbash R, Potosky AL, Harlan LC, et al. 1996. Factors associated with surgical and radiation therapy for early stage breast cancer in older women. *Journal of the National Cancer Institute* 88(11):716–726.

Bassett AA. 1985. Occult breast cancer and changing patterns of surgical practice. *Canadian Journal of Surgery* 28(4):297–298.

Becker DM, Gomez EB, Kaiser DL, et al. 1989. Improving preventive care at a medical clinic: How can the patient help? *American Journal of Preventive Medicine* 5(6):353–359.

Begg CB, Carbone PP. 1983. Clinical trials and drug toxicity in the elderly: The experience of the Eastern Cooperate Oncology Group. *Cancer* 52:1986–1992.

Bergner M, Allison CJ, Diehr P, et al. 1990. Early detection and control of cancer in clinical practice. *Archives of Internal Medicine* 150(2):431–436.

Bernabei R, Gambassi G, Lapane K, et al. 1998. Management of pain in elderly patients with cancer. *Journal of the American Medical Association* 279(23):1877–1882.

Bindman AB, Grumbach K, Osmond D, et al. 1996. Primary care and receipt of preventive services. *Journal of General Internal Medicine* 11(5):269–276.

Bleyer WA, Tejeda HA, Murphy SB, et al. 1997a. Equal participation of minority patients in U.S. national pediatric cancer clinical trials. *Journal of Pediatric Hematology/Oncology* 19(5):423–427.

Bleyer WA, Tejeda H, Murphy SB, et al. 1997b. National cancer clinical trials: Children have equal access; adolescents do not. *Journal of Adolescent Health* 21:366–373.

Blustein J. 1995. Medicare coverage, supplemental insurance, and the use of mammography by older women. *New England Journal of Medicine* 332:1138–1143.

Breen N, Figueroa JB. 1996. Stage of breast and cervical cancer diagnosis in disadvantaged neighborhoods: A prevention policy perspective. *American Journal of Preventive Medicine* 12:319–326.

Brown ML, Potosky AL, Thompson GB, Kessler LG. 1990. The knowledge and use of screening tests for colorectal and prostate cancer: Data from the 1987 national health interview survey. *Preventive Medicine* 19(5):562–574.

Burack RC, Gimotty PA. 1997. Promoting screening mammography in inner-city setting. The sustained effectiveness of computerized reminders in a randomized controlled trial. *Medical Care* 35:921–931.

Burns RB, McCarthy EP, Freund KM, et al. 1996. Black women receive less mammography even with similar use of primary care. *Annals of Internal Medicine* 125(3):173–182.

Caplan LS, Helzlsouer KJ, Shapiro S, et al., 1996. Reasons for delay in breast cancer diagnosis. *Preventive Medicine* 25(2):218–224.

Chambers CV, Balaban DJ, Carlson BL, et al. 1989. Microcomputer-generated reminders. Improving the compliance of primary care physicians with screening guidelines. *Journal of Family Practice* 29(3):273–280.

Champion VL. 1994a. Beliefs about breast cancer and mammography by behavioral stage. *Cancer* 72: 1100–1112.

Champion VL. 1994b. Strategies to increase mammography utilization. *Medical Care* 32(2):118–129.

Champion VL, Huster G. 1994. Effect of interventions on stage of mammography adoption. *Journal of Behavioral Medicine* 18(2):169–187.

Chang SW, Kerlikowske K, Napoles-Springer A, et al. 1996. Racial differences in timeliness of follow-up after abnormal screening mammography. *Cancer* 78:1395–1402.

Cheney C, Ramsdell JW. 1987. Effect of medical records' checklists on implementation of periodic health measures. *American Journal of Medicine* 83:129–136.

Chlebowski RT, Bulter J, Nelson A, et al. 1993. Breast cancer chemoprevention. Tamoxifen: Current issues and future prospective. *Cancer* 2(3 Suppl.):1032–1037.

Christakis NA, Escarce JJ. 1996. Survival of Medicare patients after enrollment in hospice programs. *New England Journal of Medicine* 335(3):172–178.

Chu J, Diehr P, Feigle P, et al. 1987. The effect of age on the care of women with breast cancer in community hospitals. *Journal of Gerontology* 42(2):185–190.

Cleeland CS, Gonin R, Baez L, et al. 1997. Pain and pain treatment in minority outpatients with metastatic cancer: The Eastern Cooperative Oncology Group Minority Outpatient Pain Study. *Annals of Internal Medicine* 127:813–816.

Cleeland CS, Gonin R, Hatfield AK, et al. 1994. Pain and its treatment in outpatients with metastatic cancer. *New England Journal of Medicine* 330:592–596.

Clementz GL, Aldag JC, Gladfelter TT, et al. 1990. A randomized study of cancer screening in a family practice setting using a recall model. *Journal of Family Practice* 30:537–541.

Cooper GS, Yuan Z, Landefeld CS, Rimm AA. 1996. Surgery for colorectal cancer: Race-related differences in rates and survival among Medicare beneficiaries. *American Journal of Public Health* 86(4):582–586.

Covinsky KE, Goldman L, Cook EF, et al. 1994. The impact of serious illness on patients' families. SUPPORT Investigators. Study to Understand Prognoses and Preferences for Outcomes and Risks of Treatment. *Journal of the American Medical Association* 272(23):1839–1844.

Cowan JA, Heckerline PS, Parker JB. 1992. Effect of a fact sheet reminder on performance of the periodic health examination: A randomized controlled trial. *American Journal of Preventive Medicine* 8:104–109.

Davis NA, Nash E, Bailey C, et al. 1997. Evaluation of three methods for improving mammography rates in a managed care plan. *American Journal of Preventive Medicine* 13(4):298–302.

Davis TC, Arnold C, Berkel HJ, et al. 1996. Knowledge and attitude on screening mammography among low-literate, low-income women. *Cancer* 78:1912–1920.

Deber RB, Thompson GG. 1987. Who still prefers aggressive surgery for breast cancer? Implications for the clinical applications of clinical trials. *Archives of Internal Medicine* 147:1543–1547.

De Waard F, Collette HJA, Rombach JJ, et al. 1984. The DOM project for the early detection of breast cancer, Utrecht, The Netherlands. *Journal of Chronic Diseases* 37:1–44.

Elixhauser A, Ball JK. 1994. Black/white differences in colorectal tumor location in a national sample of hospitals. *Journal of the National Medical Association (United States)* 85:449–458.

Farley TA, Flannery JT. 1989. Late-stage diagnosis of breast cancer in women of lower socioeconomic status: Public health implications. *American Journal of Public Health* 79(11):1508–1512.

Farrar WB. 1991. Clinical trials: Access and reimbursement. *Cancer* 67(6 Suppl.):1779S–1782S.

Farrow DC, Hunt WC, Samet JM. 1992. Geographic variation in the treatment of localized breast cancer. *New England Journal of Medicine* 326:1097–1101.

Farrow DC, Samet JM, Hunt WC. 1996. Regional variation in survival following the diagnosis of cancer. *Journal of Clinical Epidemiology* 49(8):843–847.

Fink R, Shapiro S, Roester R. 1972. Impact of efforts to increase participation in repetitive screenings for early breast cancer detection. *American Journal of Public Health* 62:328–336.

Foley JF, Moertel CG. 1991. Improving accrual into cancer clinical trials. *Journal of Cancer Education* 6:165–173.

Fox E. 1997. Predominance of the curative model of medical care: A residual problem. *Journal of the American Medical Association* 278(9):761–764.

Fox P, Amsberger P, Zhang X. 1997. An examination of differential follow-up rates in cervical cancer screening. *Journal of Community Health* 22:199–209.

Fox SA, Stein JA. 1991. The effect of physician–patient communication on mammography utilization by different ethnic groups. *Medical Care* 29(11):1065–1082.

Fox SA, Klos DS, Tsou CV. 1988. Underuse of screening mammography by family physicians. *Radiology* 166:431–433.

Fox SA, Roetzheim RG, Kington RS. 1997. Barriers to cancer prevention in the older person. *Clinics in Geriatric Medicine (United States)* 13(1):79–95.

Fox SA, Siu AL, Stein JA. 1994. The importance of physician communication on breast cancer screening of older women. *Archives of Internal Medicine* 154:2058–2068.

Fox SA, Tsou CV, Klos DS. 1985. An intervention to increase mammography screening by residents in family practice. *Journal of Family Practice* 20(5):467–471.

Francis AM, Polissar L, Lorenz AB. 1984. Care of patients with colorectal cancer. A comparison of a health maintenance organization and fee-for-service practices. *Medical Care* 22(5):418–429.

Freeman HP, Muth BJ, Kerner JF. 1995. Expanding access to cancer screening and clinical follow-up among the medically underserved. *Cancer Practice* 3(1):19–30.

Gelband H, Greene A, Kidd E. 1999. *Issues in End of Life Care for People with Cancer: Interviews with Selected Providers and Researchers.* Washington, D.C.: National Academy Press.

Gemson DH, Elinson J, Messeri P. 1988. Differences in physician prevention practice patterns for white and minority patients. *Journal of Community Health* 13:53–64.

GIVIO. 1988. Survey of treatment of primary breast cancer in Italy. *British Journal of Cancer* 57:130–134.

Glanz K, Resch N, Lerman C, Rimer BK. 1996. Black–white differences in factors influencing mammography use among employed female health maintenance organization members. *Ethnicity and Health* 1(3):207–220.

Gluck ME. 1999. A Medicare Prescription Drug Benefit. National Academy of Social Insurance, *Medicare Brief* April 1999 (1):1-13.

Goodwin JS, Hunt WC, Samet JM. 1993. Determinants of cancer therapy in elderly patients. *Cancer* 72(2):594–601.

Goodwin JS, Samet JM, Hunt WC. 1996. Determinants of survival in older cancer patients. *Journal of the National Cancer Institute (United States)* 88(15):1031–1038.

Gordon NH, Crowe JP, Brumberg DJ, Berger NA. 1992. Socioeconomic factors and race in breast cancer recurrence and survival. *American Journal of Epidemiology* 135:609–618.

Gordon NP, Rundall TG, Parker L. 1998. Type of health care coverage and the likelihood of being screened for cancer. *Medical Care* 36(5):636–645.

Grady KE, Lemkau JP, McVay JM, Reisine ST. 1992. The importance of physician encouragement in breast cancer screening of older women. *Preventive Medicine* 21:766–780.

Greenberg ER, Chute CG, Stukel T, et al. 1988. Social and economic factors in the choice of lung cancer treatment. A population-based study in two rural states. *New England Journal of Medicine* 318:612–617.

Greenfield S, Blanco DM, Slashoff RM, Ganz PA. 1987. Patterns of care related to age of breast cancer patients. *Journal of the American Medical Association* 257:2766–2770.

Greenfield S, Kaplan SH, Ware JE, et al. 1988. Patient's participation in medical care: Effects of blood sugar control and quality of life in diabetes. *Journal of General Internal Medicine* 3:448–457.

Greenwald HP. 1987. HMO membership, copayment, and initiation of care for cancer: A study of working adults. *American Journal of Public Health* 77(4):461–466.

Greenwald HP, Borgatta EF, McCorkle R, Polissar N. 1996. Explaining reduced cancer survival among the disadvantaged. *Milbank Quarterly* 74(2):215–239.

Guadagnoli E, Shapiro C, Gurwitz JH, et al. 1997. Age-related patterns of care: Evidence against ageism in the treatment of early stage breast cancer. *Journal of Clinical Oncology* 15:2338–2344.

Guadagnoli E, Weeks JC, Shapiro CL, et al. 1998. Use of breast-conserving survey for treatment of Stage I and Stage II breast cancer. *Journal of Clinical Oncology* 16(1):101–106.

Guidry JJ, Aday LA, Zhang D, Winn RJ. 1997. Transportation as a barrier to cancer treatment. *Cancer Practice* 5(6):361–366.

Guidry JJ, Aday LA, et al. 1998. Cost considerations as potential barriers to cancer treatment. *Cancer Practice* 6(3):182–187.

Guidry JJ, Greisinger A, Aday LA, et al. 1996. Barriers to cancer treatment: A review of published research. *Oncology Nursing Forum* 23(9):1393–1398.

Haidet P, Hamel MB, Davis RB, et al. 1998. Outcomes, preferences for resuscitation, and physician–patient communication among patients with metastatic colorectal cancer. SUPPORT Investigators. Study to Understand Prognoses and Preferences for Outcomes and Risks of Treatments. *American Journal of Medicine* 105(3):222–229.

Harlan L, Brawley O, Pommerenke F, et al. 1995. Geographic, age, and racial variation in the treatment of local/regional carcinoma of the prostate. *Journal of Clinical Oncology (United States)* 13:93–100.

Harris DR, Andrews R, Elixhauser A. 1997. Racial and gender differences in use of procedures for black and white hospitalized adults. *Ethnicity and Disease* 7:91–105.

Harris JR, Hellman S, Kinne DW. 1985. Limited surgery and radiotherapy for early breast cancer. *New England Journal of Medicine* 313:1365.

Hayward RA, Shapiro MF, Freeman HE, Corey CR. 1988a. Inequities in health services among insured Americans. Do working-age adults have less access to medical care than the elderly? *New England Journal of Medicine* 318:1507–1512.

Hayward RA, Shapiro MF, Freeman HE, Corey CR. 1988b. Who gets screened for cervical and breast cancer? *Archives of Internal Medicine* 148:1177–1181.

Health Insurance Association of America. 1998. http://www.hiaa.org.

Hearn J, Higginson IJ. 1997. Outcome measures in palliative care for advanced cancer patients: A review. *Journal of Public Health Medicine* 19(2)193–199.

Hedegaard HB, Davidson AJ, Wright R. 1996. Factors associated with screening mammography in low-income women. *American Journal of Preventive Medicine* 12(1):51–56.

Hewitt M. 1998. Special tabulations, 1992 National Health Interview Survey, Cancer Survivorship Section.

Hiatt RA, Pasick RJ. 1996. Unsolved problems in early breast cancer detection: Focus on the underserved. *Breast Cancer Research and Treatment* 40:37–51.

Hillman AL, Ripley K, Goldfarb N, et al. 1998. Physician financial incentives and feedback: Failure to increase cancer screening in Medicaid managed care. *American Journal of Public Health* 88(11):1699–1701.

Hillner BE, Penberthy L, Desch CE, et al. 1996. Variation in staging and treatment of local and regional breast cancer in the elderly. *Breast Cancer Research and Treatment* 40:75–86.

Hoffman C. 1998. *Uninsured in America: A Chart Book.* The Kaiser Commission on Medicaid and the Uninsured.

IOM (Institute of Medicine). 1994. *Access to Health Care in America.* Washington, D.C.: National Academy Press.

IOM. 1997. *Approaching Death: Improving Care at the End of Life.* MJ Field, CK Cassel, eds. Washington, D.C.: National Academy Press.

Irwig L, Turnbull D, McMurchie M. 1990. A randomized trial of general practitioner-written invitations to encourage attendance at screening mammography. *Community Health Studies* 14:357–364.

Janz NK, Schottenfeld D, Doerr KM, et al. 1997. A two-step intervention to increase mammography among women aged 65 and older. *American Journal of Public Health* 87:1683–1686.

Johnson FE, McKirgan LW, Coplin MA, et al. 1996a. Geographic variation in patient surveillance after colon cancer surgery. *Journal of Clinical Oncology* 14:183–187.

Johnson FE, Naunheim KS, Coplin MA, Virgo KS. 1996b. Geographic variation in the conduct of patient surveillance after lung cancer surgery. *Journal of Clinical Oncology* 14:2940–2949.

Johnson FE, Novell LA, Coplin MA, et al. 1996c. How practice patterns in colon cancer patient follow-up are affected by surgeon age. *Surgical Oncology* 5:127–131.

Kagawa-Singer M. 1997. Addressing issues for early detection and screening in ethnic populations. *Oncology Nursing Forum* 24(10):1705–1711.

Kaluzny A, Brawley O, Garson-Angert D, et al. 1993. Assuring access to state-of-the art care for U.S. minority populations: The first 2 years of the minority-based community clinical oncology program. *Journal of the National Cancer Institute* 85(23):1945–1950.

Kaplan SH, Greenfield S, Ware JE. 1989. Assessing the effects of physician–patient interactions on the outcomes of chronic disease. *Medical Care* 27:S110–127.

Katz SJ, Hofer TP. 1994. Socioeconomic disparities in preventive care persist despite universal coverage. Breast and cervical cancer screening in Ontario and the United States. *Journal of the American Medical Association* 272(7):530–534.

Kendall C, Hailey BJ. 1993. The relative effectiveness of three reminder letters on making and keeping mammogram appointments. *Behavioral Medicine* 19(1):29–34.

Kerlikowske K. 1996. Timeliness of follow-up after abnormal screening mammography. *Breast Cancer Research and Treatment* 40:53–64.

Kiefe CI, McKay SV, Halevy A, Brody BA. 1994. Is cost a barrier to screening mammography for low-income women receiving Medicare benefits? A randomized trial. *Archives of Internal Medicine* 154:1217–1224.

King ES, Rimer BK, Seay J, et al. 1994. Promoting mammography use through progressive interventions: Is it effective? *American Journal of Public Health* 84:104–106.

Kogevinas M, Porta M. 1997. Socioeconomic differences in cancer survival: A review of the evidence. *IARC Scientific Publication* 138:177–206.

Kosary CL, Ries LAG, Miller BA, et al. 1995. *SEER Cancer Statistics Review, 1973–1992: Tables and Graphs.* Bethesda, MD: National Cancer Institute, National Institutes of Health.

Lacey L, Whitfield J, DeWhite W, et al. 1993. Referral adherence in an inner city breast and cervical cancer screening program. *Cancer* 72:950–955.

Landis SE, Hulkower SD, Pierson S. 1992. Enhancing adherence with mammography through patient letters and physician prompts: A pilot study. *North Carolina Medical Journal* 53:575–578.

Lannin DR, Mathews HF, Mitchell J, et al. 1998. Influence of socioeconomic and cultural factors on racial differences in late-stage presentation of breast cancer. *Journal of the American Medical Association* 279:1801–1807.

Lantz PM, House JS, Lepkowski JM, et al. 1998. Socioeconomic factors, health behaviors, and mortality. Results from a nationally representative prospective study of U.S. adults. *Journal of the American Medical Association* 279:1703–1708.

Lantz PM, Stencil D, Lippert MT, et al. 1995. Breast and cervical cancer screening in a low-income managed care sample: The efficacy of physician letters and phone calls. *American Journal of Public Health* 85:834–836.

Lash TL, Silliman RA. 1998. Re: Prevalence of cancer. *Journal of the National Cancer Institute* 90(5):399–400.

Lazovich D, White F, Thomas DB, Moe RE. 1991. Under-utilization of breast-conserving surgery and radiation therapy among women with Stage I or II breast cancer. *Journal of the American Medical Association* 266:3433–3438.

Lee-Feldstein A, Anton-Culver H, Feldstein PJ. 1994. Treatment differences and other prognostic factors related to breast cancer survival. Delivery systems and medical outcomes. *Journal of the American Medical Association* 271(15):1163–1168.

Lerman C, Caputo C, Milller S, et al. 1992. Telephone counseling improves adherence to colposcopy among lower-income minority women. *Journal of Clinical Oncology* 10:330–333.

Levin ML, Berry JI, Leiter J. 1998. Management of terminally ill patients: Physician reports of knowledge, attitudes, and behavior. *Journal of Pain and Symptom Management* 15:27–40.

Levy MH. 1996. Drug therapy: Pharmacologic treatment of cancer pain. *New England Journal of Medicine* 335:1124–1132.

Liberati A, Apolone G, Nicolucci A, et al. 1991. The role of attitudes, beliefs, and personal characteristics of Italian physicians in the surgical treatment of early breast cancer. *American Journal of Public Health* 81:38–42.

Liberati A, Patterson WB, Biener L, McNeil BJ. 1987. Determinants of physicians' preference for alternative treatments in women with early breast cancer. *Tumori* 73:601–609.

Liff JM, Chow WH, Greenberg RS. 1991. Rural–urban differences in stage at diagnosis. Possible relationship to cancer screening. *Cancer* 67:1454–1459.

Lo B. 1995. Improving care near the end of life: Why is it so hard? *Journal of the American Medical Association* 274(20):1634–1636.

Lurie N, Manning WG, Peterson C, et al. 1987. Preventive care: Do we practice what we preach? *American Journal of Public Health* 77(7):801–804.

Lurie N, Margolis KL, McGovern PG, et al. 1997. Why do patients of female physicians have higher rates of breast cancer and cervical screening? *Journal of General Internal Medicine* 12:34–43.

Mackillop WJ, Stewart WE, Ginsburg AD, et al. 1988. Cancer patients' perception of their disease and treatment. *British Journal of Cancer* 58:355–358.

Mandel JS, Bond JH, Church TR, et al. 1993. Reducing mortality from colorectal cancer by screening for fecal occult blood. *New England Journal of Medicine* 328:1365–1371.

Mandelblatt J, Kanetsky PA. 1995. Effectiveness of interventions to enhance physician screening for breast cancer. *Journal of Family Practice* 40:162–170.

Mandelblatt J, Andrews H, Kao R, et al. 1995. Impact of access and social context on breast cancer stage at diagnosis. *Journal of Health Care for the Poor and Underserved* 6(3):342–351.

Mandelblatt J, Andrews H, Kao R, et al. 1996. The late-stage diagnosis of colorectal cancer: Demographic and socioeconomic factors. *American Journal of Public Health* 86:1794–1797.

Mandelblatt J, Andrews H, Kerner J, et al. 1991. Determinants of late stage of diagnosis of breast and cervical cancer: The impact of age, race, social class, and hospital type. *American Journal of Public Health* 81:646–649.

Mandelblatt J, Freeman H, Winczewski D, et al. 1997. The costs and effects of cervical cancer screening in a public hospital emergency room. *American Journal of Public Health* 87(7):1182–1189.

Mandelblatt JS, Ganz PA, Kahn KL. 1998. A proposed agenda for the measurement of breast cancer quality of care outcomes in oncology practice. Submitted to *Journal of Oncology*.

Mandelblatt J, Richart R, Thomas L, et al. 1992a. Is human papillomavirus associated with cervical neoplasia in the elderly? *Gynecologic Oncology* 46:6–12.

Mandelblatt J, Traxler M, Lakin P, et al. 1992b. Mammography and Papanicolaou smear use by elderly poor black women. The Harlem Study Team. *Journal of the American Geriatrics Society* 40(10):1001–1007.

Mandelblatt JS, Wheat ME, Monane M, et al. 1992c. Breast cancer screening for elderly women with and without comorbid conditions. A decision analysis model. *Annals of Internal Medicine* 116:722–730.

Mandelblatt J, Traxler M, Lakin P, et al. 1993a. Breast and cervical cancer screening of poor, elderly, black women: Clinical results and implications. *American Journal of Preventive Medicine* 9(3):133–138.

Mandelblatt JS, Traxler M, Lakin P, et al. 1993b. A nurse practitioner intervention to increase breast and cervical cancer screening for poor, elderly black women. *Journal of General Internal Medicine* 8:173–178.

Mandelblatt J, Traxler M, Lakin P, et al. 1993c. Targeting breast cancer and cervical cancer screening to elderly poor black women: Who will participate? *Preventive Medicine* 22:20–33.

Mandelblatt J, Yabroff KR, Kerner J. 1998. Access to quality cancer care: Evaluating and ensuring equitable services, quality of life and survival. National Cancer Policy Board commissioned paper.

Mann LC, Hawes DR, Ghods M, et al. 1987. Utilization of screening mammography: Comparison of different physician specialties. *Radiology* 164:121–122.

Marcus AC, Crane LA, Kaplan CP, et al. 1992. Improving adherence to screening follow-up among women with abnormal Pap smears. Results from a large clinic-based trial of three intervention strategies. *Medical Care* 30:216–230.

Mayer JA, Clapp EJ, Bartholomew S, Elder J. 1994. Facility-based inreach strategies to promote annual mammograms. *American Journal of Preventive Medicine* 10(6):353–356.

McCaffery M, Ferrell BR. 1995. Nurses' knowledge about cancer pain: A survey of five countries. *Journal of Pain and Symptom Management* 10:356–369.

McCarthy BD, Yood MU, Janz NK, et al. 1996a. Evaluation of factors potentially associated with inadequate follow-up of mammographic abnormalities. *Cancer* 77:2070–2076.

McCarthy BD, Yood MU, Boohaker EA, et al. 1996b. Inadequate follow-up of abnormal mammograms. *American Journal of Preventive Medicine* 12:282–288.

McCarthy EP, Burns RB, Coughlin SS, et al. 1998. Mammography use helps to explain differences in breast cancer stage at diagnosis between older black and white women. *Annals of Internal Medicine* 128(9):729–736.

McPhee SJ, Bird JA, Fordham D, et al. 1991. Promoting cancer prevention activities by primary care physicians. Results of a randomized, controlled trial. *Journal of the American Medical Association* 266(4):538–544.

McPhee SJ, Bird JA, Jenkins CNH, Fordham D. 1989. Promoting cancer screening. A randomized, controlled trial of three interventions. *Archives of Internal Medicine* 149:1866–1872.

McQuellon RP, Muss HB, Hoffman SL, et al. 1995. Patient preferences for treatment of metastatic breast cancer: A study of women with early-stage breast cancer. *Journal of Clinical Oncology* 13:858–868.

Michielutte R, Diseker RA, Young LD, May WJ. 1985. Noncompliance in screening follow-up among family planning clinic patients with cervical dysplasia. *Preventive Medicine* 14(2):248–258.

Mickey RM, Vezina JL, Worden JK, Warner SL. 1997. Breast screening behavior and interactions with health care providers among lower income women. *Medical Care* 35(12):1204–1211.

Miller BA, Kolonel LN, Bernstein L, et al., (eds.). 1996. *Racial/Ethnic Patterns of Cancer in the United States, 1988–1992.* Bethesda MD: National Cancer Institute.

Miller SM, Siejak KK, Schroeder CM, et al. 1997. Enhancing adherence following abnormal Pap smears among low-income minority women: A preventive telephone counseling strategy. *Journal of the National Cancer Institute* 89(10):703–708.

Mitchell JB, McCormack LA. 1997. Time trends in late-stage diagnosis of cervical cancer: Differences by race/ethnicity and income. *Medical Care* 35(12):1220–1224.

Mitchell JM, Meehan KR, Kong J, Schulman KA. 1997. Access to bone marrow transplantation for leukemia and lymphoma: The role of sociodemographic factors. *Journal of Clinical Oncology (United States)* 15:2644–2651.

Mo B. 1992. Modesty, sexuality, and breast health in Chinese-American women. *Western Journal of Medicine* 157:260–264.

Mohler PJ. 1995. Enhancing compliance with screening mammography recommendations: A clinical trial in a primary care office. *Family Medicine* 27:117–121.

Monticciolo DL, Sickles EA. 1990. Computerized follow-up of abnormalities detected at mammography screening. *American Journal of Roentgenology* 155:751–753.

Mor V, Masterson-Allen S, Goldberg RJ, et al. 1985. Relationship between age at diagnosis and treatments received by cancer patients. *Journal of the American Geriatric Society* 33:585–589.

Mosconi P, Meyerowitz BE, Liberati, et al. 1991. Disclosure of breast cancer diagnosis: Patient and physician reports. *Annals of Oncology* 2:273–280.

Moul JW, Douglas TH, McCarthy WF, McLeod DG. 1996. Black race is an adverse prognostic factor for prostate cancer recurrence following radical prostatectomy in an equal access health care setting. *Journal of Urology* 155:1667–1673.

Mouton CP, Harris S, Rovi S, et al. 1997. Barriers to black women's participation in cancer clinical trials. *Journal of the National Medical Association (United States)* 89:721–727.

Muss HB, Hunter CP, Welsey M, et al. 1992. Treatment plans for black and white women with Stage II node-positive breast cancer—The National Cancer Institute Black/White Cancer Survival Study. *Cancer* 70:2460–2467.

Myers RE, Ross EA, Wolf TA, et al. 1991. Behavioral interventions to increase adherence in colorectal cancer screening. *Medical Care* 29:1039–1050.

National Cancer Institute. 1995a. Breast and cervical cancer screening among underserved women. *Archives of Family Medicine* 4:617–624.

National Cancer Institute. 1995b. *Cancer Screening Consortium for Underserved Women.* Bethesda, MD: National Institutes of Health.

National Center for Health Statistics. 1997. *Healthy People 2000 Review.* Hyattsville, MD: Public Health Service.

National Institutes of Health. 1994. NIH guidelines on the inclusion of women and minorities as subjects in clinical research. *Federal Register* 59:14508–14513.

Nattinger AB, Gottlieb MS, Hoffman RG, et al., 1996. Minimal increase in use of breast-conserving surgery from 1986 to 1990. *Medical Care* 34(5)479–489.

Nattinger AB, Gottlieb MS, Veum J, et al. 1992. Geographic variation in the use of breast-conserving treatment for breast cancer. *New England Journal of Medicine* 326:1102–1127.

Nattinger AB, Panzer RJ, Janus J. 1989. Improving the utilization of screening mammography in primary care practices. *Archives of Internal Medicine* 149:2087–2092.

Newschaffer CJ, Penberthy L, Desch CE, et al. 1996. The effect of age and comorbidity in the treatment of elderly women with nonmetastatic breast cancer. *Archives of Internal Medicine* 156:85–90.

O'Malley AS, Mandelblatt J, Gold K, et al. 1997. Continuity of care and the use of breast and cervical cancer screening services in a multiethnic community. *Archives of Internal Medicine* 157(13): 1462–1470.

Organ Transplant Fund, Inc. 1998. http//:www.otf.org.

Ornstein SM, Garr DR, Jenkins RG, et al. 1991. Computer-generated physician and patient reminders. Tools to improve population adherence to selected preventive services. *Journal of Family Practice* 32:82–90.

Osteen RT, Karnell LH. 1994. The National Cancer Data Base report on breast cancer. *Cancer* 73:1994–2000.

Paskett ED, White E, Carter WB, Chu J. 1990. Improving follow-up after an abnormal Pap smear: A randomized controlled trial. *Preventive Medicine* 19(6):630–641.

Passik SD, Dugan W, McDonald MV, et al. 1998. Oncologists' recognition of depression in their patients with cancer. *Journal of Clinical Oncology* 16:1594–1600.

Phillips KA, Kerlikowske K, Baker LC, et al. 1998. Factors associated with women's adherence to mammography screening guidelines. *Health Services Research* 33(1):29–53.

Plawker MW, Fleisher JM, Vapnek EM, Macchia RJ. 1997. Current trends in prostate cancer diagnosis and staging among United States urologists. *Journal of Urology* 158(5):1853–1858.

Potosky AL, Breen N, Graubard BI, Parsons PE. 1998. The association between health care coverage and the use of cancer screening tests. Results from the 1992 National Health Interview Survey. *Medical Care* 36:257–270.

Ries LAG, Kosary CL, Hankey BF, Miller BA, Harras A, Edwards BK, eds. 1997. *SEER Cancer Statistics Review, 1973–1994.* NIH Pub. No. 97-2789. Bethesda, MD: National Cancer Institute, National Institutes of Health.

Riley GF, Potosky AL, Lubitz JD, Brown ML. 1994. Stage of cancer at diagnosis for Medicare HMO and fee-for-service enrollees. *American Journal of Public Health* 84:1598–1604.

Rimer B, Levy M, Kleintz MK, et al. 1987. Improving cancer patients' pain control through education. *Progress in Clinical and Biological Research* 248:123–127.

Roberts CS, Cox CE, Reintgen DS, et al. 1994. Influence of physician communication on newly diagnosed breast patients' psychologic adjustment and decision making. *Cancer* 74(1 Suppl.):336–341.

Robinson SB, Ashley M, Haynes MA. 1996. Attitudes of African-Americans regarding prostate cancer clinical trials. *Journal of Community Health* 21(2):77–87.

Rogowski J, Lillard L, Kington R. 1997. The financial burden of prescription drug use among elderly persons. *Gerontologist* 37(4):475–482.

Rojas M, Mandelblatt J, Cagney K, et al. 1996. Barriers to follow-up of abnormal screening mammograms among low-income minority women. *Ethnicity and Health* 1(3):221–228.

Rutledge DN, Hartmann WH, Kinman PO, Winfield AC. 1988. Exploration of factors affecting mammography behaviors. *Preventive Medicine* 17:412–422.

Samet JM, Hunt WC, Farrow DC. 1994. Determinants of receiving breast-conserving surgery. *Cancer* 73:2344–2351.

Samet JM, Hunt WC, Goodwin JS. 1990. Determinants of cancer stage. A population-based study of elderly New Mexicans. *Cancer* 66:1302–1307.

Satariano W. 1992. Cormorbidity and functional status in older women with breast cancer: Implications for screening, treatment, and prognosis. *Journal of Gerontolology* 47:24–31.

Savage D, Lindenbaum J, Van Ryzin J, et al. 1984. Race, poverty, and survival in multiple myeloma. *Cancer* 54(12):3085–3094.

Schapira DV, Kumar NG, Clark RA, Yag C. 1992. Mammography screening credit card and compliance. *Cancer* 70:509–512.

Schapira DV, Panies RJ, Kumar NB, et al. 1993. Cancer screening. Knowledge, recommendations, and practices of physicians. *Cancer* 71:839–843.

Schiffer CA, Dodge R, Larson RA. 1997. Long-term follow-up of cancer and leukemia group B studies in acute myeloid leukemia. *Cancer* 80(11):2210–2214.

Schleifer SJ, Bhardwaj S, Lebovits A, et al. 1991. Predictors of physician nonadherence to chemotherapy regimens. *Cancer* 67:945–951.

Schwartz JS, Lewis CE, Clancy C, et al. 1991. Internists' practices in health promotion and disease prevention. A survey. *Annals of Internal Medicine (United States)* 114:46–53.

Selby JV, Friedman GD, Quesenberry CP Jr., Weiss N. 1992. A case-control study of sigmoidoscopy and mortality from colorectal cancer. *New England Journal of Medicine* 326:653–657.

Shapiro S, Venet W, Strax P, et al. 1982. Ten-to-fourteen-year effect of screening on breast cancer mortality. *Journal of the National Cancer Institute* 69:349.

Silliman RA, Guadagnoli F, Weitberg AB, Mor V. 1989. Age as a predictor of diagnostic and initial treatment intensity in newly diagnosed breast cancer patients. *Journal of Gerontology* 44:M46–50.

Siminoff LA, Fetting JH, Abeloff MD. 1989. Doctor–patient communication about breast cancer adjuvant therapy. *Journal of Clinical Oncology* 7:1192–1200.

Simone J, Lyons J. In press. Superior cancer survival in children compared to adults: A superior system of cancer care? Salt Lake City: Huntsman Cancer Institute, University of Utah.

Skinner CS, Strecher VJ, Hospers H. 1994. Physician's recommendations for mammography: Do tailored messages make a difference? *American Journal of Public Health* 84:43–49.

Slevin ML, Stubbs L, Plant HJ, et al. 1990. Attitudes to chemotherapy: Comparing views of patients with cancer with those of doctors, nurses, and general public. *British Medical Journal* 300(6737): 1458–1460.

Smith TJ, Penberthy L, Desch CE, et al. 1995. Differences in initial treatment patterns and outcomes of lung cancer in the elderly. *Lung Cancer* 13:235–252.

Smith TJ, Swisher K. 1998. Telling the truth about terminal cancer. *Journal of the American Medical Association* 279(21)1746–1748.

Sofaer S, Davidson B, Goodman R, et al. 1990. Helping Medicare beneficiaries choose health insurance: The illness episode approach. *Gerontologist* 30(3):308–315.

Stein JA, Fox SA, Murata PJ. 1990. The influence of ethnicity, socioeconomic status, and psychological barriers on use of mammography. *Journal of Health and Social Behavior* 32:101–113.

Strull WM, Lo B, Charles G. 1984. Do patients want to participate in decision making? *Journal of the American Medical Association* 252(21):2990–2994.

Studnicki J, Schapira DV, Bradham DD, et al. 1993. Response to the National Cancer Institute alert— The effect of practice guidelines on two hospitals in the same medical community. *Cancer* 72: 2986–2992.

SUPPORT Principal Investigators. 1995. A controlled trial to improve care for seriously ill hospitalized patients. The study to understand prognoses and preferences for outcomes and risks of treatments (SUPPORT). *Journal of the American Medical Association* 274(20):1591–1598.

Taplin SH, Anderman C, Grothaus L, et al. 1994. Using physician correspondence and postcard reminders to promote mammography use. *American Journal of Public Health* 84:571–574.

Taylor KM, Margolese RG, Soskolne CL. 1984. Physicians' reasons for not entering eligible patients in a randomized clinical trial of surgery for breast cancer. *New England Journal of Medicine* 310:1363–1367.

Tejeda HA, Green SB, Trimble EL, et al. 1996. Representation of African Americans, Hispanics, and whites in National Cancer Institute cancer treatment trials. *Journal of the National Cancer Institute* 19(88):812–816.

Thompson IM, Colman CA, Brawley OW, et al. 1995. Chemoprevention of prostate cancer. *Seminars in Urology* 13:122–129.

Tierney WM, Hui SL, McDonald CJ. 1986. Delayed feedback of physician performance versus immediate reminders to perform preventive care. *Medical Care* 24:659–666.

Trowbridge R, Dugan W, Jay SJ, et al. 1997. Determining the effectiveness of a clinical practice intervention in improving the control of pain in outpatients with cancer. *Academic Medicine* 72:798–800.

Underwood SM. 1995. Enhancing the delivery of care to the disadvantaged: The challenge to providers. *Cancer Practice* 3:31–36.

U.S. Bureau of the Census. 1998. *Health Insurance Coverage:1997.* www.census.gov/hhes/hlthins/ hlthin97/hi97t2.html.

U.S. Department of Health and Human Services. 1991. *Healthy People 2000. National Health Promotion and Disease Prevention Objectives.* Publication No. (PHS)91-50213. Washington, D.C.

U.S. Department of Health and Human Services. 1996. *Guide to Clinical Preventive Services: Report of the U.S. Preventive Services Task Force.* Second Edition. Washington, D.C.

U.S. General Accounting Office. 1997. *The Health Insurance Portability and Accountability Act of 1996: Early Implementation Concerns.* GAO-HEHS-97-200R. Washington, D.C.

U.S. General Accounting Office. 1998. *Many HMOs Experience High Rates of Beneficiary Disenrollment.* GAO-HEHS-98-142. Washington, D.C.

Van Roenn JH, Cleeland CS, Gonin R, et al. 1993. Physician attitudes and practice in cancer pain management: A survey from the Eastern Cooperative Oncology Group. *Annals of Internal Medicine* 119:121–126.

Vellozzi CJ, Romans M, Rothenberg RB. 1996. Delivering breast and cervical cancer screening services to underserved women: Part I. Literature review and telephone survey. *Women's Health Issues* 6(2):65–73.

Vernon SW. 1997. Participation in colorectal cancer screening: A review. *Journal of the National Cancer Institute* 89(19)1406–1422.

Virgo KS, McKirgan LW, Caputo MC, et al. 1995. Post-treatment management options for patients with lung cancer. *Annals of Surgery* 222(6):700–710.

Waitzkin H. 1985. Information giving in medical care. *Journal of Health and Social Behavior* 26(2):81–101.

Ward SE, Goldberg N, Miller-McCauley V, et al. 1993. Patient-related barriers to management of cancer pain. *Pain* 52:319–324.

Weeks JC, Cook EF, O'Day SJ, et al. 1998. Relationship between cancer patients' prediction of prognosis and their treatment preferences. *Journal of the American Medical Association* 279(21)1709–1714, June 3.

Weinberger MW, Saunders AF, Samsa GP, et al. 1991. Breast cancer screening in older women: Practices and barriers reported by primary care physicians. *Journal of the American Geriatric Society* 39:22.

Weisman C, Celentano D, Teitelbaum M, Klassen A. 1989. Cancer screening services for the elderly. *Public Health Reports* 104:209–214.

Wells BL, Horm JW. 1992. Stage at diagnosis in breast cancer: Race and socioeconomic factors. *American Journal of Public Health* 82(10):1383–1385.

Yarnall KS, Michener JL, Broadhead WE, Tse CK. 1993. Increasing compliance with mammography recommendations: Health assessment forms. *Journal of Family Practice* 36:59–64.

Yellen SB, Cella DF, Leslie WT. 1994. Age and clinical decision making in oncology patients. *Journal of the National Cancer Institute* 86(23):1766–1770.

Zaloznik AJ. 1995. Breast cancer stage at diagnosis: Caucasians versus Afro-Americans. *Breast Cancer Research and Treatment* 34(3):195–198.

Zaloznik AJ. 1997. Breast cancer stage at diagnosis: Caucasians versus Hispanics. *Breast Cancer Research and Treatment* 42(2):121–124.

Zapka JG. 1994. Promoting participation in breast cancer screening. *American Journal of Public Health* 84(1):12–13.

Zapka JG, Berkowitz E. 1992. A qualitative study about breast cancer screening in older women: Implications for research. *Journal of Gerontology* 47:93–100.

Zapka JG, Hosmer D, Costanza ME, et al. 1992. Changes in mammography use: Economic, need and service factors. *American Journal of Public Health* 82:1345–1351.

Zapka JG, Stoddard A, Maul L, Costanza ME. 1991. Interval adherence to mammography screening guidelines. *Medical Care* 29:697–707.

4

Defining and Assessing Quality Cancer Care

This chapter provides an overview of how quality of care is defined and measured, why quality assessment is important, and how quality information is collected. Evidence of quality problems is then summarized for two common cancers for which an evidence base exists: breast and prostate cancer.

DEFINING QUALITY OF CARE

The quality of health care can be precisely defined and accurately measured, but there are many different perspectives of quality to consider. Patients tend to evaluate care in terms of its responsiveness to their individual needs and may expect and value access to, and choice of services, doctors, and treatments that maximize their ability to work and enjoy life. Physicians may view quality in terms of their ability to exercise their medical judgment to optimize outcomes for patients. From a health plan's point of view, quality might mean efficiency, appropriate use of diagnostic and therapeutic technologies, and maintenance of high levels of patient satisfaction with care. From a public health perspective, quality might be reflected in high levels of access to primary care, effective prevention, and in low morbidity and mortality rates. A challenge to assessing quality is balancing these sometimes divergent perspectives (McGlynn, 1997).

The Institute of Medicine (IOM) has defined quality as **the degree to which health services for individuals and populations increase the likelihood of desired health outcomes and are consistent with current professional knowledge** (IOM, 1990). In practical terms, poor quality can mean too much care (e.g., unnecessary tests, medications, or procedures, with associated risks and side effects); too little care (e.g., not receiving a lifesaving surgical procedure); or the wrong care (e.g., medicines that should not be given together, poor surgical techniques) (IOM, 1999). Good quality means providing patients with appropriate services in a technically competent manner, with good communication, shared decision making, and cultural sensitivity.

WHY MEASURE QUALITY OF CANCER CARE?

There are several reasons for measuring the quality of care:

- To help consumers and purchasers make informed choices about health care (e.g., selecting health care coverage that balances likely health care effectiveness and costs).
- To help clinicians and patients make informed treatment and referral decisions (e.g., evaluating mortality and quality of life trade-offs when deciding between two alternative treatments for cancer, comparing the relative success of two hospitals for a high-risk surgical procedure).
- To help clinicians and health plans improve their care (e.g., assessing levels of cancer screening or monitoring surgical complication rates).
- To determine the impact of new policies and systems (e.g., evaluating the consequences of increasing Medicare enrollment in health maintenance organizations [HMOs]).
- To provide clinical input to financial decision-making processes (e.g., determining services to be included in an insurer's benefit package).
- To guide public policy decisions (e.g., resource allocation decisions pertaining to the Medicaid or Medicare programs).

HOW IS QUALITY MEASURED?

Quality assessment is the measurement of quality by expert judgment (implicit review) or by systematic reference to objective standards (explicit review). Quality may be evaluated at any level of the health care system: for physicians and other health care professionals; for hospitals, clinics, rehabilitation centers, and other institutions; for health plans; and for communities.

Different approaches to assessing quality have different strengths and weaknesses, and some approaches work better in one setting than another. An example of implicit review is having a clinician review the medical records of a patient and expressing a judgment on whether the care was good or bad. The clinician may base an opinion on years of experience and understanding of the clinical situation for which care was provided. However, the same rating may not be given on another day, and different colleagues might give a different rating.

Explicit review provides a more systematic approach and can be based on one or more of three dimensions: structure, process, and outcomes (Donabedian, 1980). "Structural quality" refers to health system characteristics, "process quality" refers to what the provider does, and "outcome" refers to patients' health. Although producing good outcomes is the ultimate goal of the health care system, for a variety of technical reasons, using outcome measures to assess quality is not generally the most effective approach (discussed below). Instead, process measures are used.

Structural Quality

Structural quality refers to characteristics of the health care system that affect its ability to meet the needs of individual patients or communities. These characteristics include clinician characteristics (e.g., board certification, average years of experience, distribution of specialties), organizational characteristics (e.g., staffing patterns, reimbursement method), patient characteristics (e.g., insurance type, illness profile), and community characteristics (e.g., per capita hospital beds, transportation system, environmental risks). Structural measures specifically related to cancer quality could include the availability of a multidisciplinary cancer center, a bone marrow transplant unit, or psychological support services.

Structural characteristics are often necessary to provide good care, but they are usually insufficient to ensure excellent quality. The best structural measures are those that can be shown to have a positive influence on the provision of care (process quality) and on patients' health (outcomes), although this relationship has not been found for most measures (Brook et al., 1990).

Measures of structural quality have long been the key component in accreditation procedures. Various independent organizations accredit hospitals or health plans based on a set of criteria that generally focus on structural measures such as appropriate capacity for the covered patient population. In recent years, accreditation organizations have also been incorporating process and outcome measures into their accreditation procedures.

Process Quality

Process quality refers to what providers do for patients and how well they do it, both technically and interpersonally. *Technical process* refers to whether the right choices are made in diagnosing and treating the patient, and whether care is provided in an effective and skillful manner. Whether care is effective can be judged according to evidence from good studies (e.g., clinical trials) that show a link between a particular process and better outcomes. Quality is often measured according to *appropriateness criteria* or *professional standards,* but these may or may not conform to available evidence of effectiveness. The quality of evidence is itself rated according to aspects of the study's design and conduct. Reported "levels" of evidence are often used to evaluate the strength of clinical recommendations (see Box 4.1).

An intervention or service (e.g., laboratory test, procedure, medication) is considered appropriate if the expected health benefits (e.g., increased life expectancy, pain relief, decreased anxiety, improved functional capacity) exceed the expected health risks (e.g., mortality, morbidity, anxiety anticipating the intervention, pain caused by the intervention, inaccurate diagnoses) by a wide enough margin to make the intervention or service worthwhile (Brook et al., 1986). Some also distinguish a subset of appropriate care that they term *necessary* or crucial care. They consider care necessary if there is a reasonable chance of a nontrivial benefit to the patient and if it would be improper not to provide care. In their view, such care is important enough that it might be considered ethically unacceptable not to offer it (Kahan et al., 1994; Laouri et al., 1997). Criteria of appropriateness can be used to measure the *overuse* of care, which occurs when expected risks exceed expected benefits (which is a problem because of treatment complications and wasted resources), and the *underuse* of care, which occurs when people are not receiving care that is expected to improve their health.

A good example of the use of process measures can be found in the 1988 General Accounting Office (GAO) assessment of the use of seven "breakthrough" cancer treatments in the United States from 1975 to 1985 (e.g., adjuvant chemotherapy for breast cancer) (USGAO, 1988). All of the treatments had been proven to extend patients' survival in controlled experiments, and for many, the evidence had been available for several years. Data for 1985 show considerable variation in use of these innovative therapies (Table 4.1). The results illustrate the problem of a slow rate of diffusion of innovation of cancer care, but optimal levels of use of each intervention are not known. One factor that might account for some of the underuse is possible underreporting of treatments in the Surveillance, Epidemiology, and End Results Program (SEER) cancer registry data (see description of SEER Program below).

BOX 4.1 Levels of Evidence Applied to Clinical Research

The "hierarchy of evidence" applied to clinical research (i.e., when the question is whether a given treatment is effective in patients with a specific type of cancer) is well established and agreed upon. The following version is taken from the well-respected U.S. Preventive Services Task Force, proceeding from the most reliable to the least reliable type of evidence (i.e., from grade I to grade III):

I   Evidence obtained from at least one properly randomized controlled trial.
II-1   Evidence obtained from well-designed controlled trials without randomization.
II-2   Evidence obtained from well-designed cohort or case-control (epidemiologic) studies.
II-3   Evidence obtained from multiple time series with or without the intervention— dramatic results in uncontrolled experiments (e.g., the results of the introduction of penicillin treatment in the 1940s) could also be regarded as this type of evidence.
III   Opinions of respected authorities, based on clinical experience, descriptive studies and case reports, or reports of expert committees.

SOURCE: U.S. Department of Health and Human Services, 1996.

TABLE 4.1 Selected Results from 1988 GAO Report

Innovative Therapy	Percentage of Eligible Patients Treated, 1985[a]
Adjuvant chemotherapy for breast cancer (premeno- pausal node-positive)	63
Adjuvant chemotherapy for node-positive colon cancer	6
Adjuvant radiation therapy for rectum cancer	40
Chemotherapy for limited small-cell lung cancer	75
Chemotherapy for non-seminoma testicular cancer	50
Chemotherapy for Stage IIIB or IV Hodgkin's disease	90
Chemotherapy for diffuse intermediate or high grade non-Hodgkin's lymphoma	80[b]

[a]"Treated" includes the SEER treatment data fields of "given" and "planned."
[b] Ten percent decrease from 1979 to 1985.

SOURCE: USGAO, 1988.

Another way to measure process quality is to determine whether care meets evidence-based professional standards. This assessment can be done by creating a list of quality indicators describing a process of care that should (or should not) occur for a particular type of patient or clinical circumstance. Quality indicators are based on standards of care, which are found in the research literature and in statements of professional medical organizations or determined by an expert panel. The performance of physicians and health plans is assessed by calculating rates of adherence to the indicators for a sample of patients (see Chapter 6 for a discussion of quality assurance programs). Current performance can be compared to a physician's or plan's prior performance, to the performance of other physicians and plans, or to benchmarks of performance. Indicators can cover a specific condition (e.g., patients diagnosed with colon cancer who do not have metastatic disease should be offered a wide resection with anastomosis within six weeks of diagnosis), or they can be generic, covering general aspects of care regardless of condition (e.g., patients prescribed a medication should be asked about allergies to medications).

Interpersonal quality refers to whether the clinician provides care in a humane manner consistent with the patient's preferences. It includes such topics as whether the clinician supplied sufficient information for the patient to make informed choices and involved the patient in decision making. It is generally assessed using patient survey data.

Good process measures are based on research studies and supported by professional consensus. They are also flexible with respect to patient preferences. Some patients may not want what most people would consider proper care. Indicators can be constructed so that they are scored favorably if care was offered but declined. However, there has to be some recognition that a perfect score on indicators is not necessarily a feasible or even a desirable goal. For example, although chemotherapy is highly recommended after surgical resection for colon cancer involving the lymph nodes, some patients might decline treatment because they do not wish to experience its associated toxicities. Therefore, 100 percent adherence may not be a reasonable target for an indicator specifying adjuvant chemotherapy for these patients. Furthermore, such a target might also create incentives to ignore patient preferences in making treatment decisions. An alternative approach would be for an indicator to specify that chemotherapy was offered or recommended.

The best process measures are those for which there is evidence from research that better process leads to better outcomes. For example, adjuvant chemotherapy has been shown in several randomized controlled trials to improve survival after surgery for Duke's C colon cancer (NIH, 1990a); performing routine mammography identifies breast cancer at an earlier stage when it is more curable (Kerlikowske et al., 1995); perioperative chemotherapy and radiation therapy have been shown to increase survival for patients with rectal cancer (Krook et al., 1991; Moertel, 1994). Unfortunately, research has not covered all aspects of standard medical practice related to cancer (or other types of disease), so in these cases, expert consensus is used to decide which processes are important measures of quality. If there is not strong consensus supporting the value or superiority of a clinical practice, it generally is not used as a quality measure.

Several studies outside of oncology have tied process measures to outcomes. In a study of five hospitals in Los Angeles County, mortality rates were examined for patients who had coronary angiography and for whom a revascularization procedure was deemed "necessary" by explicit criteria. Those who received necessary revascularization within one year had a mortality of 9 percent, compared to 16 percent for those who did not. Those receiving "necessary" revascularization also had less chest pain at follow-up (Kravitz et al., 1995).

Other research also demonstrates the link between process and outcome. In a study of Medicare enrollees hospitalized with congestive heart failure, heart attack, pneumonia, and stroke in 1981–1982 and 1985–1986, better process quality of care was significantly associated with lower mortality rates 30 days after hospitalization. Patients who went to hospitals in the lowest 25th percentile on a set of process-of-care measures had a 39 percent increased likelihood of dying within 30 days after hospital admission compared to patients who went to hospitals in the highest 25th percentile, after adjustment for patient sickness at admission (Kahn et al., 1990).

Outcomes

Measurement of health-related outcomes is probably the most intuitively appealing approach to quality monitoring. "Outcomes" refers to the results of a health care delivery process. The three main types of outcomes are (1) clinical status, (2) functional status, and (3) consumer satisfaction. These outcomes, however, depend on myriad factors besides medical care, including characteristics of the patient and the disease process. Outcomes are thus valid measures of quality only to the extent that they have been associated with prior medical processes in well-designed studies.

Clinical Status

Clinical status is considered with the biological outcomes of disease, for example, how organ systems are functioning. Physicians have traditionally used clinical status to determine treatment success or failure. Cancer research, for example, has long used the outcome of five-year overall survival or five-year progression-free survival.

Other clinical measures might include postoperative wound infections or catheter infections. Proxy measures (sometimes called surrogate end points or intermediate outcomes) are also used. They do not measure the outcome of concern directly, but they do provide evidence or likelihood of a good outcome. For example, response rate (decrease in tumor size) is used to assess the impact of therapy, but the goal of therapy may be prolonged life. When used as a measure of quality or as an indicator of impact of therapy, it is important for there to be evidence that the proxy measures are really serving as a proxy. In other words, the effect of the intervention on the proxy should be concordant with the effect on the cancer itself (Schatzkin et al., 1996).

Functional Status

Measures of functional status assess how disease affects an individual's ability to participate in physical, mental, and social activities. They also cover the ability to meet the regular responsibilities of one's roles in society (e.g., parent, bank teller, volunteer). Health-related quality of life is similar to functional status but includes the person's sense of well-being as well as factors external to the individual such as social support.

Functional status assessment is based on the premise that many aspects of health are important to patients and will influence their treatment decisions. Such assessment could help someone choose between a treatment that would give many more years of life with major incapacitation and a treatment that would give fewer years of life with full function. For example, treatment success or failure for prostate cancer has historically been assessed by the clinical outcome of whether the patient died from prostate cancer. However, functional status measures would incorporate other treatment outcomes, such as the patient's urinary, sexual, and bowel function (Litwin et al., 1995). Functional status assessment often includes the degree to which disease limits one's ability to participate fully in activities of daily living. Depending on the type of cancer and phase of illness, such activities could include going to work or caring for children. In patients with more advanced disease, however, assessment of whether they are able to go to the market for groceries or to bathe or dress themselves may be more relevant.

Performance status is a measure of functional status often used in oncology clinical trials. The Karnofsky Performance Status (Karnofsky and Burchenal, 1949) is a rating of patients' functional status that has been used in clinical trials since 1949 (Grieco and Long, 1984). The rating is performed by a physician or nurse. It has been found to be a strong predictor of survival in some patient populations, most notably patients with lung cancer. However, it covers only one aspect of quality of life—physical performance—and, although significantly correlated with quality of life, accounts for less than 50 percent of the variability in patients' own ratings of their quality of life. Although clinician-rated measures have value, the field is moving more toward the use of patients' assessments of functional status and quality of life (Reifel and Gantz, in press), which are preferable models for quality assessment. Examples of patient-based measures include the Cancer Rehabilitation Evaluation System (CARES) (Ganz et al., 1992b; Schag and Heinrich, 1990), the Functional Living Index-Cancer (FLIC) (Schipper et al., 1984), and the Breast Cancer Chemotherapy Questionnaire (BCQ) (Levine et al., 1988).

Consumer Satisfaction

Consumer satisfaction refers to patients' feelings about the care they receive and is generally measured by patient surveys. There is a relationship between satisfaction and adherence to treatment regimens. Patients who are satisfied are more likely to take their antibiotics properly (Bartlett et al., 1984), to follow treatment recommendations (Hsieh and Kagle, 1991), and to return for follow-up visits (Deyo and Inui, 1980). Thus, the physician has an incentive to please his or her patients as part of the treatment—so that they will be more likely to follow the physician's advice. Furthermore, dissatisfaction with care can lead patients to switch clinicians and health care institutions (Reichheld, 1996; Rubin et al., 1993; Young et al., 1985).

Although consumers are the best source to evaluate their interpersonal care, one limitation of satisfaction ratings is that consumers cannot always tell if the care was appropriate or technically good (Aharony and Strasser 1993); research has not shown a consistent relationship between consumer satisfaction and technical quality of care (Cleary and McNeil, 1988; Davies and Ware, 1988; Hayward et al., 1993). A kind and caring physician may provide care that is technically poor (Aharony and Strasser, 1993). Also, consumer satisfaction may vary with expectations. For example, patients who have a history of poor access to health care may be so appreciative when they actually see a physician that they may report high satisfaction regardless of how well care was delivered. Therefore, it is best not to rely on satisfaction ratings to measure technical quality.

Clinical and functional status can be measured for more than one purpose. They are described here in the context of quality of care, in which outcomes are compared between two institutions as a sign of whether one institution is delivering better care (with the presumption that better care leads to better outcomes). However, these measures are also used clinically to track a patient's progress and in clinical trials to measure the efficacy or effectiveness of a new drug or intervention. The same measures can sometimes be used for both purposes, but certain measures are better suited for one purpose or the other. Five-year survival rates, for example, are a standard measure used in studies of new cancer treatments. However, when measuring quality of care for purposes of accountability or quality improvement, outcomes with a shorter time horizon than five years are generally needed. If two institutions are compared using five-year survival rates for colon cancer, one institution might have higher survival rates than the other. However, in the interim, there might have been a change in staff or a revamping of procedures that improved or weakened the quality of care at the hospitals, thereby making the comparison historically, but not practically, valuable.

Attributes of Good Outcomes Measurement

Outcomes measurement has become increasingly popular in the past few years, perhaps because outcomes are the most direct measure of the health of a population. For example, outcomes can be used to assess the quality of care that a health system provides to its cancer patients: outcomes can measure the survival and quality of life of women diagnosed with breast cancer and whether they are satisfied with their care. Their interpretation, however, must be tempered by the fact that many factors other than medical care influence outcomes.

Mortality trends are the principal yardstick used to measure overall progress against cancer because they capture the total effects of prevention, early detection, and treatment. The most recent assessment of mortality trends is encouraging—U.S. cancer mortality rates fell in the early 1990s for the first time since statistics have been collected (Wingo et al., 1998). It is difficult to estimate precisely the relative importance of factors contributing to this decline, but much of it stems from reduced smoking (among men) and other improvements in prevention (Cole and Rodu, 1996). Worthwhile advances in treatment may not be easily detected in overall mortality rates. Site- and stage-specific survival rates are better measures of treatment effects when adjusted for patient characteristics (e.g., prognostic factors such as age and extent of other illnesses).

The best outcome measures have certain key features or are used in a particular manner. First, they should be risk adjusted (or case-mix adjusted), in other words, adjusted for factors that influence outcomes but are beyond the health care system's control (e.g., age, socioeconomic status, comorbidities). Without such adjustment, it is impossible to determine how much of the improvement or worsening of outcomes is due to the care delivered (or not delivered) by the health care system. A radiation oncologist who receives referrals of patients with multiple medical problems is likely to have worse outcomes than one who takes only patients with early-stage disease and few comorbidities, even though the former may be a better radiation oncologist. To make comparisons in such a system, adjustments are needed for how ill the patients are. Risk adjustment is complex, and the factors to use in risk adjustment must be selected carefully to allow for accurate interpretation of the outcomes (Iezzoni, 1996).

Outcomes are only useful in quality assessment when the specific processes of care that relate to them are known. Then, if the outcomes are not as good as they should be, it is clear what aspects of care have to be addressed to try to improve them. In other words, if you do not know how an outcome relates to processes of care, you will not know what to do to improve the outcome when you find that it is poor at a particular hospital.

It also helps to measure outcomes from different perspectives. For example, palliative chemotherapy for metastatic cancer may decrease a patient's tumor burden and potentially prolong life, but it might also cause severe fatigue and weight loss, so the patient's clinical status might improve while functional status declines.

It is also important to use outcomes that can be reasonably related to the health care system—and the particular part of the system—that one is assessing. It is not reasonable to hold a provider or plan accountable for an outcome, unless the outcome is a direct result of the way care is provided. Sometimes, however, a single outcome may be influenced by many factors over many years, of which health care is only a part. Outcomes for lung cancer, for example, may reflect the quality of care provided over many years, including the quality of smoking prevention and cessation counseling for adolescents and adults. Outcomes for breast cancer may in part depend on the quality of screening and early detection. Given the frequency with which most patients change clinicians or health plans, it could be difficult to relate the quality of any one clinician or plan to some outcomes. Similarly, if one is trying to use outcomes to assess the quality of surgeons treating a sarcoma at various hospitals, it is important to distinguish whether the outcomes are related to the skill of the surgeon, competence of the surgical team, or organizational characteristics of the hospital. One might also want to consider the skill of the medical oncologist prescribing neoadjuvant chemotherapy. For breast cancer, treatment may depend upon an oncologist, a surgeon, and a radiation oncologist. It can be difficult to distribute responsibility among them.

In addition, outcomes should be measured on samples that are large enough to detect differences in quality. Adverse outcomes are often uncommon events, so large samples are needed to detect clinically meaningful differences between hospitals. To detect a difference of 2 percentage points in the rate of catheter infections between two hospitals (e.g., 5 percent for one and 7 percent for the other), each hospital would have to have at least 1,900 catheterized patients.

In summary, many challenges are inherent in using outcomes to measure quality of care. If these are not addressed, it is difficult to determine whether different outcomes observed among the patients of three physicians are attributable to the physicians themselves. Process measures have their own challenges (e.g., one must make sure that there is a proven link between the process and a desired outcome), but such measures can be quite effective in showing whether providers are doing what they should so that their patients have the best chance of achieving good outcomes. There has been more experience using process measures than outcomes measures to assess quality, and many quality assessment systems depend primarily or exclusively on process measures. However, interest in improving outcomes measurement is increasing, so that outcomes might be used along with process measures to provide more useful assessments of health care quality.

In conclusion, to assess quality of care, measures of structure, process, or outcome can be used. If outcomes measures are used, care must be taken to account for differences that might simply reflect differences in other factors, such as patient selection or case mix. If structure or process measures are used, they should be associated with the desired outcomes. In addition, to make inferences about quality, a measure must be compared to a standard.

Variations in Care

Simply comparing variations in the structure or process of care does not provide an evaluation of the quality of care, although it may point to potential quality problems that merit further inquiry. In one such study of variation, five-year survival rates during 1983–1991 varied markedly for several cancer sites. For women with breast cancer, for example, five-year survival ranged from 71.0 percent in Iowa to 79.9 percent in Hawaii (Farrow et al., 1996) (Table 4.2). These differences persisted after adjusting for age and stage. For all cancers other than ovary and bladder, one or more regions were found whose survival rates differed significantly from the overall mean. These differences persisted and were even more pronounced when the analysis was limited to patients less than 70 years of age with local-stage surgically treated disease. However, other important case-mix adjusters, such as the presence of comorbid illnesses, were not included in the model, so interpretation of these results is difficult. Thus, it is not clear whether these regional variations in survival from breast cancer reflect differences in patient populations, regional differences in quality of care, or other factors.

TABLE 4.2 Five-Year Survival Comparisons Across Nine SEER Sites, Non-Hispanic Whites, 1983–1991

Cancer Site	Range of Relative Risk of Death for All Patients Across Sites (adjusted for sex, age, and stage)	Range of Relative Risk of Death—Local Disease, Age <70 (adjusted for surgical treatment)	Range of 5-Year Survival All Patients Across Sites for All (unadjusted)
Stomach	0.89–1.21	0.69–1.32	10.0–14.9
Colon	0.90–1.10	0.87–1.15	47.1–53.3
Rectum	0.91–1.09	0.76–1.17	45.6–52.4
Lung	0.93–1.12	0.74–1.19	10.5–16.1
Breast	0.82–1.11	0.64–1.34	71.0–79.9
Uterus	0.81–1.21	0.84–1.26	73.2–84.0
Ovary	0.91–1.08	0.82–1.16	34.1–39.2
Prostate	0.84–1.12	0.70–1.20	51.9–64.0
Bladder	0.91–1.15	0.84–1.16	58.4–64.2

SOURCE: Farrow et al., 1996.

HOW IS QUALITY-OF-CARE INFORMATION COLLECTED?

Data for quality assessment can come from several sources. First, administrative records are widely available, and although they are limited in clinical detail, they can be used to show intensity or patterns of utilization. For example, they can be used to determine whether a patient with large-cell non-Hodgkin's lymphoma (NHL) received at least six months of chemotherapy and whether the patient had a white blood cell count performed before receiving chemotherapy. Second, medical records can provide greater clinical detail, the recorded medical history, the results of laboratory tests, and the treatment plan. For example, the medical record can show whether the patient with NHL was neutropenic, whether proper components of the physical examination were performed, and whether chemotherapy was administered appropriately. Third, patient surveys can provide additional useful information. Patients can report on what happened during a clinical encounter and thereby provide information relevant to the processes of care. They can also rate their satisfaction with care and provide information on outcomes such as functional status. It is generally more expensive and time-consuming to collect information from medical records and from patients than from administrative data.

Cancer registries are also a potential source of information. They collect information on type of cancer, histology, stage at diagnosis, patient age, and initial course of treatment (whether the patient received surgery, chemotherapy, and radiation therapy that would normally be prescribed as part of the initial treatment plan). Registries exist at the regional, state, national, and international levels.

There are two main national registries: the Surveillance, Epidemiology, and End Results Program of the National Cancer Institute (NCI) and the National Cancer Data Base (NCDB) (Swan et al., 1998). The SEER program was established as a result of the National Cancer Act of 1971 to assemble, analyze, and distribute information on the prevention, diagnosis, and treatment of cancer. Cancer is the only chronic disease (aside from HIV/AIDS) for which a national surveillance program exists. The program routinely collects information from designated population-based cancer registries in different parts of the country. The different areas have been chosen for their capacity to maintain a cancer reporting system as well as for their ability to report epidemiologically significant population subgroups. Currently, 14 percent of the U.S. population is represented by the nine geographic areas that make up the SEER program's database. Goals of the SEER program include the following:

- compiling (with the help of the National Center for Health Statistics) estimates of cancer incidence and mortality in the United States;
- discovering trends and unusual changes in specific cancers based on their geographic, demographic, and social characteristics;
- providing information about trends in therapy, changes in the extent of disease (stage at diagnosis), and changes in patient survival; and
- promoting studies that identify the factors that can be controlled through intervention strategies.

Health service researchers have linked SEER to Medicare administrative files to evaluate patterns of care, the use of health services, and the costs of treatment (Potosky et al., 1993; Edwards, personal communication to Maria Hewitt, November 1998). Many locations outside of the SEER program's area maintain cancer registries. The National Program of Cancer Registries of the Centers for Disease Control and Prevention (CDC) is bolstering states' capabilities to monitor cancer trends (CDC, 1998).

The National Cancer Data Base is a joint project of the Commission on Cancer (COC) of the American College of Surgeons (ACoS) and the American Cancer Society (ACS) to facilitate community, hospital, state, and national assessment of care of patients with cancer (Menck et al., 1997). It began in 1989, and 1,600 hospitals currently report data on 600,000 new cases annually to the NCDB (an estimated 58 percent of new cancer cases) (NCDB, 1998; Swan et al., 1998). NCDB collects information on patient characteristics, tumor characteristics, first course of treatment, and follow-up. Participating hospitals submit all cases seen at their hospital for a particular data year. The system appears to have a bias toward hospitals with a computerized cancer registry, and it does not provide comprehensive outpatient data. After 1996, hospitals with ACoS accreditation (about 1,450 hospitals) were required to participate; it is estimated that in the year 2000, 1,750 hospitals caring for 80 percent of U.S. cancer cases will be participating. The NCDB provides comparisons of cancer management patterns and outcomes to national norms at the hospital, community, and state levels. The NCDB can also be used to track how well the results of major clinical trials are incorporated into clinical practice. There have been questions about quality control of the data collected by individual hospital registries, and NCDB is working to improve the quality.

The NCDB and the SEER program, when compared in 1992, provided similar patient descriptors (e.g., age, race, gender), cancer characteristics (e.g., stage), and types of surgical treatment for breast, colon, lung, and prostate cancer (Mettlin et al., 1997a). The two registries had similar distributions of cancer cases, by clinical characteristics.

Registries represent an exceptionally valuable opportunity to conduct quality assessment on a broad level. They could go further in collecting data on explicit process measures, intermediate outcomes, and treatment information, as well as characteristics needed to risk-adjust the outcomes. They would also be more useful for quality assessment if they were able to reduce the time lag between provision of care and availability of data. This information could be used both to provide detailed information on quality of care and to tie the processes of care to the outcomes. These data would also be useful in quality improvement.

There are a number of other ongoing data collection initiatives assessing the quality of cancer care:

•   The American College of Radiology (ACR) conducts ongoing Patterns of Care Studies for a variety of cancers. Since 1971, ACR has collected information periodically from a national sample of radiation oncology facilities (Kramer and Herring, 1976). Patterns of Care data have been collected in 1972–1974, 1977, 1979, 1984, 1989, and 1994. Data collected at each of these periods have included structure and process information; some years have also included patient outcomes measures. For example, 1989 assessed only structure and process measures, whereas 1994, which has not yet been made publicly available, included outcomes assessments as well.

•   The National Comprehensive Cancer Network (NCCN) has developed an outcomes database that pools information across NCI-designated comprehensive cancer center participants. In 1997, NCCN began the creation of a uniform outcomes reporting system (Weeks, 1997); results of this effort are pending.

•   The American Urological Association is developing a Documented Outcomes Collection System (DOCS) to assess patient outcomes for a selected number of conditions and may collect information related to prostate cancer outcomes in the future.

EVIDENCE OF CANCER CARE QUALITY PROBLEMS

Efforts to measure quality of cancer care in the United States are in the early stages. National organizations conducting quality assessment have focused primarily on prevention and screening, although they are now moving more toward assessing the quality of diagnosis and management. Research studies on quality of cancer care have been limited, with most research concentrating on cancers with comparatively higher prevalence and more evidence supporting clinical practice. In this section, the evidence of cancer care quality problems is assessed for breast and prostate cancer.

Breast Cancer

Breast cancer is the most commonly diagnosed non-skin cancer among American women, and it is estimated that one in eight women will develop breast cancer in her lifetime (Ries et al., 1998). In 1999, 176,300 new breast cancer diagnoses are expected (ACS, 1999). Although lung cancer has surpassed breast cancer as the leading cause of cancer deaths in women, breast cancer still accounts for 43,300 deaths annually (ACS, 1999). Breast cancer remains a common illness with significant morbidity and mortality.

Among oncologic conditions, breast cancer has one of the most extensive scientific literatures to support a strong association between processes of care and outcomes. Unlike many malignancies, effective interventions exist for breast cancer that decrease mortality and improve quality of life. In addition, evidence from the literature suggests that all phases of the continuum of care have an important effect on breast cancer outcomes, including early detection, diagnostic evaluation, and treatment. This extensive clinical literature, with many well-designed randomized controlled trials, provides a firm grounding for the development of process measures in breast cancer. However, even in breast cancer, not every aspect of the continuum of care has been studied to determine its effect on outcomes. Thus, even for this heavily studied disease, some of the presumed associations between process and outcomes reflect consensus within the medical community and expert opinion and are not based upon reliable evidence.

Screening and Diagnostic Evaluation

Although there has been controversy over the age at which one should begin screening for breast cancer, data from multiple randomized trials and several meta-analyses provide evidence that screening with mammography results in diagnosis at an earlier stage and in better outcomes. Early detection of breast cancer through screening mammography has been shown to reduce mortality by 20 to 39 percent for women ages 50 years and older (Nyström et al., 1993; Roberts et al., 1990; Shapiro et al., 1988). Also, results for women age 40 to 50 have shown a trend toward reduced mortality ranging from 13 to 23 percent (Kerlikowske et al., 1995; Tabar et al., 1995). Although the associated benefits and risks are controversial, many professional and public health organizations, including both the American Cancer Society and the National Cancer Institute, currently recommend screening mammography beginning at age 40 (Eastman, 1997; Mettlin and Smart, 1994).

For screening mammography to be effective, abnormalities identified at screening must be evaluated appropriately. Mammography is one of the most technically challenging radiological procedures, and ensuring the quality of the image is difficult. Furthermore, according to radiological experts, mammograms are the most difficult radiographic images to read (USGAO,

1998a, b). Although certain mammographic images (e.g. a spiculated mass) are characteristic of cancer, no criteria allow the radiologist to absolutely differentiate benign from malignant lesions (Osuch, 1996; Talamonti and Morrow, 1996). Given this significant overlap in the appearance of benign and malignant lesions on mammography, other tests are necessary to rule out a malignancy. Ultrasound may be useful to differentiate cysts from solid masses; however, a biopsy to obtain a pathologic diagnosis is often the only way to determine whether a lesion is benign or malignant. Any persistent breast mass that is not determined to be a simple cyst either by aspiration of clear fluid or by ultrasound characteristics should have a pathologic diagnosis, either through fine needle aspiration or excisional biopsy. Biopsy is the gold standard. Fine needle aspiration can falsely identify from less than 1 percent to 35 percent of cancers as negative, but accuracy improves when it is used in conjunction with clinical exam and simultaneous mammography in a procedure referred to as triple diagnosis (Kaufman et al., 1994).

Studies of screening mammography suggest significant variation in both the technical quality of radiographic images and their interpretation. A series of evaluations by the Food and Drug Administration (FDA) in 1985, 1988, and 1992 suggested widespread variation in mammographic image quality (Houn and Finder, 1997). Although improvement was noted overall, with 86 percent of images being acceptable in 1992 compared to only 64 percent in 1985, a significant problem in image quality remained, which was felt to be attributable to differences in technique (Segal, 1994). At the urging of the FDA, the American College of Radiology developed a voluntary accrediting process for mammography facilities in 1987 to attempt to correct this problem (Houn and Finder, 1997).

Concern about the quality of mammography led Congress to pass the Mammography Quality Standards Act in 1992, which established minimum national quality standards for mammography facilities (USGAO, 1998a, b). During the first three years of FDA inspections, compliance with national standards and x-ray quality improved. Before the act took effect, 11 percent of facilities tested were unable to pass image quality tests; in 1996, the nationwide figure was 2 percent (USGAO, 1998a, b).

The FDA has established federal qualification requirements for physicians who interpret mammograms, but each facility uses its own data to monitor physicians' performance on interpretation (USGAO, 1998a, b). Wide variation in diagnostic accuracy has been observed. According to a recent study, radiologists' ability to identify breast cancer from a screening mammogram (with biopsy as the gold standard) ranged from 47 to 100 percent, with a mean of 79 percent, and their ability to correctly rule out breast cancer varied from 36 to 99 percent. This study involved 108 radiologists practicing in 50 participating facilities randomly sampled from 4,611 ACR-accredited mammography centers (Beam et al., 1996).

The quality of the breast biopsy procedure is important so that the clinicians who make treatment recommendations to women with a breast lesion or with breast cancer have accurate information. Multiple steps in the process of breast biopsy are critical to ensuring that results are accurate, including the biopsy procedure itself (which may be a fine needle aspiration, a stereotactic core biopsy, an open biopsy, or a needle localization procedure followed by a biopsy), the tissue preparation, the cytopathology interpretation, the assessment of estrogen receptor and progesterone receptor status, and the pathology report that communicates all of the findings. A few studies have addressed the quality of some of these steps. A single community-based study in New Hampshire assessed the degree of diagnostic agreement among general pathologists reading an investigator-defined set of breast tissue specimens obtained via core and excisional biopsies

(Wells et al., 1998). They found overall high agreement among the pathologists for assignment to diagnostic category (kappa coefficient = 0.71) and very high agreement for differentiation of benign versus malignant breast disease (kappa coefficient = 0.95.) Other studies have found that the adequacy of specimens obtained from fine needle aspiration and stereotactic core biopsy varies widely, as do their reported sensitivity and specificity (Acheson et al., 1997; Hayes et al., 1996; Stolier, 1997). Yet no published studies have explored the issues that affect the quality of these procedures as performed in the diverse clinical facilities across the United States.

The pathology report is the critical link between pathologist and clinician. Deficits in the pathology report may represent problems with communication or deficiencies in the pathologic evaluation itself. Several studies suggest that variation exists in the quality of pathology reports for breast cancer specimens that warrants further evaluation. In the mid to late 1980s, three reports, although conducted in different populations, suggested serious underreporting of pathology information. Less than one-quarter of biopsies, for example, had documentation of lymph node dissection (Table 4.3).

TABLE 4.3 Quality Process Deficiencies in Initial Breast Cancer Care in the 1980s

Variable (stage)	Illinois— All Ages, 1988	Virginia— Age >65, 1985–1889	NCDB— All ages, 1988
No tumor size (I and II)	Not reported	24%	23%
No estrogen receptors	11%	Not reported	Not reported
No lymph node dissection	9%	24%	18%

SOURCE: Hand et al., 1991; Hillner et al., 1996; Osteen et al., 1992.

More recent data appear to show gains in some aspects of pathology reporting; however, room for improvement remains. In 1995, the College of American Pathology in its Q-Probes Study reviewed 20 breast biopsy specimens and the corresponding pathology reports from 434 voluntarily participating surgical pathology laboratories in the United States, Canada, and Australia (Nakleh et al., 1997):

- In 92 percent of malignant cases the margin status was reported (necessary to determine if all of the malignancy was removed by the procedure), and 77 percent of reports contained the lesion size.
- Approximately 75 percent documented whether estrogen and progesterone receptor status had been evaluated.

A single-institution study of needle localization breast biopsy reported even lower rates of documentation for this important information in the pathology report (Howe et al., 1995). Only 33 percent of reports in this study commented on the margins of the lesion, and estrogen receptor status was determined for only 68 percent of the cases. Such deficits in pathology reports have been the target of quality improvement projects. Hammond and Flinner (1997) reduced the number of incomplete breast cancer pathology reports in a large urban pathology practice in Salt Lake

City from 57 of 356 in 1990 to only 2 of 190 in 1995, after instituting a template for the report that included all essential information.

These studies identify multiple steps during the diagnostic evaluation of breast cancer at which the quality of care may be affected by the quality of the procedure. Poor quality at any step could significantly impact the overall quality of care provided. Although having information on every step in the continuum of care would provide a comprehensive assessment of the quality of care, this generally is not practical. Acquiring such comprehensive data on quality would be intrusive, time-consuming, and expensive. Nevertheless, considering all of the steps necessary to a multistep process such as the diagnosis of breast cancer can be extremely valuable in trying to determine the reasons for a quality problem that has been identified (e.g., too many women diagnosed with late-stage breast cancer, a high rate of local recurrence after breast conserving surgery).

Treatment

Extensive evidence is available for process–outcomes links in the treatment of breast cancer from randomized controlled trials and meta-analyses of these trials. Surgery has been the primary treatment for localized breast cancer since Halsted popularized the radical mastectomy in 1894 (Halsted, 1894). More recently, randomized controlled trials have demonstrated equivalent survival with a modified radical mastectomy or with breast conserving surgery followed by radiation therapy (Fisher et al., 1985; Sarrazin et al., 1984; Veronesi et al., 1981). In addition, having a choice of surgery appears important to a woman's subsequent quality of life; studies have not demonstrated any difference in overall quality of life between women who received breast conserving surgery and those treated with modified radical mastectomy as long as they were *offered a choice* of primary therapy (Ganz et al., 1992a; Kiebert et al., 1991). The most recent National Institutes of Health Consensus Conference statement for the treatment of early-stage breast cancer specifies breast conserving surgery as the preferred mode of therapy for the majority of women with Stage I and II breast cancer (NIH, 1990). Compared to modified radical mastectomy, breast conserving surgery has fewer short-term complications, but may require a similar length of convalescence because of the recommended six weeks of postsurgery radiation therapy. It is not a less costly treatment.

Strong process–outcomes links also exist for treating women with local or regional breast cancer with chemotherapy or hormone therapy or both in addition to surgery and radiation. Systemic treatment with chemotherapy or hormone therapy after all identifiable cancer has been removed surgically is termed adjuvant therapy. The goal of adjuvant therapy is to decrease future recurrences and thereby improve survival. However, the issue of adjuvant therapy in breast cancer raises another important consideration: When, despite strong evidence in the literature for a process–outcomes link, is the impact on outcome so small that the process should not be considered requisite for quality care? Adjuvant systemic therapy with either chemotherapy or hormone therapy has been demonstrated in randomized controlled clinical trials to improve survival in all women with breast cancer, although the benefit in women with very favorable prognoses is extremely small (EBCT, 1992, 1998). In addition, a small but significant improvement in both overall and disease-free survival is obtained from combined treatment with chemotherapy and tamoxifen (hormone therapy), compared with tamoxifen alone, in women with estrogen receptor-positive tumors, regardless of the patient's age (Fisher et al., 1997). These studies demonstrate improved breast cancer outcomes with chemotherapy, tamoxifen, and perhaps both treatments together in all patients. However, given that the absolute benefit is extremely small in patients with a good prognosis (2 percent improvement in 10-year survival for low-risk patients), the benefits may not outweigh the risks of adjuvant treatment in these patients (Osborne et al., 1996). So although most experts would agree that all women with involved lymph nodes, large tumors, and even moderate-size tumors should receive adjuvant therapy, whether it is essential to offer treatment to women with extremely small tumors has not yet been clearly established. Thus, despite clear evidence of process–outcomes links for adjuvant therapy in breast cancer, the determination of whether all patients should be treated remains an issue of expert judgment and consensus. If adjuvant chemotherapy is administered, the quality of treatment can be evaluated by assessing whether an adequate dose of chemotherapy is given (Bonadonna, 1985).

Relatively few studies examine the full spectrum of cancer care. Hillner evaluated multiple dimensions of care for 983 nonelderly women diagnosed between 1989–1991 with early breast cancer and insured by Virginia Blue Cross/Blue Shield (BC/BS) according to a 12-point scorecard with target values set according to expert opinion (Table 4.4). Some procedures appeared to be overused (e.g., perioperative bone scans), while others were underused (e.g., breast conserving surgery, visit to medical oncologist to discuss adjuvant therapy). Claims for at least one cycle of chemotherapy were found for 83 percent of premenopausal, node-positive women.

Variations in Rates of Breast Conserving Surgery. Many studies have compared the proportion of women who receive breast conserving surgery (BCS) instead of mastectomy. The decision about which type of breast surgery to undergo depends on the size of the primary tumor, the skill and preferences of the surgeon, and the preferences of the patient. The proportion of women who would choose breast conserving surgery if they were presented with enough information to make an informed choice is not known. Since there is no benchmark for what percentage of women should receive breast conserving surgery, whether any identified variation in the rates of conservative surgery is associated with the quality of care cannot be ascertained. However, widespread differences in the percentage of women who receive the two types of surgery would suggest that some women are not able to completely exercise their choice.

The proportion of women who receive breast conserving surgery versus mastectomy as the primary surgical treatment for early breast cancer varies dramatically by region of the country, according to studies conducted in the 1980s after the results of randomized controlled trials demonstrating the equivalency of the two procedures were published. The proportion of all women 65 and older with early breast cancer who received breast conserving surgery ranged from 4 percent in Kentucky to 21 percent in Massachusetts in 1986 according to Medicare data (Nattinger et al., 1992). Across the nine areas with SEER registries, Seattle appeared to have the highest rates of breast conserving surgery in 1983–1989 with 34 percent of women with Stage I and II disease receiving BCS (Farrow et al., 1992; Lazovich et al., 1991; Samet et al., 1994). The national overall rates of breast conserving surgery among Medicare patients with nonmetastatic disease changed little between 1986 and 1990 (from 14.1 to 15.0 percent) (Nattinger et al., 1996). Although patient age, the sociodemographic characteristics of communities, hospital characteristics, and the availability of radiation therapy appear to affect the proportion of women who undergo breast conserving surgery, marked geographic variation in the use of the procedure persists even after adjusting for these characteristics (Farrow et al., 1992; Lazovich et al., 1991; Nattinger et al., 1992; Samet et al., 1994). Although the proportion of women who would undergo breast conserving surgery if all eligible women were offered the procedure is not known, the wide regional variations could indicate variation in the quality of breast cancer care (i.e., women not offered choice of procedure by their provider).

TABLE 4.4 Target and Observed Care in 1989–1991 in Virginia BC/BS Women Age <65

Issue	Expert Target (%)[a]	BC/BS Cohort (%)[a]
Evaluation		
Initial biopsy prior to total mastectomy[b]	>95	92
Treatment		
Axillary node dissection	>90	88[c]
Breast conserving surgery for local disease	50	33
Local breast radiation following lumpectomy	>95	86
Staging		
Perioperative (within 30 days) bone scan	<10	34
Perioperative (within 30 days) abdominal CT scan	<10	12
Adjuvant Chemotherapy		
If premenopausal and >1 axillary node (+), receive chemotherapy	>90	83
If postmenopausal and >1 axillary node (+), receive chemotherapy[d]	50	52
Referral		
At least one visit to a medical oncologist to discuss adjuvant therapy	>80	56
If mastectomy, at least one visit to a plastic surgeon to discuss reconstructive surgery	>60	27
Follow-Up		
Mammography within the first 18 months postoperatively	>95	79
Bone or CT scans for suspicious symptoms per year	<15	18–35

NOTE: CT = computed tomography.

[a] BC/BS cohort used local and regional summary staging.
[b] Biopsy could be aspiration cytology, core biopsy, or excisional biopsy prior to total mastectomy. A two-step surgical procedure is not implied.
[c] Based on axillary nodes reported to registry of those patients with summary staging; 11% of women with breast cancer were excluded since no staging data were reported.
[d] Chemotherapy only. Use of hormonal therapy could not be assessed.

SOURCE: Hillner et al., 1997.

A recent study by Guadagnoli et al. (1998b) using data collected from medical records and a patient survey reported much higher rates of breast conserving surgery but still substantial regional variation when comparing women treated in 18 hospitals in 1993–1995 in Massachusetts and 30 hospitals in Minnesota in 1993. Although the hospitals participating in Massachusetts were selected randomly (20 were originally selected but two refused to participate), those from Minnesota were part of a consortium formed by the Healthcare Education and Research Foundation and included about 60 percent of patients hospitalized in Minnesota. Overall, 64 percent of women in Massachusetts and 38 percent of women in Minnesota with Stage I and II breast cancer received breast conserving surgery. However, after excluding patients with contraindications to breast conserving surgery (e.g., prior BCS, tumor multifocal, tumor centrally located), the proportions of eligible women receiving breast conserving surgery increased to 74 and 48 percent, for Massachusetts and Minnesota, respectively. Importantly, 27 percent of women in Minnesota and 15 percent in Massachusetts who underwent mastectomy, even though they were eligible for breast conserving surgery, reported that their surgeon had not discussed BCS with them. This suggests that a significant proportion of the variation in rates of breast conserving surgery reflects the fact that women have not been given an informed choice of procedure.

Data compiled by Wennberg et al. (1996) in the Dartmouth Atlas of Health Care using 1992–1993 Medicare claims show that widespread variation in the proportion of women offered breast conserving surgery remains. Without stratifying on stage in this predominantly 65 and older population, the proportion of inpatient cancer surgery that was a breast conserving procedure ranged from 1.4 to 48.0 percent by Medicare hospital referral region. In light of the data from Guadagnoli et al. (1998b) that up to one-quarter of women who undergo mastectomy have not been provided information about BCS, the persistent widespread regional variation in the performance of breast conserving surgery would appear to indicate that many women are not being offered a choice.

Other studies also have found significant variation in the use of breast conserving surgery according to hospital characteristics (Nattinger et al., 1992, 1996). A study by Nattinger et al. (1996) found that 55 percent of breast conserving surgeries performed on Medicare patients occurred in only 10 percent of the hospitals submitting claims in 1986 to 1990. Increased use of BCS was associated with larger hospital size, the presence of a radiation facility, the presence of a cancer program, being a teaching hospital, not-for-profit status, and the volume of breast cancer surgeries performed at the hospital. The study by Guadagnoli et al. (1998b) also found a positive association between breast conserving surgery and the teaching status of the hospital. The odds of breast conserving surgery were 2.4 times higher for patients treated at teaching hospitals in Massachusetts, and 1.5 times in Minnesota, compared with patients treated at nonteaching facilities (Guadagnoli et al., 1998b). Interestingly, in contrast to the Nattinger et al. (1996) study, Guadagnoli et al. found no relation between BCS and hospital size or presence of a radiation facility, perhaps indicating that these factors are no longer significant once higher rates of breast conserving surgery have been achieved overall in the community.

These studies suggest that many women are not offered a choice in the type of breast surgery and that steps have to be taken to increase the implementation of recommendations to promote informed decision making. Further research is needed to determine what proportion of patients are aware that breast conserving surgery is available, whether they are given a fully informed choice of surgery, and which procedure they ultimately receive. To evaluate this aspect of quality of care, information would have to be obtained by patient self-report since this level of detail is not contained in cancer registries, claims, or medical records.

Receipt of Radiation, Adjuvant Chemotherapy, or Hormone Therapy Following Breast Conserving Surgery. Women who undergo breast conserving surgery should receive radiation therapy after surgery. Rates of radiation therapy after BCS suggest that in some parts of the United States, many women are not receiving needed radiation. In the nine SEER registry areas, the percentage of women receiving radiation therapy after breast conserving surgery in 1985–1986 had increased from 1983 to 1984, but still varied greatly (Farrow et al., 1992). Though Iowa had the greatest increase in the use of radiation therapy during this period, it still had the lowest use of all nine areas, with only 60 percent of women in 1985–1986 receiving radiation. Seattle had the highest use, with 81 percent in 1985–1986 receiving radiation therapy after breast conserving surgery. Although some women may refuse radiation therapy, one would hope that an informed discussion of the treatment options would lead many women who do not wish to receive radiation to choose mastectomy as their primary treatment. Thus, one might expect that only a small number of women would opt for breast conserving surgery without radiation.

A limitation of this study, and other studies that rely on cancer registry data, is that the validity of the data on treatment collected by the cancer registries has not been systematically evaluated. Thus, the low rates of radiation therapy after breast conserving surgery reported in this study may reflect incomplete data and not poor quality of care.

Alternatively, the low rates of radiation therapy after breast conserving surgery reported by Farrow et al. (1992) may reflect the practice in the 1980s but may not accurately describe the current quality of care in the United States. Two recently published studies of breast cancer care in selected populations suggest that the quality of care may have improved, at least for some women. Hillner et al. (1997) used 1989–1991 data from the Virginia Cancer Registry to evaluate the quality of care for 918 Virginia women age 64 or younger with Stage I–III breast cancer who had Blue Cross/Blue Shield health insurance. In this patient population, 82 percent of women who underwent breast conserving surgery received radiation therapy. In addition, 83 percent of women 50 and younger (who were assumed to be premenopausal) with node-positive disease received adjuvant chemotherapy. The authors were unable to assess the use of adjuvant hormone therapy through the claims data.

Guadagnoli et al. (1998a) compared the care received at 18 hospitals in Massachusetts by women diagnosed in 1993–1995 with Stage I or II breast cancer, with the care received at 30 hospitals in Minnesota by women diagnosed in 1993. In contrast to previous studies that relied on administrative data, these authors collected data about breast cancer treatment from medical records, patient surveys, and physician surveys. Among women treated at these institutions from 1993 to 1995, 84 percent in Massachusetts and 86 percent in Minnesota received radiation therapy after breast conserving surgery. In addition, 97 and 94 percent, respectively, of premenopausal women with node-positive breast cancer received adjuvant chemotherapy. By contrast, only 63 percent of postmenopausal women in Massachusetts and 59 percent in Minnesota who had positive lymph nodes and positive estrogen receptor status received adjuvant hormone therapy.

Another study (Young et al., 1996) used cancer registry data to examine the treatment of local breast cancer in Pennsylvania during 1986–1990, the time between that reported by Farrow et al. (1992) and by Hillner et al. (1997) and Guadagnoli et al. (1998a, b). This study found that 82 percent of women received radiation therapy after breast conserving surgery. Of note, there was substantial variation in the use of radiation therapy depending on the patient's type of insurance: 45 percent of Medicaid beneficiaries received radiation therapy, compared with 78 percent of Blue Cross/Blue Shield subscribers and 88 percent of Medicare enrollees.

An earlier study by Johnson et al. (1994), which looked only at the use of adjuvant therapy in women with Stage I and II breast cancer diagnosed in 1983–1989, also found high adherence to National Cancer Institute Consensus Conference guidelines among community hospitals participating in the Community Clinical Oncology Program (CCOP). The CCOP was initiated by the NCI in 1983 to increase community participation in clinical research (Kaluzny et al., 1995). In this study, the proportion of women with node-positive breast cancer receiving adjuvant hormone or chemotherapy was highest in 1988 after NCI released a clinical alert advising physicians of the potential benefits in women with *node-negative* disease. The proportion of women with node-negative breast cancer treated with adjuvant therapy increased from 26 percent in the quarter before the clinical alert to 54 percent in the quarter following its release. During the same period, the proportion of women with node-positive breast cancer treated with adjuvant therapy increased from 81 to 90 percent. A year after the NCI clinical alert, the percentage of node-negative patients treated remained elevated above baseline at 46 percent, while the percentage of node-positive women treated with adjuvant therapy had fallen back to the baseline rate of 79 percent. It is not known if the clinical alert had a transient spillover effect on the treatment of node-positive disease. The proportion of women receiving adjuvant therapy in this study approaches a level one would expect if all women who could benefit from adjuvant therapy were being offered treatment. These data are limited in their generalizability, however, because the facilities that chose to participate in the NCI's CCOP are more likely to have an interest in cancer treatment and more likely to adhere to NCI guidelines than the average facility in the community. Notwithstanding, these data—and those reported by Hillner et al. (1997) and Guadagnoli et al. (1998a)—demonstrate high levels of adherence to treatment standards for adjuvant therapy in breast cancer in selected patient populations, with the notable exception of the low use of hormone therapy in postmenopausal patients.

The higher rates of radiation therapy reported by Hillner et al. (1997), Guadagnoli et al. (1998a), and Young et al. (1996) compared with the earlier study of Farrow et al. (1992), may reflect a general improvement in the quality of breast cancer care in the United States. However, given the selected patient populations in the Hillner et al. (1997), Guadagnoli et al. (1998a), and Young et al. (1996) studies, these data must be interpreted cautiously, especially when attempting to generalize from these results to the entire U.S. population. The Hillner et al. (1997) study includes only women younger than 65 with private fee-for-service health insurance. Also, although the Guadagnoli et al. (1998a) study is not limited to a privately insured population, it is limited to patients treated at hospitals that agreed to participate and therefore may be providing a higher standard of care. The Young et al. (1996) study compared women with Blue Cross/Blue Shield, Medicare, and Medicaid and found that women with Medicaid received much poorer quality care. Nevertheless, these studies suggest that at least some women in the United States had access to high-quality breast cancer care by 1995. However, even among these women there is cause for concern since only 60 percent of postmenopausal women with node-positive, estrogen receptor-positive cancers received adjuvant hormone therapy.

One study conducted in 1988–1989 suggests that the dose of adjuvant therapy for women with breast cancer is inappropriately low. Schleifer et al. (1991) audited the care of 107 women with breast cancer by 29 oncologists at three university-affiliated practices. Adjuvant therapy over six months was retrospectively reviewed and patients were prospectively interviewed. More than one-half (52 percent) of patients had at least one unjustified dose reduction. The total dose intensity for women whose doses were reduced was not reported. Older women and treatment in a "clinic" versus academic or private practice were associated with nonadherence to the treatment schedule.

Other studies using breast cancer process measures suggest that the proportion of women receiving standard treatment decreases with age, although the results of the published literature are not concordant. Several studies using cancer registry data to assess care for Medicare patients have shown that elderly women do not receive the recommended treatments for breast cancer as often as younger women, even when controlling for comorbid illness. Using New Mexico Cancer Registry data from 1984 to 1986, Goodwin et al. (1993) found that while only 43 percent of women age 85 and older, and 84 percent of women age 75 to 84, received definitive treatment for localized breast cancer compared with 92 percent of women age 65 to 74 (Goodwin et al., 1993). Definitive breast cancer treatment was defined as lumpectomy or excisional biopsy followed by radiation therapy or mastectomy. Age remained significant even when controlling for women's access to transportation, physical activity levels, income, social support, ability to perform activities of daily living, mental status, and the presence of other medical illnesses. In a comparable population of women in Virginia in 1985–1989, also using cancer registry data, Hillner et al. (1996) found that although the reported number of women age 65 to 69 receiving radiation therapy after breast conserving surgery was inappropriately low at 66 percent, only 7 percent of women age 85 and older had received radiation therapy (Hillner et al., 1996). In addition, although adjuvant therapy is recommended for all patients with node-positive disease, only 44 percent of patients with positive lymph nodes received any adjuvant therapy and only 33 percent received hormone therapy. Several studies, using data on treatment collected by the SEER cancer registries, have also noted that the use of radiation therapy in women who have undergone breast conserving surgery is lower than expected and declines with age (Ballard-Barbash et al., 1996; Farrow et al., 1992; Lazovich et al., 1991). Ballard-Barbash et al. (1996) found that whereas 76 percent of women age 65–69 received radiation therapy after breast conserving surgery for Stage I or II cancer, 68 percent of 70- to 74-year-olds, 56 percent of 75- to 79-year-olds, and 24 percent of women 80 years or older were given radiation treatment (Ballard-Barbash et al., 1996). They found that although controlling for differences in comorbidity was associated with a decrease in the frequency of radiation therapy after breast conserving surgery across all age groups, the decline with age persisted.

An earlier study, using data obtained directly from the medical record in seven southern California hospitals in 1980 through 1982, also found that rates of appropriate breast cancer treatment declined with age (Greenfield et al., 1987). Greenfield et al. (1987) reviewed patients' medical records to determine whether they had received diagnostic testing, staging evaluation, and treatment that was consistent with stage-specific consensus recommendations at the time (e.g., radiation therapy after breast conserving surgery; adjuvant chemotherapy for premenopausal women with node-positive breast cancer; adjuvant hormone therapy for postmenopausal women with node-positive estrogen receptor-positive tumors). Although the proportion of women receiving the recommended diagnostic and staging evaluations did not vary with age, the proportion receiving the recommended treatment did. According to the authors, 83 percent of women age 50 to 69 received the recommended breast cancer treatment compared with 67 percent of women age 70 and older. This difference remained significant when controlling for comorbidity, stage of breast cancer, and hospital at which treatment occurred.

In contrast, in a study of postmenopausal women age 50 and older with Stage I and II breast cancer treated in 1993 at 30 hospitals in Minnesota, using data collected through patient self-report, survey of the treating physician, and the medical record, Guadagnoli et al. (1997) found that 92 percent of women with node-positive breast cancer received some form of adjuvant therapy. Although the likelihood of women with node-positive breast cancer receiving adjuvant therapy did appear to decline slightly with age, this was not statistically significant. The use of adjuvant therapy did decline in women with node-negative breast cancer, and this was true for both chemotherapy and hormone therapy: 73 percent of women 50 to 59 years old with node-negative breast cancer received adjuvant therapy compared with 67 percent of women age 60 to 69, 56 percent of women age 70 to 79, and 36 percent of women age 80 and older. However, these age-associated differences were not significant after adjusting for marital status, education, income, HMO membership, tumor size, lymphatic invasion, estrogen receptor status, grade, type of primary surgery, history of breast and other cancer, and severity of comorbid disease. The use of adjuvant hormone therapy in node-negative disease also declined to 34 percent in women age 80 and older from only 52 percent in the other age groups. Since the authors did not stratify on tumor size or estrogen receptor status, it cannot be determined if the subset of women with node-negative disease, but larger tumors, were more likely to receive adjuvant therapy, which would suggest that care was being provided in a manner consistent with the scientific evidence and medical consensus of the time.

This last study by Guadagnoli et al. (1997) reports appropriately high rates of adjuvant therapy and thus contradicts the other studies, which suggest that problems exist with the quality of care provided for elderly women with breast cancer in the United States (Ballard-Barbash et al., 1996; Farrow et al., 1992; Goodwin et al., 1993; Greenfield et al., 1987; Hillner et al., 1996; Lazovich et al., 1991). Of note, the Guadagnoli et al. (1997) study uses multiple data sources, including patient self-report, physician report, and the medical record, to obtain information about treatment. All of the authors who report poorer adherence to standard treatment in elderly patients, with the exception of Greenfield et al. (1987), used cancer registry data, which again raises the issue of the reliability of cancer registry data on processes of care. Another possible explanation for the higher rates of adjuvant therapy in the elderly in the study by Guadagnoli et al. (1997) is that the quality of care has improved over time; they report data from 1993, whereas the other studies include data from 1980–1986. Perhaps with the dissemination of the results of clinical trials performed in the 1980s, the use of adjuvant therapy and radiation therapy in the elderly after breast conserving surgery has increased appropriately. Alternatively, there may be regional variations in the quality of care that explain discrepancies in the results of these studies. Minnesota may have better-quality care for breast cancer than the rest of the United States. In any case, given the preponderance of data suggesting that compliance with standard therapy for breast cancer in older women in the United States is low, even in the face of an isolated study showing excellent quality of care in 30 hospitals in Minnesota, these results highlight potential problems in the quality of breast cancer care that warrant further investigation.

Evidence from the late 1980s suggests that some hospitals were providing poorer quality breast cancer care than others. In a study conducted in 1988 by Hand et al. (1991), the interquartile range (25th to 75th percentile) for hospitals in Illinois that did not provide radiation therapy after breast conserving surgery was 17 to 75 percent (Hand et al., 1991). For those not providing adjuvant therapy the interquartile range was 30 to 56 percent, and for those not performing an estrogen receptor test on the pathologic specimen it was 4 to 14 percent.

In conclusion, studies of processes of care that have compared rates of radiation therapy after breast conserving surgery and adjuvant therapy for locally advanced breast cancer suggest that problems do exist with the quality of care received by many women in the United States. Many women (perhaps as many as 40 percent) do not appear to be receiving indicated radiation therapy after breast conserving surgery. In addition, older women are less likely to receive radiation therapy after breast conserving surgery. Rates of radiation therapy after breast conserving surgery also vary across hospitals, suggesting that some hospitals are providing poorer-quality breast cancer care than others. Of equal concern, many women do not appear to be receiving adjuvant chemotherapy (perhaps as many as 60 percent). These findings must be interpreted with caution, however, since many of the data reported are from the 1980s and are based on cancer registry data, whose accuracy is not known.

Variations in Compliance with American College of Radiology Quality Standards. While many women who undergo breast conserving surgery do not get indicated postoperative radiation therapy, potential quality problems still exist for the women who do get radiation therapy. The 1988 breast cancer Patterns of Care study performed by the American College of Radiology suggests widespread variation in compliance with standards of quality established by the ACR, with academic centers demonstrating the greatest compliance, followed by hospital facilities, and free-standing facilities having the poorest adherence (Kutchner et al., 1996). For example, immobilization of breast cancer patients receiving radiation therapy, in order to obtain consistent irradiation of the desired target, varied from 80 percent at academic centers, to 73 percent in hospital facilities, to only 51 percent in free-standing facilities. Similarly, the use of techniques to decrease the divergence of the radiation beam into lung tissue (in order to decrease pulmonary toxicity) ranged from 93 percent at academic centers to 77 percent at hospital facilities and 67 percent at free-standing facilities. A problem identified in an earlier 1983 Patterns of Care study was the misuse of axillary radiation; 53 percent of axillary node-negative women received radiation therapy. More recent data are needed to assess the state of compliance with radiology quality standards.

Follow-Up Care

Women should have a mammogram within 18 months following definitive surgery for breast cancer. According to one study of care provided to 936 privately insured, nonelderly women diagnosed from 1989 to 1991 in Virginia, only 79 percent had received a mammogram in the first 18 months (see Table 4.4).

The use of bone scans and imaging to search for liver metastases has been shown to have a low yield in clinical Stage I and II disease in numerous studies. Despite good evidence that their use does not improve clinical outcomes or quality of life (GIVIO, 1994), they are commonly done as a standard part of initial evaluation and often in subsequent follow-up care. In the Virginia study, 34 percent of women had a bone scan and 21 percent a computed tomography scan within 36 months of definitive surgery (Hillner et al., 1997).

The intensity of follow-up care appears to vary by site of care. During the same period, Simon et al. (1996) tracked 222 women treated and followed at one university hospital for three years. In the first year, patients treated with radiation or followed by medical oncology had the most frequent visits and intensity of testing. Wide variation in practice that was not explained by patient or provider characteristics was noted.

Breast Cancer Summary

Studies of breast cancer quality of care have compared process and outcome measures to a standard across regions of United States. Rates of radiation therapy after breast conserving surgery and adjuvant therapy for locally advanced disease are lower than expected and suggest that problems may exist with the quality of care received by many women with breast cancer in the United States. Many women do not appear to be receiving indicated radiation therapy after breast conserving surgery, and in areas of the United States it appears that the percentage of women who do not receive radiation is very high. In addition, older women are less likely to receive radiation therapy after breast conserving surgery. Equally concerning, many women do not appear to be receiving adjuvant chemotherapy. Although these findings must be interpreted with caution since many of the data are from breast cancer cases diagnosed in the 1980s and collected primarily by cancer registries, they suggest that serious problems exist with the quality of care provided to women with breast cancer in the United States. To determine the quality of *current* practice, reliable process and outcome measures have to be applied to a national sample of newly diagnosed breast cancer patients and the results must be reported quickly.

Prostate Cancer

Prostate cancer is the most commonly diagnosed non-skin cancer in men. In 1999, 179,300 cases are expected to be diagnosed, and 37,000 men are expected to die from this disease (ACS, 1999). The number of new cases diagnosed has increased in recent years as a result of adoption of prostate-specific antigen (PSA) testing (Potosky et al., 1995), largely reflecting an increase in early detection rather than a true increase in incidence.

The risk of prostate cancer increases with age, with the average age at diagnosis about 65 years and the median age about 72; it is relatively rare in men younger than 50. Five-year survival rates are very high: nearly 90 percent of men diagnosed with prostate cancer will survive at least five years (ACS, 1998).

Assessing quality of care for prostate cancer detection and treatment is especially difficult. Definitive evidence supporting the efficacy of early detection for prostate cancer awaits the results of two clinical trials. NCI's Prostate, Lung, Colorectal, and Ovarian (PLCO) cancer screening trial is examining the efficacy of early detection of prostate and other cancers, and the Prostate Cancer Intervention Versus Observation Trial (PIVOT) is a randomized trial that is addressing the efficacy of primary treatment of early-stage prostate cancer by surgery, compared to conservative management. There is currently no professional consensus regarding whether routine screening for prostate cancer should be performed (Table 4.5). Without essential information about the efficacy of early detection, there is no standard against which to assess the quality of screening or primary treatment. The prevalence of adverse effects of treatment (complications) may provide some information about quality of care. Presently, there is some limited evidence of variation in the results of treatment from facility to facility, but very little is known about the reasons for this variation.

TABLE 4.5 Prostate Cancer Screening Recommendations

Organization	Recommendation
American Cancer Society	Offer annual PSA testing to men over age 50 who have at least a 10-year life expectancy. Counsel certain high-risk groups (those with a family history including two or more first-degree relatives and African-American men) to begin testing at earlier ages (e.g., 45) (von Eschenbach et al., 1997)
American Urological Association	Offer the PSA test to men over age 50 who present for evaluation of prostatic disease symptoms after counseling them on the risks and benefits of the test. For men at high risk (positive family history, African American) the recommended age is 40 (Correa, 1998)
National Cancer Institute's PDQ	Evidence is insufficient to establish whether improvements in survival are associated with prostate cancer screening by DRE, TRUS, or PSA testing
U.S. Preventive Services Task Force (1996)	Routine screening is not recommended because of insufficient evidence regarding efficacy. Men who request screening should be given information about the risks and benefits of early detection and treatment
Veterans Administration	Discuss the risks and benefits of prostate cancer screening, including PSA testing, with men over age 50; however, no specific recommendation for routine screening is indicated (Wilson and Kizer, 1998)

NOTE: DRE = digital rectal exam; PSA = prostate-specific antigen; TRUS = transrectal ultrasound.

Measuring outcomes also has limitations in prostate cancer since the illness often progresses very slowly, so that long follow-up times are necessary to show differences in survival or disease progression. Differences in rates of recurrence or survival may be a result of treatment, but if treatment is not proven to be efficacious, then observed differences in outcomes across providers may simply reflect differences in patient selection.

Diagnostic Evaluation

Clinical staging is done using all information available prior to primary treatment, including digital rectal examination (DRE), imaging, and biopsy results (American Joint Committee on Cancer, 1997). Clinical staging of prostate cancer may be reported using one of two systems: modified American staging, or TNM (tumor–node–metastasis), or American Joint Committee on Cancer staging. Current methods for clinical staging may result in a substantial proportion of cases being understaged (up to 59 percent), with a smaller proportion being overstaged (about 5 percent) (Bostwick et al., 1994). Men with regional or metastatic prostate cancer should not have radical prostatectomy (see below for further discussion of appropriate care for advanced disease), and there is the potential for inappropriate surgery if the cancer is understaged. Inappropriate surgery can have significant effects on quality of life because the potential side effects of radical prostatectomy include permanent urinary and sexual dysfunction.

Numerous studies have illustrated the prognostic usefulness of pretreatment PSA, clinical stage, and Gleason score in predicting posttreatment outcomes such as risk of recurrence (American Joint Committee on Cancer, 1997; Pisansky et al., 1997). Partin et al. (1993) have developed tabulated estimates for risk of the tumor spreading (called extracapsular extension) using the Gleason score (indicating tumor differentiation) and PSA. The goal of this approach is to attempt to improve the prediction of pathological stage for patient counseling and treatment planning. Estimates from their original tables have been improved by pooling data from patients across multiple facilities (Partin et al., 1997), but concerns about patient representativeness may limit the use of these tables as decision aids for physicians.

In addition to PSA, Gleason score, stage, and patient comorbidity can provide independent prognostic information about treatment outcomes. Experts in urology and radiation oncology at academic treatment centers around the United States agree about the importance of comorbidity assessment as part of the pretreatment workup, but there is considerable variation in the methods used for such assessment (Schuster et al., 1998). Suggested information to be used includes: Karnofsky performance status; patient self-reported activity levels; obesity; and history of cardiac disease, vascular disease, pulmonary disease, hypertension, diabetes, and surgeries. Pretreatment urinary, bowel, and sexual functioning have most commonly been assessed by patients' verbal reports. Some physicians have reported using the American Urological Association symptom score to assess obstruction; formal assessment of potency, voiding symptoms, or continence is rarely performed on a routine basis.

Although there is evidence in the literature that PSA, stage, Gleason score, and patient comorbidity provide useful prognostic information when treating patients, there is no evidence indicating whether performing these assessments prior to initiating treatment improves patient outcomes. Given the absence of process–outcomes links for the pretreatment evaluation, developing process measures for this aspect of prostate cancer care would have to be based completely on expert opinion. At present, there are no specific guidelines for the staging, workup, or pretreatment assessment of patient comorbidity.

Choice of Treatment Modality

The modality used for primary treatment of prostate cancer varies depending on stage of disease, age or life expectancy, and patient preference. Treatment of localized prostate cancer (T1 or T2) can include surgery (radical prostatectomy), radiation therapy (external beam, brachytherapy, or conformal radiation therapy), or expectant management (watchful waiting). However, surgical treatment is not recommended for patients whose life expectancy is less than 10 years because the risks of surgery outweigh the survival benefit (Talcott, 1996). In addition, conformal radiation therapy is still being studied for efficacy and side effects (compared to standard external beam radiation therapy), but it has not yet been widely adopted as standard practice among radiation oncologists. Definitive evidence is lacking about the comparative efficacy of alternative treatment modalities for treating early-stage prostate cancer. The information used to make such decisions may have varying accuracy depending on its source: for example, clinicians' assessments of posttreatment complications have been found to greatly underestimate the rate reported by patients themselves (Litwin et al., 1998). This finding may suggest that a potentially important area for quality assessment is differences across providers in the patient counseling process.

A specific recommendation from the American Urological Association's (AUA's) clinical guidelines on the management of clinically localized prostate cancer is that all alternative treatment modalities (radical prostatectomy, radiation therapy—external beam, interstitial treatment—and expectant management) should be presented to every patient (Middleton et al., 1995). Thus, a potential quality indicator could include whether these recommendations are followed by urologists.

Complications Associated with Primary Treatment of Prostate Cancer

Estimates of complications resulting from primary treatment of prostate cancer vary widely across facilities even when stratifying by treatment modality: surgery, external beam radiation, or brachytherapy (interstitial radiation treatment or seed implants) (Middleton et al., 1995). After radical prostatectomy, rates of stress incontinence range from less than 10 to 50 percent and impotence rates range from 25 to 100 percent across series reports. Complications following external beam radiation included proctitis, with rates ranging from less than 10 percent to more than 50 percent; cystitis, ranging from 0 to 80 percent; and impotence, ranging from less than 10 percent to nearly 40 percent. Similarly, complication rates reported for brachytherapy range from 0 to 75 percent for proctitis, less than 10 percent to 90 percent for cystitis, and less than 10 percent to 75 percent for impotence.

While these widely varying complication rates may reflect differences in quality of care, it is difficult to draw conclusions based on this type of information (Wasson et al., 1993). First, there may be differences in the way the data were collected, which could account for variations in rates of complications. Second, there may be systematic differences in patient case mix (disease severity and comorbidities) across facilities, and these differences must be accounted for before comparing outcomes across institutions. Even if series reports could be adjusted for case mix, there is usually little information available to link differences in results to differences in the technical process of care. Finally, these series report data from only a small number of providers, often large academic clinics. The results for such providers may not represent those of other institutions or clinics.

Effectiveness of Radiation Equipment in Treating Localized Prostate Cancer

An early American College of Radiology Patterns of Care study examined the association between types of radiation equipment (a structure measure) and localized prostate cancer treatment outcomes (Hanks et al., 1985). Facilities that used cobalt units were found to have higher stage-adjusted rates of disease recurrence than facilities that used linear accelerators or betatrons. The use of cobalt equipment was also correlated with other structural indicators: these facilities had lower percentages of patients who were staged, had lower staff–patient ratios, and were more likely to have parttime therapists, compared to national averages. From these results, the authors recommended that facilities using cobalt units should upgrade their treatment equipment, give palliative treatment only, or close. While this study helped to show that cobalt units were not as good as other types, the evidence available when the care was provided did not indicate that cobalt use was inappropriate. Therefore, this study was quite valuable in showing how to improve care, but it is not evidence of poor quality. Quality has to be judged by the level of knowledge and standards in place at the time care was delivered.

Treatment of Advanced Prostate Cancer

Treatment for advanced prostate cancer is palliative. Data from randomized controlled trials demonstrate a survival benefit as well as relief from bone pain by treatment with androgen ablation (the elimination of sources of male hormone such as testosterone), which can include orchiectomy alone, monotherapy with a luteinizing hormone-releasing hormone (LHRH) analogue, or "maximal androgen blockade" with either orchiectomy or an LHRH analogue and anti-androgen therapy (Garnick, 1996). When prostate cancer progresses on androgen ablation therapy, treatment is less effective; however, various drugs (ketoconazole or aminoglutethimide, estramustine, suramin, mitoxantrone with prednisone or steroids) can improve pain control and quality of life (Garnick, 1996). Because patients with prostate cancer that has metastasized to the bone often suffer excruciating pain, a primary focus in the care of patients with metastatic prostate cancer is control of their pain, with either narcotics, radiation therapy, or chemotherapy. So, although advanced prostate cancer is not curable, multiple treatment options exist and there is evidence in the scientific literature that they improve quality of life and, in some cases, prolong survival. Thus, there is sufficient evidence for process–outcomes links in advanced prostate cancer that process measures could be developed to evaluate the quality of care.

Prostate Cancer Summary

Prostate cancer provides a particular challenge for quality-of-care assessment: methods for early detection are available, but there is not yet definitive information about whether early detection improves survival. There are a number of treatment modalities for early-stage disease, but there is not definitive information about the efficacy of early treatment. The results of the PLCO trial will better inform decisions about whether routine screening for prostate cancer should be performed and for whom; and the results of the PIVOT trial will provide information about the efficacy of primary treatment of localized prostate cancer by surgery.

One candidate indicator for prostate cancer quality assessment is to identify whether information about alternative treatment modalities was presented to patients, as recommended by the AUA's practice guidelines (Middleton et al., 1995). A second candidate indicator may be to assess the rates of surgical treatment among men with life expectancies less than 10 years, using age 70 to represent a proxy for 10-year remaining life expectancy for the average patient (a high rate of surgical treatment in men with a life expectancy of less than 10 years would be an indicator of *poor* quality).

At present, available performance measures do not include quality indicators for prostate cancer treatment (e.g., measures of the National Committee on Quality Assurance and Foundation for Accountability). Investigators at RAND are developing candidate quality indicators based on a structured review of the literature, key informant interviews of prostate cancer experts, and focus groups with patients as part of a RAND study funded by the Bing Foundation. The next phase of this research will be to test the reliability and validity of these candidate measures in evaluating the quality of care, as well as exploring potential process–outcomes links.

KEY FINDINGS

Good indicators of quality are based on evidence from rigorous research, which is not available for most aspects of cancer care. For those aspects of care that have been evaluated, the quality of health care can be precisely defined and accurately measured. Measures of structure, process, and outcomes can all be used to assess quality. An outcomes indicator that is often used to evaluate cancer care has been five-year survival, but more timely and practical measures are becoming available to more precisely assess factors related to health care that can affect outcomes. Process measures can serve as good quality indicators when research has proved that a given process leads to better outcomes. Examples of good process measures for breast cancer include

- use of screening mammography,
- use of radiation therapy following breast conserving surgery, and
- use of adjuvant therapy among women with local or regional breast cancer.

In other cases, research suggests that one process does not have an advantage over another in terms of outcomes, so patient preferences should dictate the course of care. For many women with breast cancer, for example, optimal care involves presenting information on alternative treatments and supporting an informed choice.

Sometimes, research suggests that providing a service does not have a favorable impact on outcomes, indicating that the service should not be provided. Most elderly men with prostate cancer, for example, would not likely benefit from radical prostatectomy if their life expectancy is less than 10 years. High rates of surgery among very old men could indicate that surgery is being performed too often when there is no expected benefit (and there is potential harm from surgery).

Two national databases are available with which to assess the quality of cancer care, but each has limitations in the context of evaluating quality of care. The SEER cancer registry has been valuable when linked to Medicare and other insurance administrative files to assess quality of care for the elderly and other insured populations. It is also useful in identifying cases for in-depth studies of quality-related issues. The SEER registry, however, covers only 14 percent of the U.S. population and thus may not adequately represent the diversity of systems of care. Finding ways to capture measures of process of care, treatment information, and intermediate outcomes and improving the timeliness of reporting would enhance the registry's use in quality assessment. The National Cancer Data Base now includes information on more than one-half of all newly diagnosed cases of cancer and many of the demographic, clinical, and health system data elements needed to assess quality of care. The NCDB does not, however, include important aspects of care that take place in outpatient settings. The NCDB has not yet been widely used to assess quality of care but, if enhanced, would have great potential for doing so.

It is difficult to evaluate the quality of breast and prostate cancer care from the available evidence because

- many studies have relied on data from the 1980s, and the care evaluated does not represent current practice;
- many studies are difficult to interpret since dissimilar groups of patients are compared (e.g., insufficient controls for important clinical characteristics such as comorbidity);
- studies are confined to a small group of patients, in one or a few institutions, states, or health plans, making it difficult to generalize to all cancer patients; and
- studies are often based on data from cancer registries, which may not accurately represent some aspects of care (e.g., certain treatments may be underreported).

National studies of recently diagnosed individuals with cancer are necessary, using information sources with sufficient detail to allow appropriate comparisons. Ways must be found to produce information from these studies quickly, while they are still relevant to contemporaneous conditions.

Although the available evidence has limitations, it is suggestive of quality problems in cancer care. For women with breast cancer, many do not appear to be receiving indicated radiation therapy after breast conserving surgery. Of equal concern, many women with appropriate indications do not appear to be receiving adjuvant chemotherapy. Both treatments are known to improve outcomes. Furthermore, there is evidence of poor quality in essential aspects of the diagnostic process that is likely to compromise outcomes (e.g., inadequate biopsies, poor reporting of pathology studies). Evidence also suggests that a significant number of women with breast cancer and men with prostate cancer are not receiving information about the full range of treatment options available to them.

REFERENCES

Acheson MB, Patton RG, Howisey RL, Lane RF, Morgan A. 1997. Histologic correlation of image-guided core biopsy with excisional biopsy of nonpalpable breast lesions. *Archives of Surgery* 132:815–821.

Aharony L, Strasser S. 1993. Patient satisfaction: What we know about and what we still need to explore. *Medical Care Review* 50:49–79.

American Cancer Society. 1998. *Cancer Facts and Figures—1998*. Atlanta, GA.

American Cancer Society. 1999. *Cancer Facts and Figures—1999*. Atlanta, GA.

American Joint Committee on Cancer. 1997. *American Joint Committee on Cancer, Cancer Staging Manual*, 5th edition, ID Fleming, JS Cooper, DE Henson, et al., (eds.) Philadephia: Lippincott-Raven.

Ballard-Barbash, R, Potosky A, et al. 1996. Factors associated with surgical and radiation therapy for early stage breast cancer in older women. *Journal of the National Cancer Institute* 88(11): 716–726.

Bartlett EE, Grayson M, Barker R, et al. 1984. The effects of physician communications skills on patient satisfaction, recall, and adherence. *Journal of Chronic Diseases* 37(9–10):755–764.

Beam CA, Layde PM, Sullivan DC. 1996. Variability in the interpretation of screening mammograms by U.S. radiologists. Findings from a national sample. *Archives of Internal Medicine* 156(2):209–213.

Bonadonna G, Valagussa P. 1985. Adjuvant systemic therapy for resectable breast cancer. *Journal of Clinical Oncology* 3(2):259–275.

Bostwick DG, Myers RP, Oesterling JE. 1994. Staging of prostate cancer. *Seminars in Surgical Oncology* 10:60–72.

Brook R, Chassin M, Fink A. 1986. A method for detailed assessment of the appropriateness of medical technologies. *International Journal of Technology Assessment in Health Care* 2:53–63.

Brook R, Park R, Chassin M, et al. 1990. Carotid endarterectomy for elderly patients: Predicting complications. *Annals of Internal Medicine* 113:747–753.

Centers for Disease Control and Prevention. 1998. *The National Program of Cancer Registries AT-A-GLANCE 1998.* http://www.cdc.gov/nccdphp/dcpc/npcr/register.htm.

Cleary P, McNeil B. 1988. Patient satisfaction as an indicator of quality care. *Inquiry* 25:25–36.

Cole P, Rodu B. 1996. Declining cancer mortality in the United States. *Cancer* 78:2045–2048.

Correa RJ. 1998. American Urological Association response to AHCPR notice of assessment of PSA test. American Urological Association. Baltimore, MD.

Davies A, Ware J. 1988. Involving consumers in quality of care assessment. *Health Affairs* 7:33–48.

Deyo R, Inui T. 1980. Dropouts and broken appointments: A literature review and agenda for future research. *Medical Care* 18:1146–1157.

Donabedian A. 1980. *Explorations in Quality Assessment and Monitoring,* Volume I: *The Definition of Quality and Approaches to Its Assessment.* Ann Arbor, MI: Health Administration Press.

Early Breast Cancer Trialists' Collaborative Group. 1992. Systemic treatment of early breast cancer by hormonal, cytotoxic, or immune therapy. *Lancet* 399:1–71.

Early Breast Cancer Trialists' Collaborative Group. 1998. Tamoxifen for early breast cancer: An overview of the randomised trials. *Lancet* 351:1451–1467.

Eastman P. 1997. NCI adopts new mammography screening guidelines for women. *Journal of the National Cancer Institute* 89:538–539.

Farrow DC, Hunt WC, Samet JM. 1992. Geographic variation in the treatment of localized breast cancer. *New England Journal of Medicine* 326:1097–1101.

Farrow DC, Samet JM, and Hunt WC. 1996. Regional variation in survival following the diagnosis of cancer. *Journal of Clinical Epidemiology* 49(8)843–847.

Fisher B, Bauer M, Margolese R, et al. 1985. Five-year results of a randomized clinical trial comparing total mastectomy and segmental mastectomy with or without radiation in the treatment of breast cancer. *New England Journal of Medicine* 312:665–673.

Fisher B, Dignam J, Wolmark N, et al. 1997. Tamoxifen and chemotherapy for lymph node-negative, estrogen receptor-positive breast cancer. *Journal of the National Cancer Institute* 89:1673–1682.

Ganz PA, Schag AC, Lee JJ, Polinsky ML, Tan SJ. 1992a. Breast conservation versus mastectomy: Is there a difference in psychological adjustment of quality of life in the year after surgery? *Cancer* 69:1729–1738.

Ganz PA, Schag CA, Lee JJ, Sim MS. 1992b. The CARES: A generic measure of health-related quality of life for patients with cancer. *Quality of Life Research* 1:19–29.

Garnick MB. 1996. Prostate cancer: Screening, diagnosis, and management. *Annals of Internal Medicine* 118(10):804–818.

GIVIO. 1994. Impact of follow-up testing on survival and health-related quality of life in breast cancer patients. A multicenter randomized controlled trial. *Journal of the American Medical Association* 271(20):1587–1592.

Goodwin JS, Hunt WC, Samet JM. 1993. Determinants of cancer therapy in elderly patients. *Cancer* 72(2):594–601.

Greenfield S, Blanco DM, Elashoff RM, Ganz PA. 1987. Patterns of care related to age of breast cancer patients. *Journal of the American Medical Association* 257:2766–2770.

Grieco A, Long CJ. 1984. Investigation of the Karnofsky performance status as a measure of quality of life. *Health Psychology* 3(2):129–142.

Guadagnoli E, Shapiro CL, Gurwitz JH, et al. 1997. Age-related patterns of care: Evidence against ageism in the treatment of early stage breast cancer. *Journal of Clinical Oncology* 15:2338–2344.

Guadagnoli E, Shapiro CL, Weeks JC, et al. 1998a. The quality of care for treatment of early stage breast carcinoma. Is it consistent with national guidelines? *Cancer* 83(2):302–309.

Guadagnoli E, Weeks JC, Shapiro CL, et al. 1998b. Use of breast-conserving surgery for treatment of Stage I and Stage II breast cancer. *Journal of Clinical Oncology* 16:101–106.

Halsted W. 1894. The results of operations for cure of cancer of the breast performed at Johns Hopkins Hospital. *Johns Hopkins Hospital Bulletin* 4:497.

Hammond EH, Flinner RL. 1997. Clinically relevant breast cancer reporting. Using process measures to improve anatomic pathology reporting. *Archives of Pathology and Laboratory Medicine* 1:1171–1175.

Hand R, Sener S, Imperato J, et al. 1991. Hospital variables associated with quality of care for breast cancer patients [see comments]. *Journal of the American Medical Association* 266:3429–3432.

Hanks GE, Diamond JJ, Kramer S. 1985. The need for complex technology in radiation oncology. Correlations of facility characteristics and structure with outcome. *Cancer* 55(9 Suppl.):2198–2201.

Hayes MK, De Bruhl ND, Hirschowitz S, et al. 1996. Mammographically guided fine-needle aspiration cytology of the breast: Reducing the rate of insufficient specimens. *American Journal of Roentgenology* 167:381–384.

Hayward R, Bernard A, Rosevear J, et al. 1993. An evaluation of generic screens for poor quality of hospital care on a general medicine service. *Medical Care* 31:394–402.

Hillner BE, McDonald KM, Penberthy L, et al. 1997. Measuring standards of care for early breast cancer in an insured population. *Journal of Clinical Oncology* 15:1401–1408.

Hillner BE, Penberthy L, Desch CE, et al. 1996. Variation in staging and treatment of local and regional breast cancer in the elderly. *Breast Cancer Research and Treatment* 40:75–86.

Houn F, Finder C. 1997. The Mammography Quality Standards Act and interventional mammography procedures. *Bulletin of the American College of Surgeons* 82:14–22.

Howe JR, Monsees B, Destouet J, et al. 1995. Needle localization breast biopsy: A model for multidisciplinary quality assurance. *Journal of Surgical Oncology* 58:223–239.

Hsieh MO, Kagle JD. 1991. Understanding patient satisfaction and dissatisfaction with health care. *Health and Social Work* 16:281–290.

Iezzoni L. 1996. An introduction to risk adjustment. *American Journal of Medical Quality* 11:S8–S11.

IOM (Institute of Medicine). 1990. *Medicare: A Strategy for Quality Assurance*. Volume 1. Committee to Design a Strategy for Quality Review and Assurance in Medicare, Institute of Medicine. Lohr K, ed. Washington, D.C.: National Academy Press.

IOM. 1999. *Measuring the Quality of Health Care: A Statement by the National Roundtable on Health Care Quality*. Donaldson M, ed. Washington, D.C.: National Academy Press.

Johnson TP, Ford L, Warnecke RB, et al. 1994. Effect of a National Cancer Institute clinical alert on breast cancer practice patterns. *Journal of Clinical Oncology* 12:1783–1788.

Kahan K, Bernstein S, Leape L, et al. 1994. Measuring the necessity of medical procedures. *Medical Care* 32:357–365.

Kahn K, Rogers W, Rubenstein L, et al. 1990. Measuring quality of care with explicit process criteria before and after implementation of the DRG-based prospective payment system. *Journal of the American Medical Association* 264:1980–1983.

Kaluzny AD, Warnecke R, Lacey LM, et al. 1995. Using a community clinical trials network for treatment, prevention, and control research: Assuring access to state-of-the-art cancer care. *Cancer Investigation* 13: 517–525.

Karnofsky DA, Burchenal JH. 1949. The clinical evaluation of chemotherapeutic agents in cancer. Pp. 191–205 in MacLeod CM, ed. *Evaluation of Chemotherapeutic Agents*. New York: Columbia University Press.

Kaufman Z, Shpitz B, Shapiro M, et al. 1994. Triple approach in the diagnosis of dominant breast masses: Combined physical examination, mammography, and fine-needle aspiration. *Journal of Surgical Oncology* 56:254–257.

Kerlikowske K, Grady D, Rubin SM, et al. 1995. Efficacy of screening mammography. A meta-analysis. *Journal of the American Medical Association* 273:149–154.

Kiebert GD, de Haes JCJM, van de Velde CJH. 1991. The impact of breast-conserving treatment and mastectomy on the quality of life of early-stage breast cancer patients: A review. *Journal of Clinical Oncology* 9:1059–1070.

Kramer S, Herring DF. 1976. The Patterns of Care study: A nationwide evaluation of the practice of radiation therapy in cancer management. *International Journal of Radiation Oncology, Biology, Physics* 1(11–12):1231–1236.

Kravitz R, Laouri M, Kahan J, et al. 1995. Validity of criteria used for detecting underuse of coronary revascularization. *Journal of the American Medical Association* 274:632–638.

Krook JE, Moertel CG, Gunderson LL, et al. 1991. Effective surgical adjuvant therapy for high-risk rectal carcinoma. *New England Journal of Medicine* 324:709–715.

Kutchner GJ, Smith AR, Fowble BL, et al. 1996. Treatment planning for primary breast cancer: A Patterns of Care study. *International Journal of Radiation Oncology, Biology, Physics* 36:731–737.

Laouri M, Kravitz R, Berstein S, et al. 1997. Underuse of coronary angiography: Application of a clinical method. *International Journal for Quality in Health Care* 9:5–22.

Lazovich D, White E, Thomas DB, Moe RE. 1991. Underutilization of breast-conserving surgery and radiation therapy among women with Stage I or II breast cancer. *Journal of the American Medical Association* 266:3433–3438.

Levine MC, Guyatt GH, Gent M, et al. 1988. Quality of life in Stage II breast cancer: An instrument for clinical trials. *Journal of Clinical Oncology* 6:1798–1810.

Litwin MS, Hays RD, Fink A, et al. 1995. Quality-of-life outcomes in men treated for localized prostate cancer. *Journal of the American Medical Association* 273:129–135.

Litwin MS, Lubeck DP, Henning JM, Carroll PR. 1998. Differences in urologist and patient assessments of health related quality of life in men with prostate cancer: Results of the CaPSURE database. *Journal of Urology* 159:1988–1992.

McGlynn EA. 1997. Six challenges in measuring the quality of health care. *Health Affairs* 16(3):7–21.

Menck HR, Cunningham MP, Jessup JM. 1997. The growth and maturation of the National Cancer Data Base. *Cancer* 80:2296–2304.

Mettlin C, Smart CR. 1994. Breast cancer detection guidelines for women aged 40 to 49 years: Rationale for the American Cancer Society reaffirmation of recommendations. *CA—A Cancer Journal for Clinicians* 44:248–255.

Mettlin CJ, Menck HR, Winchester DP, Murphy GP. 1997a. A comparison of breast, colorectal, lung, and prostate cancers reported to the National Cancer Data Base and the Surveillance, Epidemiology, and End Results Program. *Cancer* 79:2052–2061.

Mettlin CJ, Murphy GP, Cunningham MP, Menck HR. 1997b. The National Cancer Data Base report on race, age, and region variations in prostate cancer treatment. *Cancer* 80:1261–1266.

Mettlin CJ, Murphy GP, Sylvester J, et al. 1997c. Results of hospital cancer registry surveys by the American College of Surgeons: Outcomes of prostate cancer treatment by radical prostatectomy. *Cancer* 80:1875–1881.

Middleton RG, Thompson IM, Austenfeld MS, et al. 1995. Prostate cancer clinical guidelines panel summary report on the management of clinically localized prostate cancer. *Journal of Urology* 154: 2144–2148.

Moertel CG. 1994. Chemotherapy for colorectal cancer. *New England Journal of Medicine* 330(16): 1136–1142.

Nakleh RE, Jones B, Zarbo RJ. 1997. Mammographically directed breast biopsies. A college of American Pathologists Q-Probes Study of clinical physician expectations and of specimen handling and reporting characteristics in 434 institutions. *Archives of Pathology and Laboratory Medicine* 121:11–18.

National Cancer Data Base. 1998.
http://www.facs.org/about_college/acsdept/cancer_dept/programs/ncdb/ncdb.html.

National Institutes of Health. 1990a. *NIH Consensus Statement. Adjuvant Therapy for Patients with Colon and Rectum Cancer.* 8:1–25. Bethesda, MD: National Institutes of Health.

National Institutes of Health. 1990b. *NIH Consensus Statement. Treatment of Early Stage Breast Cancer.* 8:1–19. Bethesda, MD: National Institutes of Health.

Nattinger AB, Gottlieb MS, Hoffman RG, et al. 1996. Minimal increase in use of breast-conserving surgery from 1986 to 1990. *Medical Care* 34:479–489.

Nattinger AB, Gottlieb MS, Veum J, et al. 1992. Geographic variation in the use of breast conserving treatment for breast cancer. *New England Journal of Medicine* 326:1102–1107.

Nyström L, Rutqvist LE, Wall S, et al. 1993. Breast cancer screening with mammography: Overview of Swedish randomised trials. *Lancet* 341:973–978.

Osborne CK, Clark GM, Ravdin PM. 1996. Adjuvant systemic therapy of primary breast cancer. Pp. 548–578 in Harris JR, Morrow M, Lippman ME, Hellman S, eds. *Diseases of the Breast.* New York: Lippincott-Raven Publishers.

Osteen RT. 1992. Breast cancer. Pp. 29–38 in Steele GD, Winchester DP, Menck HR, Murphy GP, eds. *National Cancer Data Base, 1992.* Atlanta, GA: American Cancer Society.

Osuch JR. 1996. Abnormalities on Physical Examination. Pp. 110–114 in Harris JR, Morrow M, Lippman ME, Hellman S, eds. *Diseases of the Breast.* New York: Lippincott-Raven Publishers.

Partin AW, Kattan MW, Subong EN, et al. 1997. Combination of prostate-specific antigen, clinical stage, and Gleason score to predict pathological stage of localized prostate cancer. A multi-institutional update. *Journal of the American Medical Association* 277(18):1445–1451.

Partin AW, Yoo J, Carter HB, et al. 1993. The use of prostate-specific antigen, clinical stage and Gleason score to predict pathological stage in men with localized prostate cancer. *Journal of Urology* 150:110–114.

Pisansky TM, Kahn MJ, Rasp GM, et al. 1997. A multiple prognostic index predictive of disease outcome after irradiation for clinically localized prostate carcinoma. *Cancer* 79(2):337–344.

Potosky AL, Riley GF, Lubitz JD, et al. 1993. Potential for cancer related health services research using a linked Medicare-tumor registry database. *Medical Care* 31(8):732–748.

Potosky AL, Miller BA, Albertson PC, Kramer BS. 1995. The role of increasing detection in the rising incidence of prostate cancer. *Journal of the American Medical Association* 273:548–552.

Reichheld FF. 1996. Learning from customer defections: Customers can help point out what is wrong with services. *Harvard Business Review* 74:56–69.

Reifel J, Ganz P. In press. Clinical applications of quality of life research. In *Cancer Policy.* Norwell, MA: Kluwer Academic Publishers.

Ries LAG, Kosary CL, Hankey BF, et al., eds. 1998. *SEER Cancer Statistics Review, 1973–1995.* Bethesda, MD: National Cancer Institute.

Roberts MM, Alexander FE, Anderson TJ, et al. 1990. Edinburgh trial of screening for breast cancer: Mortality at seven years. *Lancet* 335:241–246.

Rubin HR, Gandek B, Rogers WH, et al. 1993. Patients' ratings of outpatient visits in different practice settings. Results from the medical outcomes study. *Journal of the American Medical Association* 270:835–840.

Samet JM, Hunt WC, Farrow DC. 1994. Determinants of receiving breast-conserving surgery. The Surveillance, Epidemiology, and End Results Program, 1983–1986. *Cancer* 73:2344–2351.

Sarrazin D, Le M, Rouesse J, et al. 1984. Conservative treatment versus mastectomy in breast cancer tumors with macroscopic diameter of 20 millimeters or less: The experience of the Institut Gustave-Roussy. *Cancer* 53:1209–1213.

Schag CA, Heinrich RL. 1990. Development of a comprehensive quality of life measurement tool: CARES. *Oncology* 4:135–138.

Schatzkin A, Freedman LS, Dorgan J, et al. 1996. Surrogate end points in cancer research: A critique. *Cancer Epidemiology, Biomarkers, and Prevention* 5:947–953.

Schipper H, Clinch J, McMurray A, et al. 1984. Measuring the quality of life of cancer patients: The Functional Living Index—Cancer: Development and validation. *Journal of Clinical Oncology* 2:472–483.

Schleifer S, Bhardwaj S, Lebovits A, et al. 1991. Predictors of physician nonadherence to chemotherapy regimens. *Cancer* 67: 945–951.

Schuster MA, McGlynn EA, Brook RH. 1998. How good is the quality of health care in the United States? *Milbank Quarterly* 76(4):509, 517–563.

Segal M. 1994. Mammography facilities must meet quality standards. *FDA Consumer* 8–12.

Shapiro S, Venet W, Strax P, et al. 1988. *Periodic Screening for Breast Cancer—The Health Insurance Plan Project and Its Sequelae, 1963–1986.* Baltimore, MD: Johns Hopkins University Press.

Simon MS, Stano M, Severson RK, et al. 1996. Clinical surveillance for early stage breast cancer: An analysis of claims data. *Breast Cancer Research and Treatment* 40:119–128.

Stolier AJ. 1997. Stereotactic breast biopsy: A surgical series. *Journal of the American College of Surgeons* 185:224–228.

Surveillance, Epidemiology, and End Results Program. 1998. http://www-seer.ims.nci.nih.gov

Swan J, Wingo P, Clive R, et al. 1998. Cancer surveillance in the U.S.: Can we have a national system? *Cancer* 83:1282–1291.

Tabar L, Fagerberg G, Chen H-H, et al. 1995. Efficacy of breast cancer screening by age. New results from the Swedish two-county trial. *Cancer* 75:2507–2517.

Talamonti MS, Morrow M. 1996. The abnormal mammogram. Pp. 114–122 in Harris JR, Morrow M, Lippman ME, Hellman S, eds. *Diseases of the Breast.* New York: Lippincott-Raven Publishers.

Talcott JA. 1996. Quality of life in early prostate cancer: Do we know enough to treat? *Hematology/Oncology Clinics of North America* 10(3):691–701.

U.S. Department of Health and Human Services. 1996. *Guide to Clinical Preventive Services. Report of the U.S. Preventive Services Task Force.* Second Edition. Washington, D.C.

U.S. General Accounting Office. 1988. *Cancer Treatments 1975–85: The Use of Breakthrough Treatments for Seven Types of Cancer.* PIC ID No. 3068.1:1–21. Washington, D.C.

U.S. General Accounting Office. 1998a. Mammography Quality Standards Act: X-ray quality improved, access unaffected, but impact on health outcomes unknown. GAO/T-HEHS-98-164.

U.S. General Accounting Office. 1998b. Mammography services: Impact of federal legislation on quality, access, and health outcomes. GAO/HEHS-98-11.

Veronesi U, Saccozzi R, Del Vecchio M, et al. 1981. Comparing radical mastectomy with quandrantectomy, axillary dissection, and radiotherapy in patients with small cancers of the breast. *New England Journal of Medicine* 305:6–11.

von Eschenbach A, Ho R, Murphy GP, Cunningham M, Lins N. 1997. American Cancer Society guideline for the early detection of prostate cancer: Update 1997. *CA: Cancer Journal for Clinicians* 47:261–264.

Wasson JH, Cushman CC, Bruskewitz RC, et al. 1993. A structured literature review of treatment for localized prostate cancer. Prostate disease patient outcome research. *Archives of Family Medicine* 2:487–493.

Weeks JC. 1997. Outcomes assessment in the NCCN. *Oncology* 11(11A):137–140.

Wells WAS, Carney PA, Eliassen MS, et al. 1998. Statewide study of diagnostic agreement in breast pathology. *Journal of the National Cancer Institute* 90:142–145.

Wennberg JE, McAndrew CM. 1996. Pp. 128–129 in *The Dartmouth Atlas of Health Care in the United States*. Chicago: American Hospital Publishing, Inc.

Wilson NJ, Kizer KW. 1998. Oncology management by the "new" Veterans Health Administration. *Cancer* 82(10 Suppl.):2003–2009.

Wingo PA, Ries LA, Rosenberg HM, et al. 1998. Cancer incidence and mortality, 1973–1995: A report card for the U.S. *Cancer* 82(6):1197–1207.

Young PC, Wasserman RC, McAullife T, et al. 1985. Why families change pediatricians. Factors causing dissatisfaction with pediatric care. *American Journal of Diseases of Children* 139:683–686.

Young WW, Marks SM, Kohler SA, Hsu AY. 1996. Dissemination of clinical results. Mastectomy versus lumpectomy and radiation therapy. *Medical Care* 34:1003–1017.

5

Health Care Delivery and Quality of Cancer Care

The field of quality assessment in cancer care is relatively new, and investigators are just beginning to identify meaningful indicators of quality for many aspects of cancer care. Health services researchers have used established indicators to determine whether outcomes of care are affected by how care is delivered or who delivers care. Several aspects of the health care delivery system have the potential to affect quality:

- the resources or capacity of facilities (e.g., volume of services, scope of services, access to technology, nurse staffing levels, academic affiliation);
- characteristics of health care providers and systems (e.g., level of training, specialization, certification); and
- the way in which services are financed, organized, and delivered (e.g., managed care versus traditional fee-for-service [FFS] care; regionalization of services).

This chapter summarizes the literature that examines the effects of these factors on the quality of cancer care. Whereas Chapter 4 was confined to a review of the literature on breast and prostate cancer, this summary focuses on the way attributes of the health care system affect quality more generally and thus includes studies of other cancers. Many studies, for example, address the relationship between professional or institutional experience, as measured by the number of operations performed, and outcomes for individuals with cancers for which high-risk surgery is indicated (e.g., pancreatic cancer). In only three areas was there a body of literature to examine:

1. the effects of volume of cases handled by hospitals or individual physicians on outcome;
2. the effects of specialization of facilities or physicians on outcome; and
3. the effects of managed care versus fee-for-service care on process and outcome.

A brief overview of the conduct of health services research, and certain cautions about inferences from such studies, are warranted before individual studies in these areas are reviewed.

EVALUATING THE STRENGTH OF EVIDENCE FROM HEALTH SERVICES RESEARCH

Important questions about the way in which aspects of health care delivery affect outcomes usually cannot be answered with the most powerful research design, the randomized clinical trial. It would, for example, be unacceptable to most individuals recently diagnosed with cancer to be assigned randomly to an insurance plan, hospital, or doctor, although such studies are not impossible. For example, an experiment was conducted in the 1970s to assess how insurance plans and cost sharing affected health care and outcomes among the general population (Newhouse, 1998). Most of the time, however, considerations of cost and practicality lead health services researchers to conduct observational rather than experimental studies. Often cancer patients are identified retrospectively, through cancer registry data or hospital discharge records, and outcomes are compared across different health care settings or processes of care. Alternatively, individuals with cancer in different settings may be identified shortly after diagnosis and followed prospectively with systematic measurement tools designed to assess different outcomes (e.g., quality-of-life measures). Although they are generally less costly and easier to conduct, nonexperimental studies are subject to a number of potential biases that can make findings difficult to interpret. Any differences observed between study groups could be due to underlying differences in group membership rather than to the intervention or condition being evaluated. Individuals enrolled in health mainentance organizations (HMOs), for example, tend to be younger and healthier than those insured through FFS plans. Comparisons of groups that vary by insurance coverage must therefore control for differences in age and health status. However, information necessary to "adjust" the analysis to compare across groups of like individuals is not always available or may not capture all of the underlying differences.

Some unique features of cancer and its diagnosis make these "case-mix" adjustments very important, but difficult (Dent, 1998). Differential use of screening and diagnostic tests, for example, can bias the results of comparative studies of cancer survival. In a classic study of survival following treatment for lung cancer, Feinstein and colleagues (Feinstein et al., 1985) found higher survival rates for individuals treated in 1977 than in the period from 1953 to 1964. Survival was better for the entire group and for subgroups in each of the three main TNM (tumor–node–metastasis) stages. The more recent cohort, however, had undergone many new diagnostic imaging procedures, which resulted in "stage migration." Many patients who previously would have been classified in a "good" stage were assigned to a "bad" stage. The use of new diagnostic techniques allows patients with unobserved metastases to "migrate" from TNM stages with a better prognosis (e.g., Stage I or II) into those with a worse prognosis (Stages II and III). The migration would improve survival in the lower stages, because fewer patients with metastases are assigned to them. Migration would also improve survival in the higher stages, since the metastases in the newly added patients were silent rather than overt. This bias was called the Will Rogers phenomenon, after the humorist–philosopher who is said to have remarked, "When the Okies left Oklahoma and moved to California, they raised the average intelligence level in both states."

This bias has been noted in studies of changes in survival over time and in comparisons of survival across geographic areas (Farrow et al., 1995) or by hospital type (Greenberg et al., 1991). In a study by Greenberg and colleagues of patients with non-small-cell lung cancer, the significantly better mortality observed at university cancer centers than at community hospitals disappeared when functional status, instead of stage, was used to adjust the analysis. The patients diagnosed in academic cancer centers underwent more staging procedures (e.g., bone and liver scans) and tended to be assigned to a higher stage than similar patients diagnosed in community hospitals (Greenberg et al., 1991).

Another potential source of bias in observational studies is case selection. Findings from evaluations of the effect of managed care on cancer outcomes may not be generalizable if the study is limited to a convenience sample of a few plans. Techniques could be used to sample health plans, facilities within plans, and patients within facilities to obtain a nationally representative sample of patients.

Another factor that makes it difficult to interpret the available health services research literature is the possibility of "publication bias," which means that studies showing the expected relationship are more likely to be published than those that find no relationship. Evidence of this sort of bias exists for clinical trials and other types of research such as observational studies. Underreporting of negative results appears to be related to a failure on the part of investigators to submit manuscripts for publication, not to selective rejection of negative results by journal editors (Dickersin, 1997).

The next section reviews health services literature on hospital and provider characteristics and on managed care. The literature review is not exhaustive; only articles written in English were identified, and some studies of patients cared for before 1980 were excluded.

CASE VOLUME FOR HOSPITALS OR INDIVIDUAL PHYSICIANS

One structural measure that has been found to relate to outcomes for some conditions or procedures is volume, which refers to the number of times each year that a hospital (or clinician) performs a particular procedure or takes care of patients with a particular disease. Since the late 1970s, researchers have been studying this volume–outcome relationship. The area that has been studied most intensively is interventional cardiology, particularly coronary artery bypass graft (CABG) surgery (e.g., Hannan et al., 1995, 1997b) and percutaneous transluminal coronary angioplasty (PTCA, "angioplasty") (e.g., Ellis et al., 1997; Jollis et al., 1994, 1997). In all of these cases, a positive connection was found: the more procedures done per hospital (or where it was studied, per physician), the better are the outcomes, including fewer immediate deaths due to the procedures and lower complication rates. Similar findings have been reported for heart transplants (Hosenpud et al., 1994).

Volume–outcome relationships have been reported for other procedures and services, including hip replacement (Kreder et al., 1997), abdominal aortic aneurysm surgery (Hannan et al., 1992; Kantonen et al., 1997), craniotomy for cerebral aneurysm (Solomon et al., 1996), hip and knee arthroplasty (Lavernia and Guzman, 1995), carotid endarterectomy (Ruby et al., 1996), thyroidectomy (Sosa et al., 1998), colorectal surgery (Rosen et al., 1996), and HIV/AIDS treatment (Kitahata et al., 1996). In these cases, the more procedures carried out, the better are the results, in at least some dimensions.

Although most of the published studies of volume–outcome relationships have demonstrated better outcomes with higher volumes, this finding has not been universal. Conflicting results have been reported for trauma centers, for example, with at least two reports of better results with higher volumes (Konvolinka et al., 1995; Smith et al., 1990), one with poorer results with higher volumes (Tepas et al., 1998), and one study of trauma surgeon case volume showing no difference between high and low volumes (Richardson et al., 1998). A study of 28-day mortality rates for very low birth weight infants reported no difference associated with the number of such infants treated in the neonatal intensive care unit (Horbar et al., 1997).

Within a hospital, processing a high volume of one type of service can lead to organizational efficiency, establishment of multidisciplinary teams, use of guidelines, and evaluation of outcomes. These aspects of specialization can all contribute to success. Alternatively, it may be that the experience gained by individual providers is the key to improving outcomes. Variations in mortality and complications are influenced more by patient variables than by organizational factors (e.g., volume, nursing surveillance, quality of interaction among professionals) according to a recent review of studies of the effects of these factors on patient outcomes (Mitchell et al., 1997).

High-Risk Cancer Surgery

The treatment of several cancers involves surgery that is complex and has high short-term risks for patients. One common cancer in this category is non-small-cell lung cancer (NSCLC). Three others that occur infrequently are pancreatic, esophageal, and gastric cancers.

There is no effective screening procedure for NSCLC, and about one-half of NSCLC patients present with metastatic disease. About one-third of all NSCLC patients have their disease diagnosed at a stage where surgery is recommended as part of initial care. In a procedure called pulmonary resection, diseased portions of the lung are removed. Surgery is more commonly performed on younger patients and those with local or regional disease. Fewer than one in ten individuals with distant NSCLC receives surgery; these patients are more often treated with radiation (Table 5.1). The expected perioperative or 30-day mortality in university medical centers varies with the extent of the primary surgery, ranging from about 1 to 6 percent (Ginsberg et al., 1997). These absolute mortality risks are known to vary with patient characteristics (e.g., age, stage of disease, and comorbidity). A 30-day mortality rate of 17 percent after pneumonectomy (removal of part or all of the lung) was observed in an evaluation of a national sample of Medicare claims from the early 1980s (Whittle et al., 1991).

Two studies have shown a relationship between high hospital volume and lower mortality for NSCLC. Romano and Mark (1992) used hospital discharge abstracts to assess the outcome of surgery for all adults ($n = 12,439$) who underwent pulmonary resections in 1983–1986 in 499 nonfederal California hospitals. Hospital volume was defined by the total number of resections for lung cancer per year and was divided into quartiles. In-hospital mortality was 3.8 percent after wedge resection, 3.7 percent after segmental resection, and 11.6 percent after pneumonectomy. The likelihood of an in-hospital death was 40 percent lower for high-volume hospitals (more than 24 procedures per year) than for low-volume hospitals (fewer than 9 procedures per year) for both lesser resections and pneumonectomy after controlling for patient demographic characteristics and clinical comorbidity (chronic obstructive pulmonary disease, coronary artery disease, and diabetes). The distribution of procedures by volume was as follows: 24 percent in low-; 50 percent in medium-; and 26 percent in high-volume hospitals (Table 5.2).

Although volume had a significant effect, there was no difference in the risk of in-hospital death associated with teaching status. Hospitals were stratified into high, low, and non-teaching according to the number of residency programs at a facility. The effect of individual surgeon volume was not addressed. A limitation of this study is its reliance on hospital discharge data, which do not capture postdischarge events. The outcome is limited to in-hospital mortality, but this could be affected by hospital policies regarding length of stay (e.g., hospitals could have low in-hospital mortality but very high mortality following premature discharges).

TABLE 5.1 Initial NSCLC Care in Virginia, 1989–1991 (percent)

Initial Treatment Category	Total		Local		Regional		Distant	
	Age < 64 (n = 336)	Age ≥ 65 (n = 1,132)	Age < 64 (n = 71)	Age ≥ 65 (n = 331)	Age < 64 (n = 105)	Age ≥ 65 (n = 331)	Age < 64 (n = 160)	Age ≥ 65 (n = 468)
Surgery only	23.6	21.2	74.6[a]	50.4[a]	23.1	18.8	1.3	3.1
Surgery plus[b]	13.1	7.8	5.6	4.1	28.8[a]	13.8[a]	5.6	6.1
Radiation	40.0	39.4	7.0	25.8	31.7	41.9	60.0	47.0
Radiation + chemotherapy	6.9	1.2	1.4	0.6	3.8	0.6	11.3	2.0
Chemotherapy	4.2	1.6	0.0	0.0	2.9	1.1	6.9	2.9
None	12.2	28.9	11.3	19.1	8.7	23.9	15.0[a]	38.9[a]
Any surgery	36.7[a]	28.0[a]	80.2[a]	54.8[a]	51.9[a]	32.0[a]	6.9	9.1
Any radiation	59.1[a]	47.9[a]	14.0	30.5	65.4	56.0	76.2[a]	54.9[a]
Any chemotherapy	11.9[a]	3.3[a]	1.4	0.8	8.6	2.0	18.8[a]	5.1[a]

NOTE: Patients under age 65 were privately insured through Virginia Blue Cross/Blue Shield. Individuals age 65 and older were Medicare enrollees. Unstaged patients were excluded.

[a] Differences between cohorts were statistically different at $p < .00005$.
[b] "Surgery plus" is defined as surgery plus radiation, chemotherapy, or radiation and chemotherapy.

SOURCE: Hillner et al., 1998a.

TABLE 5.2 California Postoperative In-Hospital Mortality with Lung Cancer Surgery, 1983–1986

Hospital Volume (no. per year)	Lesser Resections			Pneumonectomy		
	Patients	Adjusted Mortality (%)	Adjusted Odds Ratio	Patients	Adjusted Mortality (%)	Adjusted Odds Ratio
<9	2,588	5.2	1.0	365	13.6	1.0
9–16	2,945	4.1	0.7	374	11.4	0.8
17–24	2,553	3.5	0.6	377	11.7	0.8
>24	2,822	3.4	0.6	413	9.7	0.6

SOURCE: Romano and Mark, 1992.

A study of 30-day mortality examined a broader range of conditions. Begg and colleagues (1998) chose five procedures that involve preoperative judgment, diagnostic accuracy, meticulous surgical technique, and demanding postoperative care:

1. pneumonectomy (removal of part or all of the lung),
2. pancreatectomy (removal of part or all of the pancreas),
3. esophagectomy (removal of part or all of the esophagus),
4. hepatic resection (removal of part or all of the liver), and
5. pelvic exenteration (removal of two or more pelvic organs in one operation).

Medicare claims files were linked to Surveillance, Epidemiology, and End Results program (SEER) data for care provided to the elderly from 1984 to 1993. "Curative" surgery is rarely performed for these cancers in the elderly. Of all incident cases of these cancers over the 10-year period, the number of procedures within two months of diagnosis ranged from about 1 to 7 percent of all patients diagnosed (Table 5.3).

TABLE 5.3 Medicare–SEER Patient Selection Statistics, 1984–1993

Procedure	Primary Cancer Diagnosis	Incident Cases	Procedures	Percentage
Pancreatectomy	Pancreas	19,205	742	3.9
Esophagectomy	Esophagus	6,782	503	7.4
Pneumonectomy	Lung-bronchus	103,425	1,375	1.3
Hepatic resection	Colon-rectum	126,395	801	0.6
Pelvic exenteration	Various	185,305	1,592	0.9

SOURCE: Begg et al., 1998.

Within the small set of patients undergoing surgery, a trend of decreasing 30-day mortality with increasing volume was seen for all conditions except pneumonectomy. When the volume–mortality relationship was observed, the risk of death was at least double in low-, compared to high-volume hospitals. However, the confidence intervals surrounding these estimates are wide, and the only significant difference between low- and high-volume hospital mortality is for esophagectomy (Table 5.4). The *p* values for the effects of volume (measured continuously) on mortality for each site, after adjusting for comorbidity, stage, and age were as follows:

- Esophagectomy $p < .001$
- Pancreatectomy $p = .01$
- Hepatic resection $p = .05$
- Pelvic exenteration $p = .05$
- Pneumonectomy $p = .19$

With a *p* value for statistical significance set at .05, only pneumonectomy fails to show a significant volume–outcome relationship.

The share of high-risk procedures performed in low-volume facilities appears to be quite high, especially for procedures for which the volume-outcome relationship is the strongest (e.g., esophagectomy):

- Esophagectomy   62%
- Pancreatectomy   53%
- Hepatic resection   60%
- Pelvic exenteration 36%
- Pneumonectomy   35%

TABLE 5.4 30-Day Mortality (percent) for High-Risk Cancer Surgery Among Medicare Beneficiaries, by Hospital Volume, 1984–1993

Procedure	Hospital Volume[a]		
	Low [b] (95% C.I.)	Medium[c]	High[d] (95% C.I.)
Pancreatectomy	12.9 (9.7, 16.6)	7.7	5.8 (2.5, 11.0)
Esophagectomy	17.3 (13.3, 22.0)	3.9	3.4 (0.7, 9.6)
Pneumonectomy	13.8 (10.9, 17.2)	14.1	10.7 (8.0, 14.0)
Hepatic resection	5.4 (3.6, 7.8)	3.5	1.7 (0.4, 5.0)
Pelvic exenteration	3.7 (2.3, 5.5)	3.2	1.5 (0.7, 2.8)

[a] Volume measured as total number of procedures performed between 1984 and 1993 for Medicare beneficiaries only. The volume measure underestimates total hospital volume because many procedures are also performed on younger patients.
[b] 1–5 cases.
[c] 6–10 cases. CIs not provided in publication.
[d] ≥11 cases.

SOURCE: Begg et al., 1998.

TABLE 5.5 Relative Risk of In-Hospital Mortality by Procedure and Hospital Volume Tier, Pancreatic Cancer, 1990–1995

Procedure	Hospital Volume		
	High[a]	Medium[b]	Low[c]
Resections (*n* = 496)	1.0	8.0 (<0.01)	19.3 (<.001)
Bypasses (*n* = 542)	1.0	1.9 (NS)	2.7 (<.05)
Stents (*n* = 198)	1.0	4.8 (NS)	4.3 (NS)

NOTE: NS = not significant.

[a] Relative risk is 1.0 because the high-volume hospital ($\geq$20 cases) is the reference group.
[b] 5–19 cases.
[c] <5 cases.

SOURCE: Sosa et al., 1998.

A strength of this study is its use of the SEER–Medicare-linked database instead of hospital discharge data. Investigators were able to determine survival at a landmark point, 30 days after surgery, avoiding the potential bias associated with discharge data where only in-hospital mortality can be assessed. Potential limitations were an imprecise measure of hospital volume (only volume for patients over age 65 was known) and a lack of control for patient sociodemographic characteristics other than age (e.g., race, income).

Five other studies provide evidence that high hospital case volume is predictive of better outcome for pancreatic surgery. Sosa et al. (1998) assessed the effect of hospital volume on in-hospital mortality for both palliative and curative surgical procedures for 1,236 patients with pancreatic cancer hospitalized in Maryland from 1990 to 1995. The relative risk of in-hospital mortality was significantly higher in low- compared to high-volume hospitals for resections and bypasses, but not for surgical insertion of stents (used for relief of obstruction) (Table 5.5). More than one-third (35 percent) of patients were cared for in low-, 22 percent in medium-, and 43 percent in high-volume hospitals. There was no effect of surgeon case volume on in-hospital death. Strengths of this study are its relatively large sample size, multivariate analytic techniques controlling for patient characteristics (age, gender, race, payer status, residence), comorbidity, urgency of admission, year of admission, and surgeon case volume. Stage information was not available. A potential limitation is that it relied on hospital discharge data. High-volume hospitals had shorter stays, and deaths could have occurred after discharge.

Glasgow examined all discharge summaries for 1,705 patients undergoing pancreatic resection in 298 California hospitals (those performing at least one pancreatic resection from 1990 to 1994) (Glasgow and Mulvihill, 1996). Low-volume hospitals had in-hospital death rates three times higher than high-volume centers (14.1 versus 3.5 percent) when adjustments were made for patient (age, sex, race, insurance status) and clinical characteristics (number of secondary diagnoses), admission type, and type of resection (Table 5.6). The vast majority of hospitals (88 percent) treated 10 or fewer patients per year, and more than half of the patients studied (53 percent) were treated at centers where 10 or fewer resections were performed in the five-year period.

TABLE 5.6 California Hospital Pancreatectomy Volume and Outcomes, 1990–1994

Hospital Volume (no. of cases)	No. of Hospitals	Length of Hospital Stay (days)	Total Charges ($)	Patients Discharged to Home (%)	Crude Mortality (%)	Risk-Adjusted Mortality Rate (%)
1 to 5	210	22.7	87,857	74.3	14.1	14.1
6 to 10	53	22.7	76,593	80.0	10.4	9.6
11 to 20	20	22.9	78,003	81.8	8.9	8.7
21 to 30	9	20.2	70,959	92.1	5.7	6.9
31 to 50	4	23.9	111,497	87.1	8.2	8.3
>50	2	20.5	71,585	95.1	3.5	3.5
Mean		22.3	83,479	82.1	9.9	9.9

SOURCE: Glasgow and Mulvihill, 1996.

TABLE 5.7 Volume–Outcome Effect for Pancreatectomy in New York State, 1984–1991

Hospital Volume (no. of surgeries over 7 years)	No. of Hospitals	Percentage of Total Patients	Mean Length of Stay (days)	Standardized Mortality (%)
<10	124	24	35	18.9
10–50	57	54	32	11.8
51–80	1	3	22	12.9
>81	2	19	27	5.5

SOURCE: Lieberman et al., 1995.

Employing a similar method, Lieberman et al. (1995) used hospital discharge abstracts to identify 1,972 patients having pancreatic resection in New York State between 1984 and 1991. Table 5.7 clearly shows the same higher-volume–better survival relationship, with mortality rates three times as high (18.9 versus 5.5 percent) in the low- (fewer than 10 cases) compared to the high-volume hospitals (more than 81 cases), after adjusting for patient characteristics (age, sex, race, number of secondary diagnoses), admission status, transfer status, year of surgery, and payer status. About one-quarter (24 percent) of patients were cared for in hospitals seeing fewer than 10 cases per year. The effect on outcomes of the volume of surgeries performed by physicians was also assessed and was not found to be a predictor of in-hospital mortality.

The volume–outcome association is also evident in a National Cancer Data Base (NCDB) study of 8,917 cases of pancreatic cancer in 1983–1985, and 8,025 cases in 1990 from 978 hospitals (25 percent teaching institutions) (Janes et al., 1996). The 1990 unadjusted operative mortality among patients receiving potentially curative cancer surgery was 7.7 percent in hospitals where fewer than 5 patients were seen per year and 4.2 percent in hospitals where 20 or more patients per year were treated. The trend of better outcomes with higher volumes was evident at each stage of disease. Teaching and community comprehensive hospitals had lower operative mortality (4.7 and 4.6 percent, respectively), whereas community hospitals and hospitals without

American College of Surgeons' Commission on Cancer approval had unadjusted mortality rates of 7.9 and 7.2 percent, respectively. A strength of this study is the large number of cases described and the extensive information gathered on each case (more than 160 data items for each patient). A large number of hospitals are represented in this study, and more than three-quarters of the hospitals invited to participate responded. Hospitals were asked to submit up to 25 consecutive patients treated during 1990. Results are not weighted to reflect the unequal probability of case selection (the chance of selection for a patient in a hospital with 25 or fewer cases is 100 percent, while the probability of selection for a patient in a hospital with 100 cases is 25 percent) making some findings difficult to interpret (e.g., the distribution of cases by hospital case volume). Results were not adjusted for patient or clinical characteristics.

Wade et al. (1995) assessed 30-day mortality among 369 patients treated with Whipple resection (i.e., pancreatico-duodenectomy) for pancreatic or other periampullary adenocarcinomas from 1987 to 1991 in 78 Department of Veterans Affairs (VA) hospitals. Hospitals reporting more than two compared with fewer than one resection per year had the lowest operative mortality rates (4 versus 7 percent), but this difference was not significantly lower than the mortality rate in lower-volume hospitals. Results were not adjusted for patient or clinical characteristics.

Prostate Cancer

A new study by Lu-Yao and Yao (1998) looked at the relationship between outcomes and the number (or volume) of patients receiving surgical treatment for prostate cancer from a surgeon or facility. Using Medicare claims data from 1991 to 1994 for 101,604 men having radical prostatectomy, they found that high-volume facilities had significantly better surgical outcomes than facilities treating fewer patients. High-volume facilities had more favorable rates of survival, complications, and readmission following treatment by radical prostatectomy than lower-volume facilities. High-volume facilities also had shorter lengths of stay (Table 5.8). The results suggest a dose–response relationship, where facilities in the highest-volume quartile showed the best outcomes, followed by those in the third and lower quartiles. These analyses controlled for differences across facilities in patient age, race, year of surgery, surgeon specialty, and hospital teaching status.

TABLE 5.8 Radical Prostatectomy Outcomes Among Medicare Beneficiaries, by Hospital Volume, 1991–1994

	Odds Ratio Compared to High-Volume Hospitals		
Hospital Volume	30-Day Mortality	Readmission Rate	Surgical Complication
Low	1.53	1.25	1.30
Medium-low	1.44	1.13	1.16
Medium-high	1.41	1.08	1.08
High	1.00	1.00	1.00

SOURCE: Lu-Yao and Yao, 1998.

TABLE 5.9 Adjusted Risk Ratios for Death for Breast Cancer Patients Hospitalized in New York State, by Hospital Volume, 1984–1989

Hospital Volume (no. of surgeries per year)	No. of Patients	Percentage of Total Patients	Risk Ratio	95% Confidence Interval
<10	958	2.0	1.60	1.42, 1.81
11–50	14,440	30.2	1.30	1.22, 1.37
51–150	22,230	46.4	1.19	1.12, 1.25
>151	10,262	21.4	1.00	—
Total	47,890	100.0	—	—

SOURCE: Roohan et al., 1998.

Breast Cancer Surgery

Roohan and colleagues report on the effect of hospital volume of breast cancer surgical cases on the five-year survival of 47,890 women (white and black) treated for breast cancer in New York from 1984 to 1989, identified through hospital discharge data and linked to the New York State cancer registry (Roohan et al., 1998). At five years, patients from very low-volume hospitals (1–10 surgeries per year) had a 60 percent greater risk of all-cause mortality than patients from high-volume hospitals (150+ surgeries per year), after controlling for surgery type (mastectomy, limited surgery), patient age, cancer stage, comorbidity, race, socioeconomic status (census tract level), and distance to hospital. A gradient of risk was evident by volume category. Nearly one-third of patients (32 percent) were seen in the lower-volume hospitals (i.e., those with 50 or fewer surgical cases) (Table 5.9). The authors speculate that high-volume hospitals are more likely than others to provide effective postsurgical adjuvant treatments that have been shown to improve survival, perhaps because of better coordination of or access to these services (Roohan et al., 1998).

Processes of breast cancer care were examined in a 1988 study of 5,766 newly diagnosed breast cancer patients in Illinois. Hospitals with low compared to high breast cancer case volumes were less likely to use indicated radiation therapy after partial mastectomy (for Stages I and II), but were not less likely to use hormone receptor tests (for Stages II through IV) (Hand et al., 1991).

Evidence on the Volume–Outcome Relationship from Other Countries

Studies from other countries support the finding that high volume leads to better outcomes.

Scotland. Centralized treatment at high-volume centers improved outcomes for a type of testicular cancer (non-seminomatous germ cell tumors), even when controlling for participation in a protocol (although protocol treatment explained a large part of the variation) (Harding et al., 1993).

TABLE 5.10 Summary of Studies Assessing the Volume–Outcome Relationship for Surgery for Pancreatic Cancer

Study	Study Years	Sample Size	Definition of Low and High Volume	Effect Size (mortality rate for low- vs. high-volume hospitals)	Patients in Low-Volume Hospitals (%)
Begg et al., 1998	1984–1993	742	1–5, ≥11	12.9 vs. 5.8[a]	53
Glasgow and Mulvi-hill, 1996	1990–1994	1,705	1–5, >50	14.1 vs. 3.5[b]	53
Janes et al., 1996	1990	8,917	<5, ≥20	7.7 vs. 4.2[c]	—
Lieberman, et al., 1995	1984–1991	1,972	<10, ≥81	18.9 vs. 5.5[b]	24
Sosa et al., 1998	1990–1995	1,236	<5, ≥20	14.7 vs. 1.9[d]	35
Wade et al., 1995	1987–1991	369	<1, >2	7.5 vs. 4.0[e]	—

[a] 30-day unadjusted mortality for pancreatectomy.

[b] Risk-adjusted in-hospital mortality for pancreatic resections.

[c] Unadjusted in-hospital mortality for "curative" procedures.

[d] Unadjusted in-hospital mortality for all procedures (i.e., resections, bypasses, stents).

[e] Unadjusted operative mortality for Whipple resections.

International Bone Marrow Transplant Registry. High transplant center volume was associated with lower treatment-related mortality among 1,313 transplants of human leukocyte antigen (HLA) identical sibling bone marrow for early leukemia (acute leukemia in first remission or chronic myelocytic leukemia [CML] in first chronic phase) performed from 1983 to 1988 (Horowitz et al., 1992). After adjustment for differences in patient and disease characteristics, the relative risks of treatment-related mortality (1.53, $p < .01$) and treatment failure (1.38, $p < .04$) were higher among patients who received transplants at centers doing five or fewer transplants per year than among those at larger centers. This lead to an absolute 10 percent difference in two-year survival (65 versus 55 percent) at the high- compared to low-volume centers. No differences were found among centers performing from 5 or more transplants to 40 or more transplants per year. One-quarter (24 percent) of centers performed 5 or fewer allogeneic transplants per year, and five (6 percent) performed more than 40 per year.

In summary, there is a large body of evidence to suggest that higher volume contributes to better outcomes for at least some aspects of care for some forms of cancer, especially high-risk surgery. The six studies that have assessed the way volume affects surgical outcomes of patients with pancreatic cancer are summarized in Table 5.10. Differences in how volume categories were defined, what procedures were assessed, and whether mortality comparisons were adjusted for case mix make it difficult to make simple comparisons of study findings. In general however, there is a two- to threefold increase in short-term postoperative mortality in lower- compared to higher-volume facilities. Although these differences may appear dramatic, they are not all statistically significant (e.g., differences noted by Wade et al., 1995). Furthermore, findings from observational studies must be interpreted with caution because they are subject to bias. In particular, differences in staging procedures and case mix associated with hospital volume could bias results in favor of higher-volume hospitals (e.g., referral centers tend to have a more favorable case mix). A relatively large share of individuals with pancreatic cancer are surgically treated in lower-volume hospitals. In the six studies described in Table 5.10, estimates varied from one-quarter to slightly more than one-half. Policies to shift care to higher-volume facilities would likely affect many individuals.

SPECIALIZATION

Specialization of Facilities

Although specialization is difficult to separate analytically from volume, some feel that specialized cancer care facilities can provide better care, in part because of the concentration of expertise and resources. Some areas have regionalized services, which attempt to triage care so that the most complex cases are referred to the facility with the most sophisticated level of resources. Investigators have assessed the relationship between specialization and outcomes using different measures: tertiary care status, academic affiliation, or even hospital size.

The relationship between specialization and the processes and outcomes of cancer care was recently examined in a review of 46 empirical studies reported in the literature since 1980 (Grilli et al., 1998). Almost all of the studies reviewed found lower mortality associated with care provided by specialized centers and clinicians. For breast cancer, where there were a number of methodologically sound studies, a pooled estimate of the effect of specialization showed that specialized cancer care was associated with an 18 percent reduction in five-year mortality. In general, Grilli judged the evidence far from conclusive because of major methodological flaws and speculated that publication bias favoring specialized centers may have accounted for observed trends. Grilli concludes that the widespread belief that cancer patients are better off when treated in specialized centers is *not* supported by available evidence. What follows is a review of recent studies of the effects of specialization on cancer care processes and outcomes.

Munoz and colleagues (1997) from the National Cancer Institute (NCI) assessed in detail the process of ovarian cancer treatment for 785 women selected from SEER sites in 1991. Only about 10 percent of women with presumptive Stage I and II, compared to 71 percent with Stage III and 53 percent with Stage IV disease received recommended staging and treatment. The absence of lymphadenectomy and assignment of histologic grade were the primary reasons women with presumptive Stage I and II disease did not receive recommended staging and treatment. The principal deficiency in Stage III and IV disease was withholding of platinum-based chemotherapy in older women. The only provider variable assessed was whether care was provided at a hospital with a residency program. The odds ratio for receiving appropriate care was 1.9, or almost double, if care was given at a hospital with a residency program.

Gordon and colleagues (1995) looked at the effects of regionalization of care by comparing hospital mortality, length of stay, and costs of care for pancreatic cancer at one specialty center, Johns Hopkins (271 patients), in 1988–1993 with all other hospitals throughout the State of Maryland (230 patients in 38 hospitals) using hospital discharge data. The results were striking: in-hospital mortality 2.2 versus 13.5 percent (a relative risk of 6.1 [confidence interval {C.I.}] 2.9–12.7), average length of stay (23 versus 27 days), and average total charges were 20 percent greater outside Johns Hopkins. A follow-up study by Gordon et al. (1998) attributes 61 percent of the decline in the Maryland in-hospital mortality for pancreas surgery (17.2 to 4.9 percent) between 1984 and 1995 to the increase in share of discharges at the high-volume provider, Johns Hopkins. During this period, Johns Hopkins increased its yearly share of pancreatico-duodenectomies from 21 percent to 59 percent.

Feuer et al. (1994) retrospectively compared survival of 133 patients with metastatic testicular cancer participating in a clinical trial at a large cancer center in New York (Memorial Sloan-Kettering Cancer Center) to the survival of 172 patients cared for at other hospitals identified from five SEER registries in 1978–1984. Although 89 percent of the SEER cases received chemotherapy and 95 percent of these used cisplatin regimens, the three-year survival was markedly better at the cancer center. For patients with minimal to moderate extent of disease the benefit was more striking (95 versus 73 percent three-year survival rate) than for advanced cases (52 versus 40 percent). The authors speculate that the differences could have been due to many factors including chemotherapy regimen, dose intensity, or institutional factors. Limitations of this study are its small sample size, the comparison of clinical trial participants with population controls, and inclusion of only one specialized center.

Radiation treatment planning and delivery for rectal and sigmoid cancers appeared to be better at academic than nonacademic hospitals according to a Patterns of Care study (Kline et al., 1997). The care received by 408 patients in 1989–1990 from 73 randomly selected facilities (21 academic, 24 hospital based, and 24 free standing) was audited according to consensus guidelines.

Davis et al. (1987) contrasted the survival of 3,607 Hodgkin's disease (HD) patients diagnosed in 1977–1982 and registered by SEER (community care) with that of 2,278 HD patients treated at one of 21 comprehensive cancer (university or referral) centers. Modest differences in patient age, histologic pattern, and frequency of Stage II disease between locations were seen and adjusted for in the comparisons. The mortality rate among SEER patients was higher (relative risk 1.5; 95 percent C.I. 1.3–1.7) than among those treated at comprehensive centers. The survival difference was consistently seen for all stages, histologic types, and patient ages. A strength of this study is the large number of cases of HD represented nationally. Underlying differences in the comparison groups may not have been accounted for in the analysis (e.g., comorbidity).

In a study by Lee-Feldstein et al. (1994), hospital teaching status had no effect on five-year survival of women with localized or regional breast cancer diagnosed 1988 and 1990. Three large studies suggest that relative to other hospitals, teaching hospitals are more likely to use breast conserving surgery (Ballard-Barbash and Potosky, 1996; Johantgen et al., 1995; Nattinger et al., 1992).

Several European and Canadian studies have assessed the effects of specialization on outcomes. In England, Basnett et al. (1992) compared survival of 999 women with breast cancer treated initially between 1982 and 1986 in two settings, an urban teaching hospital and a rural nonteaching one, both of which had radiation and chemotherapy capabilities. Numerous differences in process of care were seen. After adjusting for age and stage, the adjusted risks of relapse or death were worse (1.45 and 1.74, respectively) for the nonteaching hospitals. Multivariate analyses to explore the reasons for these differences were not reported. Chemotherapy was used in only 5–8 percent of women in both settings, but more often at teaching hospitals. It is difficult to attribute differences reported in this study to the teaching status of the hospital. There is also a rural–urban difference between hospitals. Furthermore, differences in staging by hospital type could confound the observed relationship.

Two studies from Scotland address the effects of referral to specialty centers on processes and outcomes. Clarke et al. (1995) determined that 92 percent of testicular cancer was referred to specialty centers between 1983 and 1990, and that the quality of care at these specialty centers varied. Harding et al. (1993) performed a population-based audit of the management of 440 men diagnosed in 1975–1989 with non-seminomatous germ cell tumors (NSGCT) in western Scotland. All but 11 patients were treated at tertiary referral centers; 235 were treated at a single unit (unit 1) and 194 at four other units (units 2–5). Independent prognostic factors for NSGCT survival were extent of tumor at diagnosis, five-year period of diagnosis (from 1975–1979 to 1985–1989), and treatment unit (unit 1 versus units 2–5). Unit 1 had the best survival rates, had treated the most patients overall (53 percent), and had treated the majority (70 percent) with the worst prognosis (e.g., metastatic disease). Receipt of care according to the nationally agreed-upon protocol treatment varied: 97 percent at unit 1 versus 61 percent at units 2–5. After adjusting for known prognostic factors and limiting the analysis to those treated according to protocol, the relative risk of death outside unit 1 was 2.8 (C.I. 1.5–5.2). The authors conclude, "These findings suggest that centralization of treatment for NSGCT improves outcome; the benefit seems to be additional to any advantage resulting from protocol treatment."

Aass et al. (1991) noted a similar trend, although not as dramatic. They studied 193 patients with metastatic testicular cancer treated at 14 Swedish or Norwegian centers between 1981 and 1986 who entered a clinical trial. If all care had been given at the lead institution, which treated 46 percent of cases, the chance of dying after controlling for known prognostic factors would have been reduced by 28 percent. A limitation of this study is the relatively small sample size.

Junor et al. (1994) reported one of the few studies addressing the benefits of multidisciplinary clinical care. In 1987, 533 cases of ovarian cancer were diagnosed and 479 records were available for audit in Scotland; 27 percent of cases were referred postoperatively to a multidisciplinary clinic. After adjusting for clinical factors and the use of platinum chemotherapy (about 50 percent of patients younger than 65 received chemotherapy), the relative risk of death was 0.73 (27 percent reduction) if patients received care at the multidisciplinary clinic.

Specialization of Physicians

Intuition would dictate that being cared for by a physician who has extensive training and experience in cancer care would improve outcomes. Only one U.S. study and several studies conducted in Great Britain or Canada have assessed the relationship between specialization of individual physicians and processes or outcomes. Specialization is defined in different ways: receipt of specialty training, professional identification as a specialist, or university affiliation.

Physician specialty affected the processes and outcomes of care of women with ovarian cancer according to a study by Nguyen and colleagues (1993), conducted as part of the U.S. National Survey of Ovarian Carcinoma. Detailed data were requested on 25 consecutive patients from 1,230 hospitals with cancer programs across the United States from 1983 and 1988. A total of 904 hospitals provided data on 5,156 patients for 1983 and 7,160 patients for 1988. About 96 percent of patients had exploratory surgery as their initial management. The breakdown of physician's specialty was 19 percent general surgeons, 25 percent gynecologic oncologists, 43 percent general gynecologists, and 13 percent other. In general, gynecologists saw patients with less advanced disease at presentation.

Differences on a number of process measures were found that could account for the mortality difference, for example, surgical staging and completeness of surgical debulking (i.e., removal of cancer), which varied with specialty. Staging and debulking were assessed for 1983 and 1988, whereas assessment of survival was limited to the 1983 cohort. The biopsy rates were highest among the gynecologic oncologists but were less than ideal (about 35 percent in Stage I to IIIB disease). Optimal tumor removal was done in about 45 percent of cases by each of the gynecology groups versus 25 percent by the general surgeons. As shown in Table 5.11, stage-stratified median survival tended to be higher for patients of gynecologists compared to general surgeons.

A limitation of this study is the lack of details about postoperative management, specifically chemotherapy, especially platinum-based regimens. The assumption was made that the primary surgeon was also in charge of the patient's postoperative care, including chemotherapy and referral to a medical oncologist, and that the ultimate survival outcome depended on the total management by the primary surgeon.

In two British studies, the effect of surgical specialty and survival was strongly noted. Kehoe et al. (1994) retrospectively assessed the survival of 1,184 women with ovarian cancer in central England between 1985 and 1987. General surgeons cared for patients with more advanced disease and poorer prognosis. According to the multivariate model, the five-year relative risk of death when a general surgeon, rather than a gynecologist, gave initial care was 1.34 (C.I. 1.05–1.71).

Woodman et al. (1997) found similar results in 691 women diagnosed with ovarian cancer in 1991–1992 in the northwest region of Britain. Compared to gynecologists, surgeons had a three-year adjusted relative risk (RR) of death of 1.58. More interestingly, case volume was not predictive of survival, but referral to a medical oncologist was strongly predictive (RR = 0.54). Given the generally low use of chemotherapy in Britain, it would be important to know the relative rates of chemotherapy in women with advanced disease, but this is not reported.

TABLE 5.11 Ovarian Cancer Survival by Physician's Specialty, 1983

Stage	Patients (*n*)	Five-Year Survival (%)			Median Survival (months)		
		GYO	OBG	GS	GYO	OBG	GS
I	1,377	88.6 ± 2.5	89.6 ± 1.1	87.8 ± 2.1	≥96	≥96	≥96
II	448	62.6 ± 5.9	60.9 ± 3.1	47.4 ± 5.5	≥84	≥96	61.7
III	1,355	25.2 ± 2.6	29.2 ± 1.9	16.8 ± 2.0	26.4	29.1	20.7
IV	1,080	10.4 ± 2.6	16.8 ± 1.8	10.9 ± 1.6	18.0	19.2	14.3

NOTE: GS = general surgery, GYO = gynecologic oncology, OBG = obstetrics–gynecology.

SOURCE: Nguyen et al., 1993.

TABLE 5.12 Five-Year Breast Cancer Survival by
Surgeon Specialty, Scotland, 1980–1988

	Specialist Surgeon (%)	Nonspecialist Surgeon (%)
Disease		
Node negative	81	77
Node positive	58	47
Age		
<50	72	64
51–64	68	57
65–74	59	54
Social indicators		
Affluent	72	64
Intermediate	66	58
Deprived	65	54

SOURCE: Gillis and Hole, 1996.

Gillis and Hole (1996) compared the survival experience of women with breast cancer diagnosed between 1980 and 1988 in western Scotland, according to whether or not their provider was a "specialist." Surgeons were characterized as specialists if they were involved in a dedicated breast clinic, organized and facilitated clinical trials, and kept separate records of patients limited to breast cancer. Such specialists provided about 25 percent of the care to the 3,786 cases. There was an absolute 9 percent difference in survival between groups at 5 years and 8 percent at 10 years. Specialty care was associated with an adjusted relative risk of death of 0.84 (C.I. 0.75–0.94). The benefit was seen for all clinical and social indicators considered (Table 5.12).

An early study by McArdle and Hole (1991) in Scotland from 1974 to 1979 found a four-fold variation in survival and surgical complications based on a surgeon's specialty volume and interest in colorectal disease or surgical oncology. Subsequent British studies have not confirmed this effect. Kingston et al. (1991) evaluated the care provided for 578 patients by 12 surgeons interested in colorectal cancer, but practicing outside academia, to university care and found no benefit from university care. Mella et al. (1997) performed a one-year audit of 3,221 patients diagnosed in 1992–1993 in Wales and Scotland. The 30-day mortality was 7.6 percent. No surgeon volume effect (using either 10 or 30 cases per year as a dichotomous variable) or specialty interest effect was noted for 30-day mortality.

A recent report from Canada compared the care of 683 patients treated by 52 surgeons for rectal cancer at five Edmonton hospitals between 1983 and 1990 (Porter et al., 1998). Five surgeons had specific fellowship training in colorectal surgery. After adjusting for known clinical factors, local recurrence and disease-specific survival were both adversely affected by being cared for by a non-specialty-trained surgeon or low-volume surgeon (fewer than three cases per year, on average). Local recurrence is an especially strong indicator of surgical technique and a much more dire (essentially untreatable) event than local recurrence in breast cancer. The relative risk for local recurrence was 2.5 (if not specialty trained) and 1.8 (if a low-volume surgeon). The relative risks against disease-free survival were 1.5 and 1.4 for non-specialty-trained or low-volume surgeons, respectively.

In England, Sainsbury et al. (1995) assessed the effect of a surgeon's volume of cases on the five-year survival of 12,861 women with breast cancer treated with "curative" surgery between 1979 and 1988 in Yorkshire, England (population 3.6 million). There was no difference in survival between patients treated by surgeons seeing <10 and 10–29 cases per year, but if the surgeons saw >30 cases per year, the adjusted risk of death at five years was 0.85 (C.I. 0.77–0.93). About 50 percent of patients were seen by high-volume (>30 cases) surgeons. After controlling for case mix and clinical variables (e.g., axillary node status, histologic grade), variation among the consultants accounted for about an absolute 8 percent difference in survival. This benefit was principally associated with the greater use of chemotherapy.

The evidence on the effects of specialization, either by hospitals or by physicians, does not present a consistent picture; most, but not all, studies show improved care with specialization. Findings from these observational studies must be interpreted with caution because they are highly subject to bias. Patients cared for by specialty providers and specialty centers differ from patients treated elsewhere, and analyses must account for these differences in case mix. Many studies do not appropriately control for important patient variables and clinical factors that likely vary by site of care. Specialty providers such as those in teaching hospitals differ from community-based providers in their use of staging procedures, which could contribute to a stage migration bias that favors specialists.

MANAGED CARE VERSUS FEE-FOR-SERVICE CARE

There is a great deal of interest in the way patients with chronic illnesses such as cancer fare within managed care organizations (see definition and discussion of managed care in Chapter 2). Theoretically, quality of care could be compromised if individuals enrolled in managed care plans could not access needed cancer care specialists or services. On the other hand, care could be enhanced if managed care plans implemented effective early detection, clinical practice guidelines, or disease management programs to a greater extent than FFS plans. Although intriguing questions have been raised, there is little evidence on which to judge the impact of managed care on the quality of cancer care. Individuals enrolled in managed care plans are generally satisfied with the care that they receive, and in one study, Medicare beneficiaries in managed care did not have high rates of switching into FFS plans after a cancer diagnosis (Riley et al., 1996). This does not necessarily mean that beneficiaries were entirely satisfied with care, but that any dissatisfaction does not seem to lead to high levels of disenrollment.

HMO enrollees as compared to those in FFS settings receive more cancer screening services (see Chapter 3). Only eight studies have looked directly at the effect of managed care on cancer care. Riley et al. (1999) recently examined treatment for early breast cancer between 1988 and 1993 among elderly women receiving care in HMO and FFS settings in 11 U.S. geographic areas. Use of breast conserving surgery was similar among women with early-stage disease enrolled in HMO and FFS plans (38 and 37 percent, respectively). Among women undergoing

BCS, HMO enrollees were significantly more likely than those in FFS plans to receive radiation therapy (69 versus 64 percent). Analyses of treatment patterns were controlled for age, race, cancer history, year of diagnosis, stage at diagnosis, tumor size, county of residence, and education at the census tract level. Investigators found aggregate comparisons of the experiences of HMO and FFS populations to obscure important variation among HMO plans. Among BCS cases, for example, radiation therapy was more commonly received by HMO enrollees overall but the pattern varied by HMO. Enrollees in some HMOs were significantly more likely than those in FFS plans to have had radiation therapy, and in other HMOs, the opposite was true. The authors conclude that variation among HMOs is likely attributable to differences in both plan and market characteristics. Plans differ in their structure, organization, benefit packages, payment policies, practice protocols, and provider relationships. Market characteristics vary along many dimensions, such as degree of competition, managed care penetration, and availability of radiation facilities. These findings illustrate how difficult it is to generalize about managed care.

In an earlier study, Potosky et al. (1997) compared HMO to FFS care among 13,358 Medicare beneficiaries diagnosed with breast cancer from 1985 to 1992 in the Seattle–Puget Sound and San Francisco Bay areas. Cancer registry data (i.e., SEER) were linked to Medicare administrative files to assess aspects of care and survival (Potosky et al., 1997). In San Francisco–Oakland, the 10-year adjusted risk of death due to breast cancer was 29 percent lower, and the overall adjusted risk of death 30 percent lower, among women belonging to an HMO (i.e., Kaiser Permanente of Northern California) compared to women insured by FFS plans (Table 5.13). A significant HMO mortality advantage was not found in the Seattle–Puget Sound area (i.e., Group Health of Puget Sound).

Women enrolled in HMOs in both areas were more likely than those covered by FFS plans to have received breast conserving surgery (BCS) and, among those having BCS, were more likely to have had radiation therapy following surgery (Table 5.13). The authors conclude that long-term survival outcomes in the two prepaid group practice HMOs were at least equal to, and possibly better than, outcomes in the FFS system. In addition, the use of recommended therapy for early-stage breast cancer was more frequent in the two HMOs. Medicare patients with breast cancer in these two established nonprofit staff- and group-model HMOs appeared to receive better quality of care than Medicare enrollees in FFS.

Strengths of this study were the large sample size; adjustments for sociodemographic (i.e., age, race, area-level educational status); and clinical factors (i.e., stage, whether the diagnosis was a single or first primary cancer, comorbidity); and the length of follow-up (10 years). The authors speculate that the observed HMO survival advantage is, in part, due to more frequent screening. HMO compared to FFS care was associated with earlier stage at diagnosis and within stage, with smaller tumors. Some of the HMO survival advantage could be artifactual if higher rates of screening within HMOs are identifying biologically less aggressive tumors, including those that would never have been detected via symptoms. The analysis controlled for stage, but not for the within-stage shift in tumor size. The findings from this study may not be generalizable to other areas or types of managed care plans (e.g., for profit, independent practice associations). The two HMOs included in the study embody core features of traditional managed care, which include an emphasis on creating long-standing relationships between patient and providers, preventive care, the practice of evidence-based medicine, less stringent utilization review with greater physician autonomy, and greater coordination of specialty care (Clancy and Brody, 1995).

In contrast to the Potosky study, no difference in the use of breast conserving surgery was found among women with HMO versus FFS insurance in a recent study conducted in Massachusetts and Minnesota (Guadagnoli et al., 1998). Guadagnoli and colleagues examined the medical records of women diagnosed with breast cancer from 1993 to 1995 cared for in a random sample of hospitals in Massachusetts and a convenience sample of hospitals in Minnesota. Among 2,135 women eligible for breast conserving surgery, 74 percent of women in Massachusetts and 48 percent of women in Minnesota underwent BCS. Investigators examined correlates of BCS and mastectomy use including sociodemographic characteristics of women (age, education, household income, urban residence), insurance status (HMO or non-HMO), characteristics of the surgeon (gender, board certification, years since graduation), and hospital characteristics (teaching status, bed size, presence of American College of Surgeons-approved cancer program, presence of a radiation facility). According to multivariate analyses, women in Massachusetts cared for in a teaching hospital were twice as likely as other women to undergo BCS (odds ratio [OR] = 2.4; C.I. 1.3–4.6). In Minnesota, younger women and residents of urban areas were more likely than others to undergo BCS. The absence of an HMO effect in Massachusetts and Minnesota in this study, in contrast to the Potosky findings, could be due to a number of factors, including the use of more recent data (1993–1995 versus 1985–1992) or the difference in managed care providers in Massachusetts and Minnesota relative to California and Washington. Unadjusted HMO versus non-HMO BCS rates were not reported for Massachusetts and Minnesota, so one cannot tell if an HMO advantage is apparent when provider and hospital characteristics are left out of the model. The Potosky finding of an HMO advantage could hypothetically be related to hospital teaching status or to other hospital or provider characteristics that were not considered in their analyses.

TABLE 5.13 Outcome and Process Odds Ratios for HMO versus FFS Care for Elderly Women with Breast Cancer (in situ, Stages I and II), by Location

End Point	San Francisco–Oakland	Seattle–Puget Sound
Outcome		
10-year overall survival[a]	0.70 (0.62–0.79)[b]	0.86 (0.72–1.03)
10-year breast cancer survival[a]	0.71 (0.59–0.87)	1.01 (0.77–1.33)
Process		
BCS	1.55 (1.35–1.77)[c]	3.39 (2.76–4.17)
XRT post-BCS[d]	2.49 (1.95–3.19)	4.62 (3.20–6.66)

NOTE: Reference group is FFS care. Outcome odds ratios less than 1 indicate greater survival, and process odds ratios greater than 1 indicate more frequent desired care.

[a] Adjusted for age, race, census tract education and income, comorbidity, and stage.
[b] Odds ratio of <1.0 means that women in HMOs were less likely to die than women in FFS.
[c] Odds ratio of >1.0 means that women in HMOs were more likely to receive the treatment than women in FFS.
[d] XRT post-BCS: x-ray therapy after breast conserving surgery. .

SOURCE: Potosky et al. (1997).

Lee-Feldstein et al. (1994), using cancer registry data, found significantly worse five-year survival among women with *localized* breast cancer treated at HMO hospitals in Orange County, California, in 1984–1990, compared to women treated at teaching hospitals, small community hospitals, and large community hospitals. Patients treated at an HMO facility had a 63 percent increased risk of dying, compared with the reference group treated in small hospitals, when age, tumor size, number of positive lymph nodes, and type of treatment (e.g., breast conserving surgery with radiation versus no radiation) were controlled for. The excess deaths among HMO patients with localized disease were limited to 1984 through 1987. Only 380 HMO patients with localized disease were available for analysis, and the confidence interval around the point estimate (i.e., OR = 1.63) ranges from 1.16 to 2.30. No HMO mortality disadvantage for women with *regional* disease was found. The unexpected finding of a 45 percent increased risk of death for patients having a total mastectomy compared to those having BCS, when no difference is expected, has raised questions about the validity of this study (Hillner et al., 1998b). Furthermore, survival comparisons between HMO and non-HMO hospitals did not control for comorbidity, race, and socioeconomic status. Clinical and socioeconomic variables are likely to differ by type of hospital and are strongly related to survival of women with breast cancer (Charlson et al., 1987; Eley et al., 1994; Greenwald, 1992). Methodologic flaws of this study limit its interpretation.

Retchin and Brown (1990) assessed the effect of being insured by an HMO in two different studies related to care for colorectal cancer in the elderly. The first study examined pre- and postoperative care processes for 330 patients diagnosed from 1983 to 1986 as part of an evaluation of the Medicare demonstrations in prepaid care. Some differences in use of diagnostics tests were observed, but findings are difficult to interpret because analyses were largely descriptive in nature, with few controls for clinical or sociodemographic characteristics. A more recent study of 813 patients diagnosed in 1989 compared perioperative care and outcomes within 19 geographically dispersed HMOs to FFS care (Retchin et al., 1997). There were some differences in processes of care; for example, compared to those covered by FFS plans, HMO enrollees had shorter lengths of stay and received fewer tests and services. There was no evidence that HMO members experienced different outcomes (e.g., hospital readmissions, in-hospital deaths, admissions within one year of discharge). A limitation of this study is the lack of control in some comparisons for sociodemographic characteristics, stage, and other clinical factors.

Greenwald and Henke (1992) compared care and outcomes by HMO status among Medicare beneficiaries with prostate cancer diagnosed from 1980 to 1982 in the Seattle area. Patients in Group Health of Puget Sound ($n = 131$) relative to 1,032 FFS patients had less surgery, more radiation therapy, and—after adjustment for stage, urban location, and age—better survival. The relatively small sample from one HMO, the age of the data, and a lack of adjustment for clinical prognostic factors in the analysis limit the value of this study.

Vernon and colleagues (1992) evaluated the effect of insurance status on the care of 330 patients with colorectal cancer diagnosed from 1984 to 1989 and seen by the same set of providers in one group practice in Houston, Texas. No systematic differences were found in the care offered to HMO and FFS patients (e.g., type of primary treatment). Limitations of this study include the small sample size and a lack of adjustments for differences in the HMO and FFS study populations (e.g., HMO members were younger).

In summary, relatively few studies have compared cancer care under managed care and FFS financing and delivery arrangements. Most of these studies have involved comparisons of

FFS care with care in a staff- or group-model HMO. These studies show processes and outcomes of care in these settings that are equal to or better than those in FFS settings.

The findings of many of the studies of managed care can be challenged on methodological grounds—retrospective cross-sectional designs, small sample sizes, nonrandom potentially biased selection of cases, and inadequate use of control variables to adjust for underlying differences in patient populations served in HMOs and FFS. Furthermore, most of the studies have been limited to large staff- or group-model HMOs that now represent only about 15 percent of managed care enrollment (http://www.aahp.org). Five of the eight studies reviewed evaluated the care of patients diagnosed before 1990. Most of these studies included an analysis of mortality, so long follow-up times were necessary; however, the processes of care that may have contributed to differences in outcomes have in all likelihood changed. Recent evidence points to significant variation among HMOs in the quality of cancer treatment (Riley et al., 1999). Carefully designed, large studies are needed to assess how features of managed care plans and market areas affect the quality of cancer care.

KEY FINDINGS

Among the first questions many individuals ask after receiving a diagnosis of cancer care are, "Where should I go for care?" and "What kind of doctor should I see?" Health services research has not fully addressed these important questions. There is very limited evidence on the way structures and technical processes of care affect cancer care outcomes, and the strength of available evidence is weakened by methodological shortcomings of the research. Only a handful of studies were available for this review on the effects of managed care or on the effects of the volume and specialization of facilities or physicians on cancer care quality. Many of the available studies on these topics were done outside the United States, making inferences to care in the United States difficult. Most of the published literature includes mortality as the main outcome measure and has long periods of follow-up. Consequently, most of the studies apply to patients who were diagnosed with cancer in the early to late 1980s.

A large body of evidence supports a relationship between high surgical case volume and better survival for several cancers for which high-risk surgery is indicated (e.g., pancreatic cancer, non-small-cell lung cancer). Several studies show very large effects, with low-volume hospitals having postsurgical mortality rates two to three times those of high-volume hospitals. A dose–response effect is also evident to support the finding that as volume increases, so do good outcomes. The observational studies described, however, must be interpreted cautiously because they are prone to biases that favor large centers (e.g., greater use of diagnostic tests can contribute to a stage migration bias; patients at high-volume centers tend to be healthier than at smaller hospitals).

Studying the effect of institutional specialization on outcomes is difficult because specialization is often closely tied to the size of a facility and the volume of services. Nevertheless, a number of studies have attempted to identify differences in outcomes of facilities according to various measures of specialization—for example, whether they are cancer centers, university affiliated, or designated as research centers or have residency training programs. There does appear to be a consistent trend of improved outcomes associated with specialization, however defined.

In most of these studies, however, facility size was not controlled for in the analysis, which makes it difficult to know whether improvement is truly an effect of specialization. Other limitations of the available research in this area are the small number of institutions included in the studies and a lack of information on whether underlying differences in patient populations across facilities are taken sufficiently into account. Furthermore, the potential for publication bias is significant in these kinds of studies (e.g., specialty centers would be likely to publish only positive results). At this time the evidence is insufficient, and well-designed studies are needed to understand the relationship between institutional specialization and outcomes.

Very little can be said about the effects of physician specialization on outcomes of cancer care. Only one U.S. study was found that compared the outcomes of patients cared for by physicians with different levels of training. The one U.S. study and several studies conducted outside the United States appear consistently to show improved outcomes with specialization, but the definitions of specialization varied widely. For three of the studies, the outcomes of patients with ovarian cancer were compared according to whether their provider was a general surgeon or a gynecologist. Other studies used different definitions of specialization (e.g., training, interest, practices such as keeping separate records for cancer patients). Here again, the evidence is insufficient, and well-designed studies are needed to understand the importance of physician specialization.

Few studies compared cancer care under managed care with fee-for-service care, and studies are usually limited to group- or staff-model HMOs that have a relatively small share of the total managed care enrollment. The limited body of evidence suggests that processes and outcomes of care in these managed care settings are equal to or better than those in fee-for-service settings. Recent evidence suggests that there is significant variation in quality of care among HMOs.

There are a number of data systems in place that could substantially improve the quality of information available to provide additional insights into which structures and technical processes of care may lead to better patient outcomes. The National Cancer Data Base, for example, could be used more extensively to address quality issues if a nationally representative sample of facilities and providers was used. The SEER–Medicare-linked database appears to be an underutilized resource with which to evaluate aspects of care that affect outcomes for Medicare beneficiaries. Existing data systems, however, must be enhanced so questions about quality of care can be answered comprehensively on a national scale. An effective system would have to capture information about

- the person with cancer (e.g., age, race or ethnicity, socioeconomic status, insurance coverage);
- the condition (e.g., stage, grade, histological pattern, comorbid conditions);
- the treatment including significant outpatient treatments (e.g., adjuvant therapy);
- the providers (e.g., specialty training);
- where care was delivered (e.g., community hospital, cancer center);
- the type of delivery care system (e.g., managed care versus fee for service); and
- the outcomes (e.g., relapse, complications, death, satisfaction, quality of life).

It may be costly and difficult to obtain all of the desirable data elements for all individuals in any one data system, so existing databases could be used effectively to identify a sample of patients for augmented data collection in targeted studies. Linking available databases is another option for expanding the set of variables for analysis. For example, linking information about hospitals or other facilities that provide care with patient-level databases would allow the analyses of important structural components of care. To improve the timeliness of data, data collection has to be standardized and automated to provide relatively quick turnaround of information. It is important to assess the following aspects of care, which could affect quality, but also will present analytic challenges: multidisciplinary care teams, referral patterns to specialists, second opinions, and the communication skills of health providers.

REFERENCES

Aass N, Klepp O, Cavallin-Stahl E, et al. 1991. Prognostic factors in unselected patients with nonseminomatous metastatic testicular cancer: A multicenter experience. *Journal of Clinical Oncology* 9:818–826.

Ballard-Barbash R, Potosky A, et al. 1996. Factors associated with surgical and radiation therapy for early stage breast cancer in older women. *Journal of the National Cancer Institute* 88(11):716–726.

Basnett I, Gill M, Tobias JS. 1992. Variations in breast cancer management between a teaching and a non-teaching district. *European Journal of Cancer* 28A:1945–1950.

Begg CB, Cramer LD, Hoskins WJ, Brennan MF. 1998. Impact of hospital volume on operative mortality for major cancer surgery. *Journal of the American Medical Association* 280(20):1747–1751.

Charlson ME, Pomei P, Ales KL, MacKenzie CR. 1987. A new classifying prognostic comorbidity in longitudinal studies: Development and validation. *Journal of Chronic Diseases* 40:373–383.

Clancy CM, Brody H. 1995. Managed care: Jekyll or Hyde? *Journal of the American Medical Association* 273:338–339.

Clarke K, Howard GC, Elia MH, et al. 1995. Referral patterns within Scotland to specialist oncology centres for patients with testicular germ cell tumours. The Scottish Radiological Society and the Scottish Standing Committee of the Royal College of Radiologists. *British Journal of Cancer* 72:1300–1302.

Davis S, Dahlberg S, Myers MH, et al. 1987. Hodgkin's disease in the United States: A comparison of patient characteristics and survival in the Centralized Cancer Patient Data System and the Surveillance, Epidemiology, and End Results Program. *Journal of the National Cancer Institute* 78:471–478.

Dent DM. Cancer surgery: Why some survival benefits may be artefactual. *British Journal of Surgery* 85(4):433–434.

Dickersin K. 1997. How important is publication bias? A synthesis of available data. *AIDS Education and Prevention* 9(Suppl. A):15–21.

Eley JW, Hill HA, Chen VW, et al. 1994. Racial differences in survival from breast cancer. Results of the Cancer Institute Black/White Cancer Survival Study. *Journal of the American Medical Association* 272(12):947–954.

Ellis SG, Weintraub, D Holmes, et al. 1997. Relation of operator volume and experience to procedural outcome or percutaneous coronary revascularization at hospitals with high interventional volumes. *Circulation* 95(11):2479–2484.

Farrow D, Hunt W, Samet J. 1995. Biased comparisons of lung cancer survival across geographic areas: Effects of stage bias. *Epidemiology* 6(5):558–560.

Feinstein AR, Sosin DM, Wells CK. 1985. The Will Rogers phenomenon: Stage migration and new diagnostic techniques as a source of misleading statistics for survival in cancer. *New England Journal of Medicine* 312(25):1604–1608.

Feuer EJ, Frey CM, Brawley OW, et al. 1994. After a treatment breakthrough: A comparison of trial and population-based data for advanced testicular cancer. *Journal of Clinical Oncology* 12:368–377.

Gillis CR, Hole DJ. 1996. Survival outcome of care by specialist surgeons in breast cancer: A study of 3786 patients in the west of Scotland. *British Medical Journal* 312:145–148.

Ginsberg RJ, Vokes EE, Raben A. 1997. Non-small cell lung cancer. Pp. 858–910 in Devita VT, Hellman S, Rosenberg SA, eds. *Cancer: Principles and Practice of Oncology.* Fifth Edition. Philadelphia: Lippincott-Raven.

Glasgow RE, Mulvihill SJ. 1996. Hospital volume influences outcome in patients undergoing pancreatic resection for cancer. *Western Journal of Medicine* 165:294–300.

Gordon TA, Bowman HM, Tielsch JM, et al. 1998. Statewide regionalization of pancreaticoduodenectomy and its effect on in-hospital mortality. *Annals of Surgery* 228:71–78.

Gordon TA, Burleyson GP, Tielsch JM, Cameron JL 1995. The effects of regionalization on cost and outcome for one general high-risk surgical procedure. *Annals of Surgery* 221:43–49.

Greenberg ER, Baron JA, Dain BJ, et al. 1991. Cancer staging may have different meanings in academic and community hospitals. *Journal of Clinical Epidemiology* 44(6):505–512.

Greenwald HP. 1992. *Who Survives Cancer?* Berkeley, CA: University of California Press.

Greenwald HP, Henke CJ. 1992. HMO membership, treatment, and mortality risk among prostatic cancer patients. *American Journal of Public Health* 82:1099–1104.

Grilli R, Minozzi S, Tinazzi A, et al. 1998. Do specialists do it better? The impact of specialization on the processes and outcomes of care for cancer patients. *Annals of Oncology* 9:365–374.

Guadagnoli E, Weeks J, Shapiro C, et al. 1998. Use of breast-conserving surgery for treatment of Stage I and Stage II breast cancer. *Journal of Clinical Oncology* 16(1):101–106.

Hand R, Sener S, Imperato J, et al. 1991. Hospital variables associated with quality of care for breast cancer patients. *Journal of the American Medical Association* 266(23):3429–3432.

Hannan EL, Kilburn H Jr., O'Donnell JF, et al. 1992. A longitudinal analysis of the relationship between in-hospital mortality in New York State and the volume of abdominal aortic aneurysm surgeries performed. *Health Services Research* 27(4):517–542.

Hannan E, Siu A, Kumar D, et al. 1995. The decline in coronary artery bypass graft surgery mortality in New York State. *Journal of the American Medical Association* 273(3):209–213.

Hannan EL, Racz M, Ryan TJ, et al. 1997a. Coronary angioplasty volume–outcome relationships for hospitals and cardiologists. *Journal of the American Medical Assocation* 19:277(11):892–898.

Hannan EL, Siu AL, Kumar D, et al. 1997b. Assessment of coronary artery bypass graft surgery performance in New York. Is there a bias against taking high-risk patients? *Medical Care* 35(1):49–56.

Harding MJ, Paul J, Gillis CR, Kaye SB. 1993. Management of malignant teratoma: Does referral to a specialist unit matter? *Lancet* 341:999–1002.

Hillner B, McDonald K, Desch C, et al. 1998a. A comparison of patterns of care of nonsmall cell lung carcinoma patients in a younger and Medigap commercially insured cohort. *Cancer* 83(9):1930–1937.

Hillner BE, Smith TJ. 1998b. The quality of cancer care: Does the literature support the rhetoric? National Cancer Policy Board commissioned paper.

Horbar JD, Badger GL, Lewit EM, et al. 1997. Hospital and patient characteristics associated with variation in 28-day mortality rates for very low birth weight infants. Vermont Oxford Network. *Pediatrics* 99(2):149–156.

Horowitz MM, Przepiorka D, Champlin RE, et al. 1992. Should HLA-identical sibling bone marrow transplants for leukemia be restricted to large centers? *Blood* 79:2771–2774.

Hosenpud J, Breen T, Edwards E, et al. 1994. The effect of transplant center volume on cardiac transplant outcome: A report of the United Network for Organ Sharing scientific registry. *Journal of the American Medical Association* 271(23):1844–1849.

Janes RH Jr., Niederhuber JE, Chmiel JS, et al. 1996. National patterns of care for pancreatic cancer. Results of a survey by the Commission on Cancer. *Annals of Surgery* 223:261–272.

Johantgen ME, Coffey RM, Harris DR, et al.. 1995. Treating early-stage breast cancer: Hospital characteristics associated with breast-conserving surgery. *American Journal of Public Health* 85(10): 1432–1434.

Jollis J, Peterson E, DeLong E, et al. 1994. The relation between the volume of coronary angioplasty procedures at hospitals treating Medicare beneficiaries and short-term mortality. *New England Journal of Medicine* 331(24):1625–1629.

Jollis J, Peterson E, Nelson CL, et al. 1997. Relationship between physician and hospital coronary angioplasty volume and outcome in elderly patients. *New England Journal of Medicine* 95(11):2267–2270.

Junor EJ, Hole DJ, Gillis CR. 1994. Management of ovarian cancer: Referral to a multidisciplinary team matters. *British Journal of Cancer* 70:363–370.

Kantonen I, Lepantalo M, Salenius JP, et al. 1997. Mortality in abdominal aortic aneurysm surgery—The effect of hospital volume, patient mix, and surgeon's case load. *European Journal of Vascular and Endovascular Surgery* 14(5):375–379.

Kehoe S, Powell J, Wilson S, Woodman C. 1994. The influence of the operating surgeon's specialisation on patient survival in ovarian carcinoma. *British Journal of Cancer* 70:1014–1017.

Kingston RD, Walsh S, Jeacock J. 1991. Curative resection: the major determinant of survival in patients with large bowel cancer. *Journal of the Royal College of Surgeons of Edinburgh* 36:298–302.

Kitahata NM, Koepsell TD, Deyo RA, et al. 1996. Physicians' experience with the acquired immunodeficiency syndrome as a factor in patients' survival. *New England Journal of Medicine* 334(11): 701–706.

Kline RW, Smith AR, Coia LR, et al. 1997. Treatment planning for adenocarcinoma of the rectum and sigmoid: A Patterns of Care study. *International Journal of Radiation Oncology, Biology, Physics* 37:305–311.

Konvolinka CW, Copes WS, Sacco WJ. 1995. Institution and per-surgeon volume versus survival outcome in Pennsylvania's trauma centers. *American Journal of Surgery* 170(4):333–340.

Kreder HJ, Deyo RA, Koepsell T, et al. 1997. Relationship between the volume of total hip replacements performed by providers and the rates of postoperative complications in the State of Washington. *American Journal of Bone and Joint Surgery* 79(4):485–494.

Lavernia CJ, Guzman JF. 1995. Relationship of surgical volume to short-term mortality, morbidity, and hospital charges in arthroplasty. *Journal of Arthroplasty* 10(2):133–140.

Lee-Feldstein A, Anton-Culverm H, Feldstein P. 1994. Treatment differences and other prognostic factors related to breast cancer survival. *Journal of the American Medical Association* 271(15): 1163–1168.

Lieberman MD, Kilburn H, Lindsey M, Brennan MF. 1995. Relation of perioperative deaths to hospital volume among patients undergoing pancreatic resection for malignancy. *Annals of Surgery* 222:638–645.

Lu-Yao G, Yao S. 1998. Relationships between surgical volume, outcomes, and length of stay—A national study of patients undergoing radical prostatectomy. Abstract submitted to *American Society of Clinical Oncology.*

McArdle CS, Hole D. 1991. Impact of variability among surgeons on postoperative morbidity and mortality and ultimate survival. *British Medical Journal* 302:1501–1505.

Mella J, Biffin A, Radcliffe AG, et al. 1997. Population-based audit of colorectal cancer management in two UK health regions. *British Journal of Surgery* 84:1731–1736.

Mitchell PH, Shortell SM. 1997. Adverse outcomes and variations in organization of care delivery. *Medical Care* 35(11 Suppl.):NS19–NS32.

Munoz KA, Harlan LC, Trimble EL. 1997. Patterns of care for women with ovarian cancer in the United States. *Journal of Clinical Oncology* 15:3408–3415.

Nattinger AB, Gottlieb MS, Veum J, et al. 1992. Geographic variation in the use of breast-conserving treatment for breast cancer. *New England Journal of Medicine* 326(17):1102–1107.

Newhouse JP. 1998. *RAND Health Insurance Experiment (in Metropolitan and Non-Metropolitan Areas of the United States), 1974–1982.* 2nd ICPSR version. Santa Monica, CA: RAND [producer]. Ann Arbor, MI: Interuniversity Consortium for Political and Social Research [distributor].

Nguyen HN, Averette HE, Hoskins W, et al. 1993. National survey of ovarian carcinoma. Part V. The impact of physician's specialty on patients' survival. *Cancer* 72:3663–3670.

Porter GA, Soskolne CL, Yakimets WW, Newman SC. 1998. Surgeon-related factors and outcome in rectal cancer. *Annals of Surgery* 227:157–167.

Potosky AL, Merrill RM, Riley GF, et al. 1997. Breast cancer survival and treatment in health maintenance organization and fee-for-service settings. *Journal of the National Cancer Institute* 89: 1683–1691.

Retchin SM, Brown B. 1990. Management of colorectal cancer in Medicare health maintenance organizations. *Journal of General Internal Medicine* 5:110–114.

Retchin SM, Penberthy L, Desch C, et al. 1997. Perioperative management of colon cancer under Medicare risk programs. *Archives of Internal Medicine* 157:1878–1884.

Richardson JD, Schmieg R, Boaz P, et al. 1998. Impact of trauma attending surgeon case volume on outcome: Is more better? *Journal of Trauma* 44(2):266–271.

Riley GF, Feuer EJ, Lubitz JD. 1996. Disenrollment of Medicare cancer patients from health maintenance organizations. *Medical Care* 34(8):826–836.

Riley GF, Potosky AL, Klabunde CN, et al. 1999. Stage at diagnosis and treatment patterns among older women with breast cancer: An HMO and fee-for-service comparison. *Journal of the American Medical Association* 281(8):720–726.

Romano PS, Mark DH. 1992. Patient and hospital characteristics related to in-hospital mortality after lung cancer resection. *Chest* 101:1332–1337.

Roohan P, Bickell N, Baptiste M, et al. 1998. Hospital volume differences and five-year survival from breast cancer. *American Journal of Public Health* 88(3):454–457.

Rosen L, Stasik JJ, Reed JF, et al. 1996. Variations in colon and rectal surgical mortality. Comparison of specialties with a state-legislated database. *Diseases of the Colon and Rectum* 39(2):129–135.

Ruby ST, Robinson D, Lynch JT, Mark H. 1996. Outcome analysis of carotid endarterectomy in Connecticut: The impact of volume and specialty. *Annals of Vascular Surgery* 10(1):22–26.

Sainsbury R, Haward B, Rider L, et al. 1995. Influence of clinician workload and patterns of treatment on survival from breast cancer. *Lancet* 345:1265–1270.

Smith RF, Frateschi L, Sloan EP, et al. 1990. The impact of volume on outcome in seriously injured trauma patients: Two years' experience of the Chicago Trauma System. *Journal of Trauma* 30(9):1066–1075.

Solomon RA, Mayer SA, Tarmey JJ. 1996. Relationship between the volume of craniotomies for cerebral aneurysm performed at New York State hospitals and in-hospital mortality. *Stroke* 27(1):13–17.

Sosa JA, Bowman HM, Gordon TA, et al. 1998. Importance of hospital volume in the overall management of pancreatic cancer. *Annals of Surgery* 228(3):429–438.

Tepas JJ 3rd, Patel JC, DiScala C, et al. 1998. Relationship of trauma patient volume to outcome experience: Can a relationship be defined? *Journal of Trauma* 44(5):827–830.

Vernon SW, Hughes JI, Heckel VM, et al. 1992. Quality of care for colorectal cancer in a fee-for-service and health maintenance organization practice. *Cancer* 69 (10):2418–2425.

Wade TP, El-Ghazzawy AG, Virgo KS, et al. 1995. The Whipple resection for cancer in U.S. Department of Veterans Affairs hospitals. *Annals of Surgery* 221(3):241–248.

Whittle J, Steinberg EP, Anderson GF, Herbert R. 1991. Use of Medicare claims data to evaluate outcomes in elderly patients undergoing lung resection for lung cancer. *Chest* 100:729–734.

Woodman C, Baghdady A, Collins S, Clyma JA. 1997. What changes in the organization of cancer services will improve the outcome for women with ovarian cancer? *British Journal of Obstetrics and Gynaecology* 104:135–139.

6

Cancer Care Quality Assurance

Individuals with cancer (or at risk of cancer) have relatively few direct or indirect ("surrogate") indicators of quality available to help them choose doctors, hospitals, and health plans or to evaluate the merits of alternative courses of treatment. This situation is changing as the science of measuring health care quality matures and begins to focus on consumer-oriented indicators for the treatment of chronic diseases. No national comprehensive quality monitoring system exists in the United States, but there is a patchwork of federal and private efforts to assess quality, each with different purposes, perspectives, and audiences. Much of the recent impetus for quality assessment stems from the desire of large employers, business groups, and government programs to purchase managed care products for employees on the basis of quality, as well as cost.

An important aspect of quality is accountability, which can be applied to many aspects of health care. Providers can, for example, be held accountable for professional competence, legal and ethical conduct, financial performance, accessibility of services, public health promotion, and community benefit (Emanual and Emanual, 1996). There have also been calls to hold managed care organizations and other insurers publicly accountable for the "reasonableness" of their decisions by making rationales for limit-setting decisions (e.g., decisions regarding coverage for new technologies) explicit and publicly available (Daniels and Sabin, 1997; 1998a). Many parties may wish to hold providers accountable, and "accountors" may at the same time be "accountees" (Darby, 1998). A hospital, for example, may require physicians to adhere to clinical practice guidelines, while the hospitals themselves, in turn, are subject to oversight from government regulators and professional groups. At least three types of forces exert pressure on the health care system to foster accountability (although the degree to which they influence the system is quite variable) (Darby, 1998; Donaldson, 1998):

1. The *public sector* relies on the regulatory, oversight, and purchasing actions of government at the federal, state, and local levels to ensure quality. Government health agencies also conduct disease surveillance to monitor public health and develop tools to assess quality, often in partnership with the private sector. The courts are often the final arbitrators in disputes about possible medical negligence and the appropriateness of care.

144

2. The *market* relies on the use of quality data by health care purchasers and consumers in choosing plans and providers. The underlying assumption is that quality is a market force on a par—or nearly so—with cost.

3. The *professional community* relies on the actions of private-sector accreditation groups, trade associations and health plans, hospitals, and other providers to ensure quality. The profession assumes leadership for policing itself and demonstrating quality to outside parties.

Although these categories are convenient for describing the forces at work, they are not entirely independent, and in fact, the number of public and private collaborative efforts is increasing. For instance, the President's Advisory Commission on Consumer Protection and Quality in the Health Care Industry (1998) recommended that two complementary bodies be formed on health care quality—one lodged in the public sector to promote interagency coordination among federal agencies (Quality Interagency Coordination Health Care Task Force), and the other in the private sector to improve health care quality measurement and reporting (National Forum for Health Care Quality Measurement and Reporting). The goals of the Quality Forum are to (http://www.uhfnyc.org/intro/qfpc.htm):

- ensure system-wide capacity to evaluate and report on the quality of care,
- promote and inform consumer choice and further consumer understanding and use of quality measures,
    - enable providers to use data to improve performance,
    - allow meaningful quality comparisons of health care providers and plans,
    - promote competition on the quality of health care services,
    - use broad representation to marshal market forces for quality, and
- reduce the burdens on providers and health plans by enabling them to collect consistent data that avoids duplication.

This chapter first considers the individual consumer's point of view in describing the strengths and weaknesses of the tools and information available to help understand accountability in cancer care and the quality of such care. Next, the forces that affect accountability are described, using the three categories listed above. Finally, some of the specific activities that are in place to try to measure and improve the quality of health care (and cancer care, specifically) are described.

QUALITY ASSURANCE: AN INDIVIDUAL CONSUMER PERSPECTIVE

Choosing Insurers

Most people are healthy when they first select a health plan or source of care and so do not focus specifically on the quality of cancer care. Then too, even if consumers wanted to comparison shop for a health plan on the basis of quality, many have no real choice of health plan. Most individuals under age 65 are insured through their employer, and less than half of employees (41 percent) who are offered insurance at work can choose among two or more plans (Long and Marquis, 1998). Furthermore, most new cases of cancer occur among those age 65 and older who receive care within Medicare's fee-for-service (FFS) system, where consumer-oriented quality measures are generally less available.

Consumer-oriented quality initiatives have focused largely on helping people choose among managed care plans. For those with the opportunity to opt into managed care or switch plans, there is a wealth of information that, over time, is beginning to address meaningful issues for those with chronic illnesses such as cancer (see descriptions of the National Committee for Quality Assurance [NCQA] and the Foundation for Accountability [FACCT] later in this chapter).

A new generation of consumer surveys about health plans is now available that go beyond simple ratings of satisfaction (Cleary et al., 1997). Consumers are asked to report on specific experiences in obtaining health care, for example, difficulty in obtaining referrals. If a plan is large enough, cancer-specific ratings—or at least the experience of individuals with chronic illness or functional limitations—could be provided to those making health plan choices. Here too, standardized measures are being developed to allow managed care and FFS comparisons (http://www.ahcpr.gov/qual/cahpfact.htm). The Health Care Financing Administration (HCFA) has posted on the internet (www.medicare.gov) some results of these consumer satisfaction ratings for Medicare beneficiaries in health plans, along with comparative plan ratings on indicators such as mammography use. HCFA plans to survey those who have disenrolled from health plans to provide information to beneficiaries on why people leave health plans (*Medicine & Health*, 1999).

Most individuals with a new diagnosis of cancer find themselves in an insurance system that they must live with, at least in the short term. At this point, many people have little flexibility in terms of their insurance plan, although they are usually able to choose among physicians within their plan and among institutions covered by their insurer.

Choosing Physicians and Hospitals

In choosing a physician, one basic piece of information is whether the physician is certified by a cancer specialty board, which requires completion of an approved training program and passing a rigorous written and oral exam about cancer care. Other potential indicators of physician quality of relevance to consumers might include: history of disciplinary action, hospital admitting privileges, volume of cancer patients treated, number and credentials of support staff, and the personality and demeanor of the provider and staff. Not all of this information is readily available, and as described in Chapter 5, good evidence is lacking to support the link between these indicators and outcomes of care. There are, for example, very few studies of the effects of physician specialization on outcomes of care, so although board certification has some intuitive appeal as a quality measure, the effect of certification on outcomes of care is virtually unknown.

For hospitals, there are several indicators of the range of services available (e.g., research programs), structure (e.g., size as indicated by annual hospital discharges), and to a limited extent, the quality of cancer-related services (e.g., appropriate use of diagnostic tests):

• The American College of Surgeons' Commission on Cancer (see below) has standards for approving hospitals.
• The National Cancer Institute (NCI) designates cancer centers for support of cancer research, and these centers are affiliated with a wide range of small and large hospitals. Treatment at participating hospitals means patients could have access to clinical trials (see Chapter 3).

•   The Joint Commission on Accreditation of Heathcare Organizations (JCAHO) is the lead organization in accrediting hospitals in the United States. JCAHO has recently instituted an outcomes-based performance system that includes specific oncology measures and may, over the coming years, improve the relevance of JCAHO certification to individuals with cancer (see below).

Although various organizations collect information related to the quality of hospital-based cancer care, the consumer usually can find out only whether or not a hospital is approved or accredited. The overwhelming majority of hospitals that voluntarily submit to an inspection or review are approved or accredited, but the details of hospital performance on various indicators are not yet publicly available. Even if the information were available, it would be difficult for consumers to evaluate a particular hospital's quality because there are few established links between hospital attributes and quality (see Chapter 5). Standards can, however, help to ensure that hospitals meet minimum infection control, safety, and security standards. If a hospital fails to meet the criteria set forth by professional groups, consumers are justified in searching out more detail about potential problems before agreeing to use the facility.

The news media and the popular press may also be sources of consumer information about the quality of health plans and hospitals. A few widely circulated magazines have sponsored national surveys of consumers regarding their satisfaction with care, and of providers regarding their assessments of the quality of sites of care, that they have used to rank services on the basis of quality. *Consumer Reports* has, for example, evaluated managed health care plans, and each year *U.S. News & World Report* ranks hospitals, including hospital-based cancer centers (Box 6.1), a feature that has been very popular with consumers and has been used by the high-ranking centers in marketing (Memorial Sloan-Kettering Cancer Center, 1998). While the *U.S. News & World Report* ranking includes indicators for which there is some evidence linking them to good health outcomes (i.e., volume of services, nurse to patient bed ratio), the ranking system itself has not been validated externally and the methodology has been criticized (Teasley, 1996).

BOX 6.1 *U.S. News and World Report* Annual Ranking of Cancer Centers

With a circulation of more than 2 million, the *U.S. News & World Report* annual ranking of hospital-based cancer programs is perhaps the most widely read source of information on the quality of cancer care. In 1997, 998 hospital-based cancer care programs were ranked according to measures of structure, process, and outcome:

• reputation score among board-certified oncologists;
• severity-adjusted cancer mortality rate;
• membership in the Council of Teaching Hospitals;
• availability of cancer-related technology;
• number of cancer discharges; and
• nurse to patient bed ratio.

The authors of the ranking system concluded that there are a few extremely "good" hospitals, many hospitals providing "competent" care, and a few hospitals at the bottom of the curve.

SOURCE: Comarow, 1997; Ehrlich et al., 1997.

Choosing Treatment Options

Most consumers do not have the scientific background to evaluate their treatment options, but they can still participate intelligently in decisions about their care. Specifically, they can

- seek independent second opinions;
- use information resources such as the patient-oriented version of the NCI's Physician Data Query (PDQ) system, which can be accessed by computer and describes (in nontechnical language) treatment options by type of cancer. Information is also available through telephone services operated by both NCI and the American Cancer Society (ACS) (Murphy et al., 1997);
- enter systems of care that employ a comprehensive approach to cancer treatment and management. (Programs that emphasize patient education, adherence to evidence-based protocols, and use of multidisciplinary teams of providers have been shown to contribute to greater patient satisfaction and better health outcomes (Wagner et al., 1996); and
- make use of an array of available consumer-oriented products that enable individuals with cancer to electronically access health educational materials, communicate with their providers and with individuals with cancer, and make more fully informed treatment decisions (CancerDesk, 1999; Gustafson et al., 1993).

Use of Quality Information by Consumers

There is evidence that the available quality information is not viewed by many consumers as relevant to their decision making (Hibbard and Jewett, 1997b). In one national survey, three-quarters of Americans said that they would opt to see a surgeon they know rather than one they do not, even if the alternative had much higher quality ratings. Also, although many Americans perceive great differences in the quality of care among health plans, hospitals, and doctors, relatively few are now using quality data to make health care choices (Kaiser Family Foundation, 1996). In many cases, consumer-oriented information is just not available for all of the decisions that a person with cancer may have to make—selecting a doctor, choosing among treatments, or finding a home health service, rehabilitation program, or hospice. The type of information needed about the quality of cancer care services can vary greatly by individual. The services important to the high-risk patient or person who has not yet been diagnosed are quite different from those important to a long-term cancer survivor.

Barriers to the use of quality information include the complexity of the task of evaluating health care quality, difficulties in understanding such information (e.g., high rates of functional illiteracy, non-English speakers), a lack of familiarity among the public with the workings of the health care system (e.g., most Americans do not understand the concept of managed care) and the way in which the organization of care might influence quality, and importantly, a paucity of user-friendly information (Hibbard et al., 1997b).

If large numbers of consumers do not use quality information directly, decisions at the intermediary level may offer important guidance to consumers (Hibbard et al., 1997c). Having a "thumbs-up" or "thumbs-down" rating from an influential group such as the American Association of Retired Persons (AARP) might be more useful for some consumers than detailed quality report cards. Awareness of quality issues in cancer care will likely increase as cancer advocacy groups promote measurement of aspects of care of particular relevance to individuals with cancer and disseminate information to raise awareness of quality issues. The National Coalition for Cancer Survivorship has, for example, published "principles of excellence" in cancer care (Box 6.2).

BOX 6.2 National Coalition for Cancer Survivorship: Imperatives for Quality Cancer Care

Principle 1

People with cancer have the right to a system of universal health care. This access should not be precluded because of preexisting conditions, genetic or other risk factors, or employment status.

Principle 2

Quality cancer care should be available in a health care system whose standards and guidelines are developed in consideration of treating the whole person with cancer. Health care plans must regard the cancer patient as an autonomous individual who has the right to be involved in decisions about his or her care.

Principle 3

Standards of cancer care should be driven by the quality of care, not only by the cost of care, and should include participation in clinical trials and quality-of-life considerations.

Principle 4

All people diagnosed with cancer should have access to and coverage for services provided by a multidisciplinary team of care providers across the full continuum of care. Health care plans should be held accountable for timely referral to appropriate specialists when symptoms of cancer or its recurrence may be present.

Principle 5

People with cancer should be provided a range of benefits by all health care plans that include primary and secondary prevention; early detection; initial treatment; supportive therapies to manage pain, nausea, fatigue, and infections; long-term follow-up; psychosocial services; palliative care; hospice care; and bereavement counseling.

Principle 6

People with histories of cancer have the right to continued medical follow-up with basic standards of care that include the specific needs of long-term survivors.

Continued

BOX 6.2 Continued

Principle 7

Long-term survivors should have access to specialized follow-up clinics that focus on health promotion, disease prevention, rehabilitation, and identification of physiologic and psychosocial problems. Communication with the primary care physician must be maintained.

Principle 8

Systematic long-term follow-up should generate data that contribute to improvements in cancer therapies and decreases in morbidity.

Principle 9

The responsibility for appropriate long-term medical care must be shared by cancer survivors, their families, the oncology team, and primary care providers.

Principle 10

The provision of psychosocial services must be safeguarded and promoted. Persons diagnosed with cancer should receive psychosocial assessments at critical junctures along the continuum of cancer care to determine the availability of needed support and their ability to seek information and advocate on their own behalf.

Principle 11

Psychosocial research is integral to comprehensive cancer care, and as such, psychosocial outcome measures should be included in all future clinical trials. The importance of this research and its application and transfer to oncology care plans should be recognized and encouraged.

Principle 12

Cancer survivors, health care providers, and other key constituency groups must work together to increase public awareness; educate consumers, professionals, and public policy makers; develop guidelines and disseminate information; advocate for increased research funding; and articulate for and promote survivors' rights.

SOURCE: NCCS, 1995.

QUALITY ASSURANCE: A MARKET APPROACH

Although individual consumers may not yet wield much clout in the health care marketplace, large private-sector purchasers are already doing so. Most nonelderly Americans receive their health care insurance through an employer, and employers choose health care plans for their employees on the basis of price, benefits, quality, and service. A common metric for quality is essential if health plans are to compete on the basis of value. Information on the quality of care provided in managed care plans is sometimes made available to employers, consumers, and other purchasers in the form of report cards, using a standardized format to make comparisons possible across health plans.

Most employers currently make health care purchasing decisions on the basis of price, not quality (Darby, 1998). When quality enters the decision-making process, some evidence suggests that employers are more likely to consider consumer satisfaction and accreditation status than clinical performance measures (Hibbard et al., 1997a). Some very large employers (e.g., Digital, Xerox) have been addressing quality of care concerns for years, and employers are increasingly banding together increasingly to form large coalitions to gain purchasing clout and to push for uniform quality assessment among health plans. Purchasers may use quality information to identify high-value plans with which to contract, to steer employees into higher-performing plans, or as leverage when establishing rates for premiums (Darby, 1998).

The Pacific Business Group on Health (PBGH), for example, is a nonprofit coalition of large health care purchasers in California and Arizona representing, as of 1996, 2.5 million insured individuals employed by 33 private- and public-sector organizations. PBGH collects and analyzes health plan performance data to produce report cards for consumers; promotes shared treatment decision making between providers and consumers; and collects, analyzes, and reports plan-level consumer satisfaction ratings (Castles et al., 1999; President's Advisory Commission, 1998). PBGH is also developing several disease-specific quality assessment programs, including one for breast cancer. PBGH was the first purchasing coalition to impose a condition on contracting plans whereby it would withhold 2 percent of the premium until the plans achieved specific goals for improving customer satisfaction and quality of care. The Alliance, a health insurance purchasing cooperative in Denver, subsequently adopted a similar approach (Darby, 1998).

An informal group of large employer organizations including PBGH, called the Leapfrog group, is promoting "evidence-based hospital referral," the channeling of patients to certain hospitals for selected conditions and procedures (e.g., coronary angioplasty, bypass surgery) for which clear evidence exists that a higher volume of procedures or teaching status is associated with better outcomes. The PBGH is asking California HMOs with whom it has contracts to use new performance standards for physician groups, hospital precertification, and enrollee education to advance "evidence-based hospital referral" (Bodenheimer, 1999).

QUALITY ASSURANCE: THE PUBLIC-SECTOR APPROACH

Oversight through accreditation and licensing is one of the oldest systems of quality assurance employed by the federal government (e.g., accrediting hospitals providing care for Medicare beneficiaries) and states (e.g., licensing physicians). Although traditionally focused on regulation and oversight to ensure at least a minimal level of acceptable quality, government bodies are increasingly turning to market-based approaches. State-sponsored initiatives in Minnesota, Maryland, and Pennsylvania, for example, publish reports that allow consumers to compare health plans on various aspects of quality (Darby, 1998).

Health Care Financing Administration

Many of the federal health care accountability systems are housed within the Health Care Financing Administration (HCFA), the principal payer for health care. HCFA has two main quality-of-care strategies: (1) As part of its certification activities, it requires fee-for-service providers, HCFA-contracting health maintenance organizations (HMOs), and clinical laboratories to meet Medicare standards; (2) it undertakes quality improvement initiatives in cooperation with its peer review organization (PRO) programs.

On the regulatory front, HCFA is revising its rules to certify Medicare providers in four areas: home health, hospital care, hospice care, and end-stage renal disease, placing more emphasis on clinical performance and patients' experience with care. The proposed home care rule, for example, would require Medicare home health agencies to use a standard system called the Outcomes and Assessment Information Set (OASIS) to measure quality and patient satisfaction with care (Darby, 1998). HMOs contracting with HCFA must now report clinical performance data (i.e., Health Plan Employer Data and Information Set [HEDIS] data) and information on patients' experience and satisfaction with plans (i.e., results from a new Consumer Assessment of Health Plans Survey). HCFA is also implementing the Quality Improvement System for Managed Care to require participating health plans to show improvement in the health care they provide. Minimum service levels for improvement measures such as mammography will be set, along with targets specific to a geographic region. Initially, the focus will be on preventive and acute care services. A similar system is being developed for fee-for-service care (Voelker, 1997).

Relatively few Medicare beneficiaries are enrolled in managed care plans (13 percent as of 1997), and efforts are underway to gather performance information from providers in the FFS environment. Medicare beneficiaries are beginning to have more choices in type of health coverage beyond fee-for-service and HMOs. With the Medicare+Choice program, beneficiaries will be able to select new insurance options including preferred provider organizations (PPOs) and medical savings accounts. Many believe that HCFA will lead the effort to converge on a single set of quality measures applicable across delivery systems (Darby, 1998).

In 1992, HCFA established the Health Care Quality Improvement Program, which promotes partnerships between PROs and hospitals, health plans, and physicians to improve quality. Each state has a PRO that evaluates whether care given to Medicare patients is reasonable, necessary, and provided in the most appropriate setting. Funding for PROs in 1997 was $183 million. HCFA maintains a quality-of-care surveillance system to provide information to PROs about Medicare health care utilization, patterns, and trends to help PROs target their quality improvement activities. Among the indices tracked are rates of radical prostatectomy among men 70 years or older (see examples of PRO activities in Box 6.3). As of 1998, more than 700 quality improvement projects were underway, some of which were national in scope and disease specific. The Cardiovascular Cooperative Project, for example, is a national, data-based effort to improve care for Medicare patients hospitalized for heart attacks (President's Advisory Commission, 1998). PROs appear to have been effective in improving the care of patients with acute myocardial infarction, according to a recent quasi-experimental assessment (Marciniak, 1997).

HCFA is also actively involved in the development of clinical performance measures to assess quality. As part of HCFA's Outcomes Project, for example, it is identifying multiple domains of processes and outcomes of care for breast cancer, collecting and summarizing the existing evidence supporting performance measures in each of these domains, and identifying multiple sources of performance data (Katherine Kahn and Marge Pearson, RAND, personal communication to Mark Schuster, 1998).

BOX 6.3 HCFA's Peer Review Organizations— Examples of Cancer Care Quality Monitoring

Radical Prostatectomy (RP) in Men 70 and Older. RP should generally not be used for men 70 and older, given the risks and benefits of the procedure. The PRO overseeing Medicare quality assurance in Kentucky and Indiana identified five "outlier" hospitals in each state with high rates of RP for older men (20–22 percent of prostate cancer admissions among elderly males). Provider education and monitoring of RP led to significant declines in RP in outlier hospitals, and in Kentucky, the rate of RP among older men was reduced to statewide norms (ML Daffron, personal communication to Maria Hewitt, February 18, 1998).

Breast Conserving Surgery. The PRO overseeing Medicare quality in Delaware found that rates of breast conserving surgery (BCS) rose from 16 to 80 percent from 1993–1994 to 1996–1997 among Medicare beneficiaries with Stage I or II breast cancer. Among women eligible for BCS for whom mastectomy was performed, documentation of patient choice of mastectomy rose from 50 to 72 percent of cases (Cochran, 1997).

Cancer Pain Management. The Minnesota PRO evaluated hospital adherence to the Agency for Health Care Policy and Research and American Pain Society guidelines on pain management. According to a review of 271 charts of patients admitted for specific cancers (e.g., metastasis to bone and spinal cord, liver, intestine, peritoneum), hospitals excelled at documenting some form of a patient's initial self-assessment of pain (93 percent of patients). Most hospitals, however, did not utilize effective means of communicating pain intensity (26 percent of patients). Pain reassessment was found to be inconsistent among hospitals. The PRO is planning interventions to improve compliance with pain management guidelines (Stratis Health, 1997).

Determinants of Use of Adjuvant Cancer Therapy. The Colorado PRO matched cancer registry data with Medicare A and B claims data to assess factors associated with the use of adjuvant therapy for Stage I or II breast cancer and Stage III colon cancer. Underuse of adjuvant therapy was found among those age 65 and older, particularly for chemotherapy following Stage III colon cancer. The principle factor associated with failure to use adjuvant therapies was advancing age, which did not appear to be explained by comorbidities (Byers et al., 1998).

Satisfaction with Breast Cancer Treatment. The Colorado PRO conducted focus groups among minority and non-minority group women and a telephone survey of women age 65 and older regarding their care for breast cancer. Women's satisfaction with cancer care was high, but areas in which doctors could provide more information to their patients were in the discussion of what to expect from surgery and the potential physical and emotional outcomes of surgery (Crane et al., 1997).

SOURCES: Byers et al., 1998; Cochran, 1997; Crane et al., 1997; Daffron, 1998; Stratis Health, 1997.

Most state Medicaid agencies monitor utilization, outcomes, consumer satisfaction, and disenrollment, through either chart review or client survey. Some have engaged in collaborative quality improvement initiatives with health plans, providers, public health agencies, and community organizations in areas such as pediatric immunization and prenatal care. Medicaid agencies are also beginning to incorporate quality-based performance indicators and specifications into their contracting strategies. Some use quality information to assess potential contractors, whereas others (e.g., Massachusetts) hold contractors accountable for measurable service improvements that are spelled out in a set of contractual terms and purchasing specifications (e.g., provision of member satisfaction data, clinical indicator data from HEDIS, and voluntary disenrollment rates) (Darby, 1998).

Public Health Monitoring

Another set of important quality assurance activities involves public health monitoring. Here, cancer registries, surveillance systems, and national survey data are used to monitor the epidemiology of cancer, the prevalence of risk factors, and the use of preventive health services. The adequacy of the nation's public health programs and services is, in part, judged by whether or not public health goals are met—for example, those established as part of the Centers for Disease Control and Prevention's (CDC's) Healthy People 2000 initiative, which highlights cancer as a priority area. The cancer objectives call for decreases in site-specific death rates (e.g., breast, colorectal); improved primary preventive health practices (e.g., reducing cigarette smoking, reducing dietary fat intake); improved early cancer detection (e.g., increased use of breast, colorectal, and cervical cancer screening); and ensuring that cancer screening and diagnostic tests meet quality standards (i.e., Pap tests, mammograms). As of 1997, progress had been made for 12 of the 17 cancer objectives, but in many cases the improvements have been slight (NCHS, 1997).

State public health agencies are building links with local health plans and providers to monitor public health goals. Plans for the Missouri Health Indicator Set, for example, include integrating public health records on births, deaths, hospital discharges, and cancer (Darby, 1998). Some States (e.g., New York, Pennsylvania) track hospital admissions and outcomes associated with certain procedures in an effort to monitor quality. New York, for example, has since the late 1980s collected standardized clinical data for coronary artery bypass surgery (CABS) patients, producing and publishing risk-adjusted mortality rates for hospitals and surgeons, and using these data to facilitate quality improvement efforts. The program has led to declines in statewide mortality (Chassin et al., 1996, 1998; Hannan et al., 1994).

Agency for Health Care Policy and Research

The Agency for Health Care Policy and Research (AHCPR) is the lead agency within the federal Department of Health and Human Services (DHHS) charged with supporting research on health care quality, cost, financing, and access (see Chapter 7). AHCPR has developed a number of practice guidelines (e.g., a 1994 practice guideline on cancer pain, which will be updated in 1999). Although no longer developing new practice guidelines, AHCPR in collaboration with the American Medical Association and the American Association of Health Plans has developed a national guideline clearinghouse accessible by Internet (www.guideline.gov). The website contains information on available guidelines, compares and contrasts the recommendations of guidelines, and allows communication among those involved in guideline development and dissemination (Stephenson, 1997).

QUALITY ASSURANCE: THE HEALTH CARE PROFESSIONAL APPROACH

Health care providers have established systems to monitor themselves and to demonstrate quality to parties outside the profession. Several organizations have incorporated quality measures into their voluntary accreditation programs (e.g., the JCAHO), developed quality monitoring systems (e.g., the National Committee for Quality Assurance), or have published standards with which to judge cancer care providers (e.g., American College of Surgeons' Commission on Cancer).

Joint Commission on Accreditation of Healthcare Organizations

The nonprofit Joint Commission on Accreditation of Healthcare Organizations, the oldest and largest standard-setting and accrediting body in health care, has broadened its institutional coverage from solely hospitals to a wide array of delivery systems including health plans, integrated delivery networks, PPOs, home care organizations, nursing homes and other long-term care facilities, behavioral health care organizations, ambulatory care providers, and clinical laboratories. JCAHO evaluates and accredits more than 16,000 health care organizations in the United States. Application for JCAHO accreditation is voluntary. About 80 percent of U.S. hospitals participate, representing about 96 percent of all inpatient admissions.

For accreditation, JCAHO conducts an on-site quality assessment every three years. It covers such topics as patient rights, patient care, patient education, continuity of care, ongoing efforts to improve quality, safety plans, information management, and infection control. Although JCAHO (and other accrediting organizations) has traditionally focused on structural measures of quality—such as whether a hospital has appropriate capacity for the covered patient population—it now incorporates process and outcomes measures into its accreditation criteria.

JCAHO instituted the ORYX system in 1997, which requires organizations seeking JCAHO accreditation to select from among 60 performance measurement systems and two specific indicators on which they will report their care. Hospitals and long-term care facilities are being instructed to begin reporting with these indicators during early 1999. One of the systems is JCAHO's Indicator Measurement System (IMS), which has specifications for 42 quality-of-care indicators (including 5 for cancer care; Table 6.1), and others are being developed. About 40–50 hospitals currently use the IMS reporting system (Chris McCravy, IMSystem, personal communication to Maria Hewitt, 1998). With institutions choosing their own indicators, making comparisons across institutions will be challenging. It should allow for comparisons with prior years within the same institution, benchmarks, and goals. JCAHO will soon rely on the American College of Surgeons' Commission on Cancer survey findings for cancer programs within JCAHO-accredited organizations (see below).

TABLE 6.1 Oncology Indicators of the JCAHO's IMSystem

	Data	Staging	Breast Cancer	Lung Cancer	Colon or Rectum Cancer
Focus	Availability of data for diagnosis and staging	Use of staging by managing physicians	Use of tests critical for prognosis and clinical management of female breast cancer	Effectiveness of preoperative diagnosis and staging	Comprehensiveness of diagnostic workup
Numerator	Patients undergoing resection for primary cancer of the lung, colon or rectum, or female breast for whom a surgical pathology consultation report is present in the medical record	Patients undergoing resection for primary cancer of the lung, colon or rectum, or female breast with stage of tumor designated by a managing physician	Female patients with Stage I or greater primary breast cancer who, after initial biopsy or resection, have estrogen receptor analysis results in the medical record	Patients with non-small-cell primary lung cancer undergoing thoracotomy with complete surgical resection of tumor	Patients undergoing resection for primary cancer of the colon or rectum whose preoperative evaluation by a managing physician included examination of the entire colon
Denominator	Patients undergoing resection for primary cancer of the lung, colon or rectum, or female breast	Patients undergoing resection for primary cancer of the lung, colon or rectum, or female breast	Female patients with Stage I or higher primary breast cancer undergoing initial biopsy or resection	Patients with non-small-cell primary lung cancer undergoing thoracotomy	Patients undergoing resection for primary cancer of the colon or rectum

SOURCE: IMSystem, 1997.

National Committee for Quality Assurance

The National Committee for Quality Assurance (NCQA) accredits managed care plans and has produced a widely used report card monitoring system called the Health Plan Employer Data and Information Set (HEDIS). As the name implies, HEDIS measures were initially designed to provide information to large purchasers about the quality of care offered to employees. More recently, the audience for results from HEDIS has broadened, and HEDIS indicators are often reported in consumer-oriented report cards.

HEDIS is a performance measurement tool designed to assist purchasers and consumers in evaluating managed care plans and holding plans accountable for the quality of their services. Because HEDIS has standard measures and uniform data reporting requirements, comparisons can be made across various health plans and their organizational structures (e.g., staff-model HMOs, point-of-service plans). The most recent iteration, HEDIS 3.0, assesses plans in eight domains: (1) effectiveness of care, (2) accessibility and availability of care, (3) satisfaction with care, (4) cost of care, (5) stability of the health plan, (6) informed health care choices, (7) use of services, and (8) descriptive information about the plan. In addition to the standard set of measures, a set of measures not used in current scoring is being tested for future iterations of HEDIS (Box 6.4). NCQA has appointed an Oncology Measurement Advisory Panel to review quality measures relevant to cancer care.

**BOX 6.4 Selected Cancer-Specific (or Cancer-Relevant)
HEDIS 3.0 Measures**

Effectiveness of Care

- Advising smokers to quit
- Cervical cancer screening
- Breast cancer screening
- Number of people in the plan who smoke*
- Smokers who quit*
- Colorectal cancer screening*
- Follow-up after an abnormal Pap smear*
- Follow-up after an abnormal mammogram (within 60 days)*
- Stage at which breast cancer was detected*
- Assessment of how breast cancer therapy affects the patient's ability to function*

Access to or Availability of Care

- Adults' access to preventive ambulatory health services
- Problems in obtaining care*

Satisfaction with the Experience of Care

- Member satisfaction
- Disenrollment*
- Satisfaction with breast cancer treatment*

Health Plan Stability

- Provider turnover

Health Plan Descriptive Information

- Provider board certification or residency completion
- Arrangements with public health, educational, and social service organizations

*Denotes testing set measures.

SOURCE: NCQA, 1998a.

The HEDIS cancer quality indicators have targeted early detection and diagnosis, not care received after cancer is diagnosed. NCQA's focus on early detection in cancer quality assessment appears to be related to its belief that "early detection remains the most effective way of improving the outcomes of breast cancer" (McGlynn, 1996). Treatment-related indicators are being evaluated—for example, assessment of the effect of breast cancer therapy on a woman's ability to function and patients' satisfaction with breast cancer treatment. NCQA has halted further work on the indicator related to the stage at which breast cancer is detected, because the incidence of breast cancer cases in most health plans is too low to make meaningful comparisons of stage at diagnosis across health plans (Schuster et al., 1998).

HEDIS is a voluntary system, although managed care plans are finding it increasingly necessary to participate to compete for patients. Some evidence suggests that most large employers are using HEDIS data to evaluate the managed care plans with which they contract (Hibbard et al., 1997a). In 1996, more than 330 plans—more than half of the plans in the United States, representing more than three-quarters of all commercial managed care enrollees—reported HEDIS measures on their enrollees. NCQA produces Quality Compass, a CD-ROM-based system that makes it possible for consumers to obtain comparative HEDIS ratings for HMOs in communities throughout the United States. A subset of Quality Compass measures appears on the World Wide Web. A health plan can refuse to disclose its HEDIS profile to the public. In 1997, less than half of plans (45 percent) permitted public reporting of the data (Bodenheimer, 1999).

American Accreditation Health Care Commission, Inc./URAC

The American Accreditation Health Care Commission, Inc./URAC (AAHC/URAC) accredits PPOs, point-of-service plans, and other open-panel plans. These plans represent a large segment of the private insurance market, yet they have relatively little in the way of a quality measurement infrastructure (Darby, 1998).

Foundation for Accountability

Although many indicators of quality that are relevant to purchasers are also relevant to consumers, the perspective of consumers is gaining a separate voice in several quality initiatives. The nonprofit Foundation for Accountability's (FACCT's) principal mission is to ensure that information on quality is effectively communicated to and used by consumers. FACCT has developed a quality assessment framework that uses categories designed to be descriptive of issues of concern to consumers: the basics, staying healthy, getting better, living with illness, and changing needs (www.facct.org; Lansky, 1998). FACCT has been developing new measures and selecting existing measures for use by others in assessing quality. One of the areas for which FACCT has been compiling a set of measures is breast cancer (Table 6.2). FACCT's breast cancer quality measures are the most comprehensive of any of the organizations that currently have breast cancer performance measures and include indicators of the process of care, patient satisfaction, and outcomes. These measures are currently being field-tested to determine the feasibility of their use.

American College of Surgeons' Commission on Cancer

Although not a formal accreditation program, The American College of Surgeons' Commission on Cancer surveys and approves hospitals, treatment centers, and other facilities according to established standards. The goal of the program is to improve the quality of patient care through multidisciplinary cancer programs that are concerned with prevention, early diagnosis, pretreatment evaluation, staging, optimal treatment, rehabilitation, surveillance, psychosocial support, and the hospice concept (http://www.facs.org). The Commission on Cancer has approved 1,500 programs, which are estimated to provide care for 80 percent of the nation's newly diagnosed patients (Carol Cook, Administrative Coordinator, American College of Surgeons, personal communication to Maria Hewitt, February, 1999).

TABLE 6.2 FACCT Breast Cancer Quality Indicators

Measure	Performance Value	Instrument or Data Source
Steps to Good Care		
Mammography	Proportion of women age 52–69 who have had a mammogram within two years	Doctor's billing or claims records (NCQA's HEDIS 3.0 breast screening measure used)
Early-stage detection	Proportion of patients whose breast cancer was detected at Stage 0 or Stage I	Patient records from cancer registry
Information about radiation treatment options	Proportion of Stage I and II patients who indicate that they had adequate information about their radiation treatment options before deciding about treatment	One question in patient satisfaction survey completed three to six months after diagnosis
Breast conserving surgery	Proportion of Stage I and II patients who undergo BCS	Patient records from cancer registry or claims records
Radiation therapy following breast conserving surgery	Proportion of BCS patients who receive radiation treatment after surgery	Patient records from cancer registry or claims records
Experience and Satisfaction		
Patient satisfaction with care	Mean score for patients' level of satisfaction with breast cancer care, including the technical quality, interpersonal and communication skills of their cancer doctor, their involvement in treatment decisions, and the timeliness of receiving information and services	32-item patient satisfaction survey completed three to six months after diagnosis
Results		
Experience of disease	Mean score for patients on CARES-SF survey, which assesses patients' quality of life and experience in living with breast cancer	59-item CARES-SF patient survey completed 12–15 months after diagnosis
Five-year disease-free survival (cancer treatment center measure)	Probability of disease-free survival for a group of patients, Stages I–IV, who were diagnosed during previous five years	Patient records from cancer registry

NOTE: CARES = Cancer Rehabilitation Evaluation System.

SOURCE: Foundation for Accountability, 1998.

An approved cancer program must provide specific state-of-the art diagnostic and treatment services in all medical disciplines that a person with cancer may need. The standards applied to institutions are not limited to surgery. Adherence to accepted clinical practice guidelines (e.g., AHCPR's Management of Cancer Pain) and the provision of discharge planning are, for example, among the standards used to evaluate programs.

A major initiative of the Comission on Cancer, in collaboration with the American Cancer Society, is the National Cancer Data Base (NCDB), which currently collects data routinely from 1,600 hospitals in all 50 states on all the patients with cancer they treat. With the program now in its sixth year, more than half of U.S. patients newly diagnosed with cancer are included. Basic demographic information about the patient, type and stage of cancer, and nature of the treatment given are reported electronically. Aggregate data from the country are available publicly. In addition, each hospital is given back its own data in summary form, which it can use to compare with national data ("benchmarking"). The national data allow problem areas to be pinpointed (e.g., widespread use of an inappropriate treatment for a particular type of cancer) and the observation of trends over time in such characteristics as stage at diagnosis, percentage of patients who have complete staging information, and type of treatment given. Results of NCDB analyses are published regularly in professional journals (NCDB, 1999).

In addition to routine data collection, each year two Patient Care Evaluation (PCE) studies are carried out, focusing on specific cancer types or general treatment issues. More extensive data are collected for these special studies, allowing a more detailed analysis of how patients are treated, with the data again fed back to hospitals so that they can see how they compare in the national spectrum. Specific information on each disease is included. For example, the breast cancer section of the report featured quality benchmarks such as completeness of disease staging according to the American Joint Committee on Cancer (AJCC), percentage utilization of breast conservation surgery for early breast cancers, and percentage of patients undergoing BCS who also received adjuvant radiotherapy. The NCDB expects an increase in hospital participation in the coming years, and it will make outcomes data available on-line. NCDB estimates that three out of every four U.S. patients with cancer will be reported on by the year 2000 (American College of Surgeons, 1999).

The findings of the American College of Surgeons' Commission on Cancer survey will soon be used as part of JCAHO's accreditation process for JCAHO-accredited organizations that house a cancer center. The collaboration is an attempt to increase the visibility of approved cancer programs, share information on standards and survey process, and increase consumer access to health care organization performance information. Reports will allow approved programs to benchmark their performance with that of other programs (ACS/CoC, 1998).

Association of Community Cancer Centers

To promote quality improvement among cancer centers, the Association of Community Cancer Centers (ACCC), a membership organization for cancer centers, has published "Standards for Cancer Programs," a description of an "ideal" cancer program (ACCC, 1997) (see Box 6.5). The standards are based on expert opinion rather than a systemic review of evidence. ACCC has not undertaken a study of the extent to which these standards have been met.

BOX 6.5 Association of Community Cancer Centers— Standards for Cancer Programs

Program Leadership
- Administrative structure is in place to ensure efficient, appropriate, and effective management of the cancer program and services.

Cancer Committee
- An interdisciplinary standing Cancer Committee provides program leadership.

Medical Director
- The program has a designated medical director on a part- or full-time basis.
- The authority of the medical director is defined and documented by the sponsoring organization of the program.
- The medical director is subject to a minimum of annual performance review.

Cancer Registry
- A cancer registry will be maintained to meet and preferably exceed the minimum requirements of the Commission on Cancer of the American College of Surgeons.

Continuous Performance Improvement
- Patient care is monitored and evaluated for the quality of services. Continuous performance improvement (CPI) plans are generated from quality review data, including attributes of timeliness, appropriateness of care, clinical outcomes of disease-free survival, and effective management of disease and treatment sequelae.

Staff Support
- A structured program for staff support is available (e.g., educational and professional skill development opportunities).

Multimodality Treatment
- Multimodality and interdisciplinary cancer case reviews are conducted on a regular basis to ensure patients' access to consultative services by all disciplines.
- Tumor conference case review is prospective in nature. Prospective is defined as prior to treatment or any time a clinical treatment plan is reviewed for further evaluation.

Patient Advocacy and Survivorship
- Information and programs specific to patients' advocacy and survivorship issues are available to cancer patients and their families.

Cancer Education and Resource Program
- Education and resource programs are developed and provided for primary care providers, cancer patients and families, and the community.

Continued

BOX 6.5 *Continued*

Cancer Prevention and Detection

- Cancer prevention and detection programs are available to reduce the risk of developing cancer, teach self-examination and symptom identification techniques, provide screening guidelines, and communicate the availability of community resources (e.g., screening mammography) for early detection.

Clinical Research

- Cancer patients are provided access to clinical research programs including treatment and cancer prevention and control trials.

Ethics

- Oncology professionals will uphold a professional code of ethics and conduct as defined by the appropriate governing professional organization.
- Oncology professionals will uphold a professional code of ethics, conduct, and confidentiality as defined by the policies and procedures of their respective employers.
- A mechanism for ethics consults should be available.

Interdisciplinary Team

- There is an interdisciplinary team approach to planning, implementing, and evaluating the care of cancer patients and their families.

Nutritional Support Services

- A clinical dietitian is available to work with patients and their families, especially those identified as at risk for having nutritional problems or special needs. The dietitian provides dietary guidelines on reducing cancer risk through program materials and services to the community.

Oncology Nursing Services

- Nursing care of the cancer patient is provided by nurses with specialized knowledge and skill in oncology.

Pastoral Care

- Pastoral care services are available to meet the needs of patients and their families.

Pharmacy Services

- Pharmacy services will purchase, store, and prepare cytotoxic agents in a safe and efficient manner.
- The dispensing of investigational drugs will meet all federal regulations.
- Pharmacy services will store and maintain all investigational cytotoxic agents in a safe and efficient manner.
- Pharmacy and oncology nursing services will prepare extravasation guidelines and drug kits for use by the nursing department.
- Pharmacy services will maintain current information on the safe handling of cytotoxic agents and prepare information for employees involved in preparation and administration of these agents.

Continued

BOX 6.5 *Continued*

Rehabilitation Services
- Comprehensive rehabilitation services are available to cancer patients and their families.

Psychosocial Services
- Social work services are provided by licensed social workers prepared at the master's level and experienced in meeting the psychosocial needs of patients and their families.
- Psychosocial services are directed by written policies and procedures.

Pain Management
- Acute and chronic cancer pain management guidelines are available to assist professional staff in alleviating patient suffering and improving quality of life.

Oncology Unit
- An inpatient oncology unit is designed for the care of patients with cancer and their families.

Ambulatory Oncology Services
- An outpatient facility or office is available and dedicated to outpatient cancer care.
- A radiation oncology facility is available for treatments.
- Integration of oncology services for optimal treatment planning, evaluation, and follow-up.

Home Care
- A home health agency or referral relationship exists to provide professional services to cancer patients and their families in the home.

Hospice
- A hospice program exists to provide professional and volunteer services to patients with cancer in the terminal stage of disease and their families. Bereavement for families is provided for a minimum of six months.

SOURCE: Association of Community Cancer Centers, 1997.

QUALITY IMPROVEMENT WITHIN HEALTH CARE ORGANIZATIONS

Several techniques are available for using internal quality assessments to improve quality within an organization. Ideally, information on quality shows where to focus efforts for improvement. Traditional quality assurance programs focus on retraining or removing clinicians who stand out as performing below group norms. By contrast, continuous quality improvement (CQI) programs (also known as total quality management [TQM] programs) focus on improving the quality of care delivered by all clinicians, with the goal of raising the average level of quality in an organization. CQI assumes that most examples of poor quality are due to correctable systematic problems rather than to individual incompetence or irresponsibility. It often incorporates routine collection and monitoring of information to assess quality so that the organization can identify and respond to problems in a timely fashion. CQI generally uses interdisciplinary teams both to identify inefficiencies that increase errors and to institute checks that make errors easier to prevent and catch (Berwick, 1989; Kritchevsky and Simmons, 1991). For example, a group of cardiothoracic surgeons practicing in three states used CQI and other techniques to improve their practices and found a 24 percent reduction in their combined mortality rates (O'Connor et al., 1996).

A hospital that finds medication errors might review the many steps involved in the process by which physicians, nurses, pharmacists, and others provide medications to patients. Solutions might include having nurses and pharmacists double-check doses, using standardized doses for patient weight ranges to reduce calculation errors, and having a standard location for documentation of all drug allergies (Leape et al., 1995). Prevention of medication errors is particularly important for cancer chemotherapy, and efforts have been initiated to improve safeguards (Cohen et al., 1996).

While there are concrete examples of the success of some CQI efforts, some health care experts do not believe that the movement has made a sizable impact on the U.S. health care system (Blumenthal et al., 1998).

Practice Guidelines

Practice guidelines are systematically developed recommendations about some or all aspects of decision making for a particular condition or clinical situation (IOM, 1990). The development of guidelines usually involves a review of the relevant research and clinical literature. The best guidelines make explicit the methods used to develop them, including how evidence was used to support recommendations. Clinical practice guidelines can be judged according to several attributes, for example, their validity, reliability, and clarity (Table 6.3).

TABLE 6.3 Institute of Medicine List of Desirable Attributes of Clinical Practice Guidelines

Attribute	Description
Validity	Lead to health and cost outcomes projected for them
Reliability/reproducibility	Given the same evidence and methods, another set of experts would produce essentially the same statement
Applicability	Explicitly state the population to which they apply
Flexibility	Identify specific exceptions
Clarity	Use unambiguous language and precise definition of terms
Multidisciplinary process	Involve participation by representatives of key affected groups
Scheduled review	Indicate when they should be reviewed
Documentation	All procedures, participants, evidence, assumptions, and analytic methods must be documented and described

SOURCE: IOM, 1990.

There are two general types of guidelines: *path* or algorithm guidelines, which include branch points and if–then statements to guide decision-making according to a standard of care, and *boundary* guidelines, which are used to define the appropriate use of a new (and generally expensive) technology. Guidelines are not intended to dictate a rigid approach to care; rather, they give options that clinicians should be aware of, even if they choose a different strategy for a particular patient. Guidelines are partly an outgrowth of the boom in scientific information that makes it difficult for individual physicians to keep up with medical advances.

Practice guidelines have been developed by government agencies (e.g., AHCPR), specialty organizations (e.g., American Society of Clinical Oncology), and cancer centers. The National Comprehensive Cancer Network (NCCN), a consortium of 15 leading cancer centers, has assembled expert panels to review evidence and develop guidelines on the treatment of 15 of the most common cancers (Marwick, 1997; McGivney, 1998). Many other hospitals and health care systems have developed their own guidelines (e.g., use of antiemetics, use of single daily dose antibiotics for infection), but they are generally not available to other institutions (see Table 6.4—for this review, cancer screening guidelines were not considered).

The Advisory Board Company, a private consulting group, has launched an Oncology Roundtable to provide cancer centers with information on "best" practices in the following areas: patient-focused oncology (i.e., ensuring convenient access, informed decision making, compassionate care, quality service); breast cancer management; prostate cancer management; and pain management (Advisory Board, 1998).

Disease management programs incorporate a systematic approach for the management of specific chronic disorders (e.g., asthma, diabetes), which often include adherence to clinical guidelines. The goal of these programs is to improve quality of care and outcomes, integrate and coordinate care, and track and manage costs associated with chronic illnesses. Memorial Sloan-Kettering Cancer Center has, for example, established 17 disease management teams to develop treatment pathways, track resource consumption, and identify appropriate patient education materials for cancers (McDermott, 1997). Nearly 100 clinical paths have been developed at the M.D. Anderson Cancer Center as part of its disease management program (Morris, 1996; Morris et al., 1996).

Practice guidelines are available for only a small fraction of oncology practice, but for some cancers, several guidelines are available. When to create a practice guideline can be difficult to gauge. The impetus to create a guideline often comes from evidence of widespread variation in practice; however, this is often a sign that there is little evidence upon which to construct a guideline. Guidelines based on sound evidence rather than expert opinion are most likely to succeed in influencing provider practice. Sometimes practice guidelines can be issued too late, after providers have already changed behavior in light of new evidence. A major recommendation of the 1979 National Institutes of Health (NIH) Consensus Development conference on treatment of primary breast cancer—that few Halsted radical mastectomies should be done—was found in subsequent reviews of medical practice to be moot since the procedure was being performed very infrequently (Kanouse et al., 1989). If the intent of a guideline is to inform and possibly change physician behavior, priority should be given to developing guidelines for which there is practice variation, despite good evidence to support a standard set of practices (U.S. Congress, 1994).

TABLE 6.4 Selected Oncology Guidelines, by Sponsoring Group

Group	Guidelines	Comment
National Comprehensive Cancer Network (NCCN)	Path or algorithm guidelines for all common cancers	Evidence-based, with consensus; when no consensus possible, options listed Intended for mandatory use for all participating cancer centers No set date for implementation No set benchmarks for care Adopted in the community for use outside of NCCN cancer centers No data yet on compliance or outcomes
American Society of Clinical Oncology (ASCO)	Boundary guidelines for new technologies Hematopoietic growth factors Outcomes important enough to justify treatment Antiemetics Surveillance of breast and colorectal cancer patients Path or algorithm guidelines for specific diseases Management of non-small-cell lung cancer Metastatic prostate cancer	Evidence-based with consensus demanded before approval Adopted by the community but no data available on compliance or outcomes Likely that all future guidelines will be boundary guidelines for new technologies, with overlap of ASCO and NCCN methods and topics
Society for Surgical Oncology	Path guidelines for management of common surgical problems	Consensus panels
American Urology Association	Path guidelines for common urology problems Localized prostate cancer	Consensus based on evidence
University of California Cancer Care Consortium (UC and PONA, Inc.)	Path guidelines for most solid tumors	PONA did systematic reviews, consulted with UC faculty for consensus

Organizations Whose Guidelines Are not Available (proprietary)

Kaiser Permanente Salicknet, Inc. Value Health Science, Inc. Multiple others	Path guidelines for management of common oncology problems	Consensus based on evidence; not available outside the corporation

SOURCE: Smith and Hillner, 1998.

Variation in practice often reflects uncertainty and points to a need for rigorous clinical research. There are, for example, no randomized clinical trials comparing best supportive care versus second-line chemotherapy for patients with non-small-cell lung cancer. (There are limited Phase II data from single institutions.) An American Society of Clinical Oncology (ASCO) guideline on this topic noted that no benefit could be proven in either survival or quality of life, so no recommendation could be made for or against second-line chemotherapy (ASCO, 1997). Without evidence to discourage it, the aggressive use of chemotherapy is common. In a survey of practices for dying patients, more than 50 percent of ASCO members stated that they would give second-line chemotherapy to a 43-year-old woman with progressive non-small-cell lung cancer, nearly 20 percent would give third-line chemotherapy, and a substantial number would give fourth-line chemotherapy (Ezekiel Emanuel, personal communication to Tom Smith, 1998).

Multiple guidelines on the same topic are not always consistent. Breast cancer screening guidelines, for example, differ in the recommended age at which routine mammography screening should begin. That there are differences in practice guidelines is not surprising given the many factors that can affect the ultimate conclusions of a guideline. Guideline recommendations may vary because of differences in the composition of guideline panels, the way evidence from the literature is reviewed, the interpretation of evidence, and the procedures to reach agreement on recommendations. The interpretation of data depends on values and perspectives. Some patients and practitioners will think that a small and statistically non-significant improvement in six-month disease-free survival associated with the use of high-dose chemotherapy in lymphoma is sufficient evidence of clinical benefit, whereas others will not.

Guideline panel membership appears to have a strong effect on shaping recommendations. There is, for example, evidence of a user bias in which physicians who perform a given intervention are more likely to judge it as beneficial. When faced with the same evidence from the literature on the effectiveness of carotid endarterectomy, a panel of surgeons rated 70 percent of indications as appropriate, whereas a multidisciplinary group found only 38 percent of indications to be appropriate (Leape et al., 1992). Panels in the United Kingdom and the United States with the same physician mix came to different conclusions when assessing the appropriateness of treatment for coronary disease, in part because the U.K. panelists seemed to require a higher standard of scientific evidence than did their U.S. counterparts (Brook et al., 1988).

One of the hallmarks of a good guideline is having clear documentation of the methods used to arrive at recommendations. The ASCO text that supports the guideline on the provision of follow-up services for patients with breast cancer can be critiqued for not documenting the basis of the guideline's recommendations. Evidence from a well-designed randomized clinical trial indicated that outcomes for women with breast cancer were similar whether follow-up care was provided by a general practice doctor or a specialist surgeon, but the ASCO guideline reinforced the ASCO board's policy that all patients with cancer have the right to see a cancer specialist at all times (Grunfeld et al., 1996). In this case, group opinion and a desire to be consistent with ASCO policy took precedence over the available literature in framing the recommendation, but the guideline does not make this explicit.

The guideline process is a dynamic one, which must incorporate new information as it becomes available. New evidence from the largest clinical trial on follow-up care for individuals with colorectal cancer will, for example, have to be considered as available guidelines are revised. The current NCCN guidelines, for example, recommend annual chest x-ray, annual colonoscopy, and regular computed axial tomography scans, all strategies that do not improve survival according to new evidence (Schoemaker et al., 1998).

How successful guidelines are in informing and changing practice depends in large part on how they are developed, disseminated, and implemented. Personal involvement in the process of change encourages adherence, and evidence suggests that physicians are more likely to ascribe credibility to information from sources they know and respect (U.S. Congress, 1994). Guidelines with greatest likelihood of success include those with internal development, specific educational intervention, patient-specific reminders at the time of consultation, and a system to hold the provider accountable for adherence (Table 6.5) (Grimshaw and Russell, 1993; Smith and Hillner, 1998). Guidelines that have a lower chance of success are those issued by a national group with no ties to local practitioners, those that rely on publication in a journal to disseminate findings, and those that limit implementation to general reminders about the recommendations. In general, changes in practice are more likely if implementation efforts are more active and intensive, if they involve multiple- rather than single-pronged approaches, and if the efforts are tailored to the specific context and problems addressed by a particular guideline (U.S. Congress, 1994). Clear benchmarks, or targets, for good practice are needed to implement and evaluate guidelines (Schoenbaum et al., 1995).

Some clinical practices are more amenable to change than others. Cancer screening practices, for example, can be increased by using computer and manual reminders, as well as a variety of other administrative mechanisms. Guidelines for the use of x-rays, blood tests, and pharmaceuticals have also been implemented successfully. Interventions to change practice have been less successful for more complex clinical decisions, such as choosing between medical and surgical treatments or managing complex medical problems (U.S. Congress, 1994).

TABLE 6.5 Framework for Analysis of Clinical Practice Guideline Success

Likelihood of Success	Development	Dissemination	Implementation	Accountability
High	Internal	Specific educational intervention	Patient-specific reminder at time of encounter	Practice monitored, feedback given
Above average	Intermediate	Continuing education	Patient-specific feedback	Practice monitored
Below average	External/local	Mailing targeted groups	General feedback	None
Low	National/external	Publication in journal	General feedback	None

SOURCE: Grimshaw and Russell, 1993, modified by Smith and Hillner, 1998.

What Evidence Is There That Cancer Practice Guidelines Have Been Successful?

There have been a modest number of successful clinical practice guideline efforts, as well as a number of documented failures. In some areas, improvements in guideline compliance have been demonstrated, but often the improvement in practice has not been substantial.

The Community Hospital Oncology Program. The Community Hospital Oncology Program (CHOP) represents an early attempt to improve oncology by disseminating locally developed practice guidelines. From 1982 to 1984, 17 CHOP programs located throughout the country implemented site-specific guidelines for staging, medical management, nursing, and rehabilitation. Community practice for breast, rectal, and small-cell lung cancer was evaluated in 1985–1986 after the program had been fully implemented. There was no evidence of diffusion of guideline principles to the majority of practicing physicians, even·those who were involved in their development (Table 6.6).

TABLE 6.6 Conformance to Accepted Standards of Care

Cancer	Standard (%)	Conformance (%)
Breast		
Clinical staging	100	33
Medical oncology consultation if node-positive	100	73
Radiation oncology consultation	100	27
Rectal		
Staging	100	67
Radiation therapy consultation	100	27
Small-Cell Lung Cancer		
Radiation oncology consultation	100	50

SOURCE: Ford et al., 1987.

Some CHOPs developed more intense programs to encourage compliance that included tumor boards, educational efforts, peer pressure, and administrative action. The CHOPs that were able to ensure staging did so by requiring completion of forms before specimens were submitted to pathology or denying privileges if forms were not completed. As the authors note, these measures were successful but did not require guidelines. The authors conclude that for clinical practice guidelines, "leadership and organizational commitment appear to be the necessary ingredients."

Even though the guidelines were developed locally, it is likely that the program failed to change provider behavior because there was no plan for implementation and no system to hold providers accountable for change (Katterhagen, 1996).

ASCO Guideline on Use of Hematopoietic Growth Factors. Hematopoietic growth factors are effective when administered to prevent or treat neutropenia (an abnormally small number of a type of blood cell), which may occur following chemotherapy, but they do not improve outcomes for those with febrile neutropenia (fever associated with neutropenia). The growth factors are expensive to use ($200 to $300 per dose), but there is little harm to patients if they are administered inappropriately. Their administration can be a significant source of income to a physician. Guidelines issued by ASCO in 1994 on the use of hematopoietic growth factors led to some reduction in their inappropriate use, but serious overuse of these substances persisted. This finding was based on physicians' self-reported use of hematopoietic growth factors on surveys conducted before, and shortly after, the 1994 guideline was issued and again following the publication of a guideline update in 1996. Response rates to the surveys were roughly 60 percent. Inappropriate use of hematopoietic growth factors was sharply reduced in one managed care organization by the institution of a simple accountability system. Before administering growth factors, physicians had to call the administrator and report the indication for its use (J.E. Katterhagen, personal communication to Thomas Smith, 1998).

AHCPR Cancer Pain Management Guidelines. Recent studies suggest that as many as one in four cancer patients is given inadequate pain relief (Rischer and Childress, 1996). Adherence to the 1994 AHCPR guideline on cancer pain management, following its widespread dissemination, was assessed in seven acute care hospitals in Utah in 1995 and again in 1996 (Rischer and Childress, 1996). On most process measures, care improved, but outcomes (e.g., pain scores) were not assessed (Table 6.7). A limitation of this study is the absence of a concurrent control group that was not exposed to the guideline dissemination intervention. Without such a group, one cannot attribute improvements to the guidelines. The program to improve pain management according to the AHCPR guideline has been implemented throughout Utah.

TABLE 6.7 Compliance with Core Guidelines

Guideline	Pre[a]	Post[b]	p Value
Opioids Prescribed	99	100	1.000
Initial Pain Assessment			
Rating Scale Used	64	79	.090
Ongoing Pain Assessment			
Pain rating scale repeated at regular intervals	27	74	<.001
Efficacy reported	83	97	.011
Analgesic Use			
Pain medicines on regular schedule	70	91	.003
Bowel Treatment Plan			
Laxatives ordered	66	69	.857
Education of Family or Patient			
Education about cancer pain	6	34	<.001
Written education	16	26	.238
Patient Satisfaction Evaluated (not actual patient satisfaction)	24	97	<.001

NOTE: Ten patients were assessed at each of seven hospitals; $n = 70$.

[a] Pre = before guideline was issued.
[b] Post = after guideline was issued.

SOURCE: Rischer and Childress, 1996.

American Urologic Association Early Prostate Cancer Guideline. The American Urologic Association recommended in 1995 that patients with localized prostate cancer be offered surgery, radiation, or surveillance as treatment options. To assess compliance with the guideline in the military health system (i.e., those covered by CHAMPUS), men who had received radical prostatectomy before and after the guideline was published were asked in a survey to report whether or not they had been offered treatment options. The guideline was mailed to each practitioner within the system. The average number of treatments offered increased following publication of the guideline (Thompson et al., 1995). A limitation of this study is that it included only men undergoing radical prostatectomy, not all men with prostate cancer.

Evidence on the Impact of Guidelines in Canada and Europe

Canada. Adherence to breast cancer guidelines in British Columbia as assessed in 1991 was very high for radiation therapy, with 95 percent of women receiving radiation therapy following breast conserving surgery. However, only 77 percent of women received adjuvant chemotherapy when indicated, and 68 percent received tamoxifen when indicated (Olivotto, 1997). Adherence to guidelines was higher at cancer centers than among community oncologists. Improvements in disease-free and overall survival coincided with implementation of the guidelines, but other factors such as the regionalization of cancer care services and the presence of strong opinion leaders may account for good outcomes.

Italy. In an effort to improve community-based cancer care in Italy, guidelines on the treatment of breast, colorectal, and ovarian cancer were sent to practitioners in 1977. The effects of the educational program were evaluated in 1987 (Grilli et al., 1991). The familiarity of practitioners with the breast cancer guidelines was poor: roughly one-half knew of the breast cancer guideline, one-third knew of the colon cancer guidelines, and one-quarter knew of the ovarian cancer guidelines (estimates are weighted averages of respondents to a survey of providers). Compliance with the recommendations of the guidelines was poor in several areas as shown by chart audit. For women with breast cancer, for example, only 37 percent had full staging, and only 61 percent had a bilateral mammogram at the time of surgery (Table 6.8). Better compliance was observed among physicians with high-volume practices. The authors note that the results were "disappointing" and that efforts to improve cancer care with a "guidelines diffusion" approach appear to have had a negligible effect on cancer treatment.

France. Cancer care guidelines developed and disseminated through a regional cancer center in Lyon, France, appear to have succeeded in improving cancer care. Guidelines on breast and colon cancer were developed by a task force in 1993 and then reviewed by all practitioners in the region. In 1994, the guidelines were widely available via different media—paper, computer disk, and on-line at the cancer center. A comparison of randomly selected patients with breast and colon cancer treated in 1993 and 1995 showed marked improvements in care. From 1993 to 1995, adherence to the recommended overall treatment sequence increased from 19 to 54 percent for breast cancer and from 50 to 70 percent for colon cancer (Table 6.9). The guidelines were reviewed again in 1995 and disseminated to a wider network of hospitals and providers through continuing education meetings and mailed reminders to physicians. Compliance measured from 1994 to 1996 also improved (Ray-Coquard et al., 1998). The success of the guideline program was attributed in part to the local development of the guidelines, their wide dissemination, and the reliance on peer pressure to change practice behavior (Ray-Coquard et al., 1997). The studies lacked a concurrent control group that was not exposed to the guideline intervention, so it is unclear whether improvements were due to the guideline program or to a generally increased awareness in the medical community.

Scotland. As part of its national health plan, Scotland has initiated comprehensive efforts to improve cancer care. On a national basis, it has limited reimbursement for cancer services to practitioners who agree to use evidence-based guidelines and submit their results to external scrutiny. Full results of the first three years of this program will be available in 1999 (Smith et al., 1998).

Effects of Local Guideline Implementation on Costs

Whether implementing guidelines increases or decreases costs depends on the medical interventions involved. Guidelines aimed at currently overused services will likely reduce some spending, whereas those aimed at underused services could increase spending. Some guidelines might shift spending from inappropriate to more appropriate care, leading to better value but not necessarily lower costs (IOM, 1992). Although the intention of guidelines is usually to improve care, an added benefit may be increased efficiency and cost savings. There are several anecdotal accounts of cost savings associated with local implementation of practice guidelines, often with attendant improvements in care:

• Implementing surgical care guidelines for patients with gynecologic cancer in one surgical practice improved clinical outcomes, decreased hospital length of stay, decreased costs, and kept patient satisfaction high. A team approach to guideline development and accountability systems accounted for the program's success (Morris et al., 1997).
• Implementing surgical care guidelines for patients undergoing radical prostatectomy in hospital practice decreased length of stay, while maintaining high scores on patient satisfaction and quality of life (Litwin et al., 1996).
• Implementing clinical pathways and treatment protocols in one cancer group practice led to greater efficiency (increases in number of patient encounters, decreases in costs) and increased participation in clinical research (Feinberg and Feinberg, 1998).
• Implementing a clinical practice guideline for endoscopic sinus surgery at an academic medical center led to improved short-term outcomes (i.e., fewer unplanned admissions) and lower costs (Stewart et al., 1997).
• Implementing critical pathways for cancer care within a managed care organization reduced length of stay and costs for patients treated for respiratory cancer and for those undergoing chest procedures and bowel surgery (Patton and Katterhagen, 1997).

In summary, several organizations have developed oncology practice guidelines to promote treatment that conforms to the best medical evidence available. Guidelines for many aspects of cancer care are not available, in part because the evidence base upon which to judge best practice does not exist. The oncology guidelines that have been put into practice have not been uniformly successful in changing physician behavior or clinical outcomes. Aspects of guideline development and implementation affect success, and the most successful guidelines are those with internal development, specific educational interventions, patient-specific reminders at the time of consultation, and a system to hold providers accountable for adherence. Studies of the impact of oncology guidelines have often not included a concurrent control group that was not exposed to the guideline intervention, which makes it difficult to attribute change to guideline implementation.

TABLE 6.8 Compliance with National Guidelines in Italy as Measured by Chart Audit, 1987

Recommendation	Compliance (%)
Breast Cancer	Gold standard: 100%
Bilateral mammography	61
Clinical stage	37
Pathological stage	60
Evaluation of axillary lymph nodes	89
Avoidance of radical mastectomy if $T < 2.0$ cm	84
Radiotherapy after quadrantectomy	65
Adjuvant chemotherapy started at <4 weeks	52
Polychemotherapy if <50, + lymph nodes	71
Chemotherapy delivered at full dosage	86
Colon Cancer	
CEA levels and liver ultrasound	40
TNM staging	78
Search for intra-abdominal metastasis	67
Information on resection borders	48
Evaluation of regional lymph nodes	66
Miles resection in lower rectal cancer	68
Radiotherapy in rectal and rectosigmoid cancer	11
No adjuvant chemotherapy in colon cancer	79
If chemotherapy, 5-FU-containing regimen	90
Ovarian Cancer	
Full information on tumor grading	30
Staging including abdominal echography	75
Histologic type according to standard classifications	89
Chest x-ray	97
Evaluation of residual tumor	45
Disease stage according to standard classification	85
Alkylating agent as part of chemotherapy for early disease	18
Cisplatin-containing regimens for advanced disease	34
Monitoring of toxicity while on chemotherapy	91
Monitoring of nephrotoxicity while on chemotherapy	84

NOTE: CEA = carcinoembryonic antigen; 5-FU = 5-fluorouracil; TNM = tumor–node–mestastasis.

SOURCE: Grilli et al., 1991.

TABLE 6.9 Compliance Rates of Medical Decisions with Guidelines, Lyon, France

Type of Procedure	Compliant with Clinical Practice Guidelines (%)		
	1993	1995	*p* Value
Breast Cancer			
Initial evaluation	75	86	.09
Surgery	96	92	.26
Chemotherapy	71	85	.01
Radiotherapy	72	93	<.001
Hormonal therapy	83	94	.01
Follow-up	31	80	<.001
Overall treatment sequence	19	54	<.001
Colon Cancer			
Initial evaluation	100	100	
Surgery	100	99	.56
Chemotherapy	56	78	.02
Follow-up	62	54	.69
Overall treatment sequence	50	70	.009

SOURCE: Ray-Coquard et al., 1998.

KEY FINDINGS

Information about quality cancer care is becoming more available to individuals with cancer (or at risk for cancer), but it is not yet easily accessible to or understandable for consumers. A number of potential quality indicators can be listed, but most have not been evaluated to assess their ultimate value to consumers. It is unclear, for example, how the following indicators affect an individual's experience of care or health care outcomes:

- a physician's board certification,
- a hospital's approval status determined by the American College of Surgeons' Commission on Cancer, and
- a health plan's accreditation status and HEDIS scores.

By the time a diagnosis of cancer is made and individuals have a clear reason to seek quality cancer care, it is often too late to switch health plans. Even if they could, however, many individuals do not have access to alternative plans. Individuals may use available quality indicators to choose doctors and hospitals within their plans, and perhaps to choose alternative courses of treatment, but evidence suggests that individual consumers can exert only a modest market pressure for quality improvement through access to better information about the quality of cancer care.

Quality assurance systems are often not apparent to consumers, but they have the potential to greatly affect care. Some large employer groups are beginning to hold health plans to quality performance goals. HCFA is requiring health plans, hospitals, and other providers to produce standardized quality reports, and state Medicaid programs are beginning to include quality provisions in their contracts with providers. The development of better standards and performance measures for cancer care could provide a way for large employers or groups of purchasers to exert influence on the quality of cancer and other health care.

A variety of mechanisms are being used to improve health care from the inside: total quality improvement initiatives, disease management programs, and implementation of clinical practice guidelines all have the potential to improve care. The experience with oncology practice guidelines has been mixed, with some examples of success but others of ineffectiveness in changing provider behavior or outcomes. Many guideline efforts have failed because of limitations in the way they were developed or implemented.

There are numerous health care accountability systems in place, but they fail to constitute a coordinated system for ensuring quality health care in general, and they do not yet embody a comprehensive, organized effort for cancer care. Given the diversity of the U.S. health care system, such fragmentation is not unexpected, but it could be remedied through a combination of public regulation and cooperation between public- and private-sector purchasers of care. Although much of the impetus for quality accountability has come from the private and professional sectors, government-sponsored programs have promoted public health accountability by maintaining cancer surveillance systems and monitoring the use of cancer screening tests among the U.S. population. The elderly are disproportionately affected by cancer, and cancer care quality indicators have in some areas been integrated into programs designed to ensure appropriate treatment for Medicare beneficiaries. The Agency for Health Care Policy and Research has assumed an important convening role in tracking clinical practice guidelines and supporting the basic health services research needed to form the basis of future guidelines.

Comprehensive improvements in health care quality and in the ability of consumers to make health care decisions that are fully informed on the basis of quality will likely occur only through collaborative efforts of the public and private sectors (President's Advisory Commission, 1998). As large health care purchasers, both sectors have a stake in improving the quality of care, and both sectors have knowledge and experience concerning quality measurement and reporting. Each sector has unique strengths. Private-sector organizations have the capacity to act quickly in response to rapid changes in the health care system. The public sector can provide established channels and safeguards to ensure representative action and open proceedings. Such an approach has recently been recommended by the President's Advisory Commission on Consumer Protection and Quality in the Health Care Industry, and some initial steps have being taken to implement a public–private collaborative effort (President's Advisory Commission, 1998). A concerted public–private collaboration on the development and reporting of performance standards for cancer and other care could provide a framework for changing incentives in the system so that they aim at publicly accountable measures of quality.

REFERENCES

The Advisory Board. 1998. *The Oncology Roundtable.* The Advisory Board Company, Washington D.C.
American College of Surgeons. 1999. National Cancer Data Base: Future plans. http://www.facs.org

American College of Surgeons, Commission on Cancer. 1998. *News from the Commission on Cancer* 9(3):4.

American Society of Clinical Oncology. 1997. Clinical practice guidelines for the treatment of unresectable non-small-cell lung cancer. *Journal of Clinical Oncology* 15(8):2996–3018.

Association of Community Cancer Centers. 1997. *Standards for Cancer Programs.*

Berwick D. 1989. Continuous improvement as an ideal in health care. *New England Journal of Medicine* 320:53–56.

Blumenthal D, Kilo CM. 1998. A report card on continuous quality improvement. *Milbank Quarterly* 76(4):625–648.

Bodenheimer T. 1999. The American health care system: The movement for improved quality in health care. *New England Journal of Medicine* 340(6):488–492.

Brook RH, Park RE, Winslow CM, et al. 1988. Diagnosis and treatment of coronary disease: Comparison of doctor's attitudes in the U.S.A. and the U.K. *Lancet* 1(8588):750–753.

Byers T, Bott R, Palmer L, et al. 1998. Age is the prinicipal determinant of the use of adjuvant cancer therapy: Findings from a study of cancer care in Colorado. Denver, CO: Colarado Foundation for Medical Care.

CancerDesk. 1999. *New Approaches to Advancing the Health of the Nation: Health Information Technology Institute.* Mitretek Systems. http://www.mitretek.org/hiti/mission/index.html.

Castles AG, Milstein A, Damberg CL. 1999. Using employer purchasing power to improve the quality of perinatal care. *Pediatrics* 103(1 Suppl. E):248–254.

Chassin MR, Gavin RW. 1998. The urgent need to improve health care quality. Institute of Medicine National Roundtable on Health Care Quality. *Journal of the American Medical Association* 280(11):1000–1005.

Chassin MR, Hannan EL, DeBuono BA. 1996. Benefits and hazards of reporting medical outcomes publicly. *New England Journal of Medicine* 334:394–398.

Clark E, Stovall E, Leigh S, et al. 1995. *Imperatives for Quality Cancer Care: Access, Advocacy, Action, and Accountability.* Silver Springs, MD: National Coalition for Cancer Survivorship.

Cleary PD, Edgman-Levitan S. 1997. Health care quality: Incorporating consumer perspectives. *Journal of the American Medical Association* 278(19):1608–1612.

Cochran R. 1997. *Breast Conserving Therapy: A White Paper. Discussion of the Treatment of Carcinoma of the Breast among Delaware Medicare Beneficiaries.*

Cohen MR, Anderson RW, Attilio RM, et al. 1996. Preventing medication errors in cancer chemotherapy. *American Journal of Health-System Pharmacy* 53(7):737–746.

Comarow A. 1997. 1997 Annual guide to America's best hospitals: Inside the rankings. *U.S. News & World Report.*

Crane L, Cyran E, Hopewell E. 1997. *Breast Cancer Treatment Satisfaction Study.* Denver: Colorado Foundation for Medical Care.

Daffron ML. 1998. Quality Improvement Specialist, Health Care Excel, Terre Haute, Indiana. Personal communication to Maria Hewitt, February 18, 1998.

Daniels N, Sabin J. 1997. Limits to health care: Fair procedures, democratic deliberation, and the legitimacy problem for insurers. *Philosophy & Public Affairs* 26(4):302–350.

Daniels N, Sabin J. 1998a. The ethics of accountability in managed care reform. *Health Affairs* 17(5):50–64.

Daniels N, Sabin J. 1998b. Last chance therapies and managed care. Pluralism, fair procedures, and legitimacy. *Hastings Center Report* 28(2):27–41.

Darby M. 1998. *Health Care Quality: From Data to Accountability.* Washington, D.C.: National Health Policy Forum.

Donaldson MS. 1998. Accountability for quality in managed care. *Journal of Quality Improvement* 24(12):711–725.

Ehrlich RH, Hill CA, Winfrey KL. 1997. The 1997 Index of Hospital Quality. Chicago: National Opinion Research Center, University of Chicago.

Emanuel EJ, Emanuel LL. 1996. What is accountability in health care? *Annals of Internal Medicine* 124(2):229–239.

Feinberg B, Feinberg I. 1998. Overall survival of the medical oncologist: A new outcome measurement in cancer medicine. *Cancer* 82(10 Suppl.):2047–2056.

Ford LG, Hunter CP, Diehr P, Frelick RW, Yates J. 1987. Effects of patient management guidelines on physician practice patterns: The Community Hospital Oncology Program experience. *Journal of Clinical Oncology* 5(3):504–511.

Foundation for Accountability (FACCT). 1998. Measures to access quality of breast cancer care in a healthcare organization. http://www.facct.org.

Grilli R, G Apolone, S Marsoni, et al. 1991. The impact of patient management guidelines on the care of breast, colorectal, and ovarian cancer patients in Italy. *Medical Care* 29(1):50–63.

Grimshaw JM, Russell TI. 1993. Effect of clinical guidelines on medical practice. *Lancet* 342:1317–1322.

Grunfeld E, Mant D, Yudkin P, et al. 1996. Routine follow-up of breast cancer in primary care: Randomised trial. *British Medical Journal* 313:665–669.

Gustafson D, Wise M., McTavish F, et al. 1993. Development and pilot evaluation of a computer-based support system for women with breast cancer. *Journal of Psychosocial Oncology* 11:69–93.

Hannan EL, Kilburn H Jr, Racz M, et al. 1994. Improving the outcomes of coronary artery bypass surgery in New York. *Journal of the American Medical Association* 271:761–766.

Hibbard JH, Jewett JJ, Legnini MW, Tusler M. 1997a. Choosing a health plan: Do large employers use the data? *Health Affairs* 16(6):172–190.

Hibbard JH, Jewett JJ. 1997b. Will quality report cards help consumers? *Health Affairs* 16(3):218–228.

Hibbard JH, Slovic P, Jewett JJ. 1997c. Informing consumer decisions in health care: Implications from decision-making research. *The Milbank Quarterly* 75(3):395–415.

IMSystem. 1997. *Oncology Indicators: Indicator Information Forms, Code Tables, Report Prototype.* Joint Commission on Accreditation of Healthcare Organizations.

IOM (Institute of Medicine). 1990. *Clinical Practice Guidelines: Directions for a New Program.* Field MJ, Lohr K, eds. Washington, D.C.: National Academy Press.

IOM. 1992. *Guidelines for Clinical Practice: From Development to Use.* Field MJ, Lohr K, eds. Washington, D.C.: National Academy Press.

Kaiser Family Foundation–Agency for Health Care Policy and Research. 1996. *Americans as Health Care Consumers: The Role of Quality Information.*

Kanouse DE, Winkler JD, Kosecoff J, et al. 1989. *Changing Medical Practice Through Technology Assessment: An Evaluation of the NIH Consensus Development Program.* Ann Arbor, MI: Association for Health Services Research and Health Administration Press.

Katterhagen G. 1996. Physician compliance with outcome-based guidelines and clinical pathways in oncology. *Oncology Hunting* 10(11 Suppl.):113–121.

Kritchevsky SB, Simmons BP. 1991. Continuous quality improvement. Concepts and applications for physician care. *Journal of the American Medical Association* 266(13):1817–1823

Lansky D. 1998. Measuring what matters to the public. *Health Affairs* 17(4):40–41.

Leape LL, Park RE, Kahan JP, et al. 1992. Group judgments of appropriateness: The effect of a panel composition. *Quality Assurance in Health Care* 4(2):151–159.

Leape LL, Bates DW, Cullen DJ, et al. 1995. Systems analysis of adverse drug events. ADE Prevention Study Group. *Journal of the American Medical Association* 274(1):35–43.

Litwin MS, Smith RB, Thind A, et al. 1996. Cost-efficient radical prostatectomy with a clinical care path. *Journal of Oncology* 155:989–993.

Long SH and Marquis MS. 1998. How widespread is managed competition? *Center for Studying Health System Change: Data Bulletin: Results from the Community Tracking Study*, Number 12, Summer.

Marciniak TA, Ellerbeck EF, Radford MJ, et al. 1998. Improving the quality of care for Medicare patients with acute myocardial infarction: Results from the Cooperative Cardiovascular Project. *Journal of the American Medical Association* 279(17):1351–1357.

Marwick C. 1997. National Comprehensive Cancer Network drafts consensus guidelines from top oncologists. *Medical Outcomes & Guidelines Sourcebook.*

McDermott KC. 1997. Practice tips from Memorial Sloan-Kettering Cancer Center, New York, NY: Disease management provides a comprehensive approach to managing healthcare delivery. *Oncology Nursing Forum* 24(1):21–22.

McGivney WT. 1998. The National Comprehensive Cancer Network: Present and future directions. *Cancer* 82(10 Suppl.):2057–2060.

McGlynn EA. 1996. Choosing chronic disease measures for HEDIS: Conceptual framework and review of seven clinical areas. *Managed Care Quarterly* 4:54–77.

Medicine & Health. 1999. 53(4):2.

Memorial Sloan-Kettering Cancer Center. 1998. http://www.mskcc.org.

Morris M. 1996. Implementation of guidelines and paths in oncology. *Oncology* 10(11 Suppl.):123–129.

Morris M, Jameson S, Murdock S, Hohn DC. 1996. Development of an outcomes management program at an academic medical center. *Best Practices and Benchmarking in Healthcare* 1(3):118–125.

Morris M, Levenback C, Burke TW, et al. 1997. An outcomes management program in gynecologic oncology. *Obstetrics and Gynecology* 89(4):485–492.

Murphy G, Morris L, Lange D. 1997. *Informed Decisions: The Complete Book of Cancer Diagnosis, Treatment, and Recovery.* Atlanta: American Cancer Society.

National Cancer Data Base. 1999. Annotated Bibliographies and Cancer Statistics by Disease Site. http://www.facs.org/about_college/acsdept/cancer_dept/programs/ncdb/ncdb.html.

National Center for Health Statistics. 1997. *Healthy People 2000 Review.* Hyattsville, MD: Public Health Service.

National Coalition for Cancer Survivorship. 1995. *Imperatives for Quality Cancer Care: Access, Advocacy, Action, and Accountability.* November 13, 1995.

National Committee for Quality Assurance. 1998a. HEDIS 3.0. Health Plan Employer Data and Information Set.

National Committee for Quality Assurance. 1998b. The State of Managed Care Quality. http://www.ncqa.org/news/report98.htm.

O'Connor G, Plume S, Olmstead E, et al. 1996. A regional intervention to improve the hospital mortality associated with coronary artery bypass graft surgery. *Journal of the American Medical Association* 275:841–846.

Olivotto IA, Coldman AJ, Hislop TG, et al. 1997. Compliance with practice guidelines for node-negative breast cancer. *Journal of Clinical Oncology* 15(1):216–222.

Patton MD, Katterhagen JG. 1997. Critical pathways in oncology: Aligning resource expenditures with clinical outcomes. *Journal of Oncology Management* 16–21.

President's Advisory Commission on Consumer Protection and Quality. 1998. *Health Care Quality Protection and Improvement.* Washington, D.C.

Ray-Coquard I, Philip T, De Laroche G, et al. 1998. Impact of a clinical guidelines program on medical practice in a French cancer network. *Proceedings of the American Society of Clinical Oncology* 17:421a(Abstract).

Ray-Coquard I, Philip T, Lehmann M, et al. 1997. Impact of a clinical guidelines program for breast and colon cancer in a French cancer center. *Journal of the American Medical Association* 278(19):1591–1595.

Rischer JB, Childress SB. 1996. Cancer pain management: Pilot implementation of the AHCPR guideline in Utah. *Journal of Quality Improvement* 22(10):683–700.

Schoemaker D, Toouli J, Black R, Giles L. 1998. Yearly colonoscopy, CT liver and chest x-ray do not influence 5-year survival of colorectal cancer patients. *Gastroenterology* 114(1):7–14.

Schoenbaum SC, Sundwall DN, Bergman D, et al. 1995. *Using Clinical Practice Guidelines to Evaluate Quality of Care: Issues*. Rockville, MD: U.S. Department of Health and Human Services.

Schuster MA, Reifel JL, McGuigan K. 1998. Assessment of the quality of cancer care: A review for the National Cancer Policy Board of the Institute of Medicine. National Cancer Policy Board commissioned paper.

Smith T, Hillner B. 1998. Ensuring quality cancer care: Clinical practice guidelines, critical pathways, and care maps. Draft submitted to National Cancer Policy Board, Washington, D.C.

Stephenson J. 1997. Revitalized AHCPR pursues research on quality. *Journal of the American Medical Association* 278(19):1557.

Stewart MG, Hillman EJ, Donovan DT, Tanli SH. 1997. The effects of a practice guideline on endoscopic sinus surgery at an academic center. *American Journal of Rhinology* 11(2):161–165.

Stratis Health. 1997. *Stratis Health–Medicare Health Care Quality Improvement Project: Cancer Pain Assessment and Management in the Hospital Setting*. Bloomington, MN.

Teasley CE. 1996. Where's the best medicine? The hospital rating game. *Evaluation Review* 20(5):568–579.

Thompson I, Optenberg S, Segura J, et al. 1995. AUA prostate cancer clinical guidelines have a significant impact upon patient care in a national study population. *J Urology* 59:257 (abstract).

U.S. Congress, Office of Technology Assessment. 1994. *Identifying Health Technologies That Work: Searching for Evidence*. Washington, D.C.

Voelker R. 1997. HCFA focuses on new plans for quality care. *Journal of the American Medical Association* 278(19):1559.

Wagner EH, Austin B, Von Korff M. 1996. Organizing care for patients with chronic illness. *Milbank Quarterly* 74(4):511–544.

7

Health Services Research in Cancer Care

WHAT IS HEALTH SERVICES RESEARCH?

Health services research is a multidisciplinary field that investigates the structure, processes, and effects of health care services (Box 7.1). Such research informs critical decisions by government officials, corporate leaders, clinicians, health plan managers, and consumers making choices about health care or health insurance. The National Cancer Policy Board (NCPB), in an effort to understand how resources for research are applied to questions regarding the quality of cancer care, undertook a review of the status of cancer-related health services research. This chapter first describes publication trends in cancer-related health services research and then summarizes support for health services research within the following organizations:

Federally Sponsored Research

- Department of Health and Human Services
    National Institutes of Health (National Cancer Institute)
    Agency for Health Care Policy and Research
    Health Care Financing Administration
    Centers for Disease Control and Prevention
- Department of Defense
- Department of Veterans Affairs

Privately Sponsored Research

- American Cancer Society
- Foundations (e.g., Robert Wood Johnson Foundation)

Although these organizations are not the only sponsors of cancer-related health services research, they represent the major funding sources for such research. Excluded from this review is health services research supported by health plans, insurers, pharmaceutical companies, and other private organizations. Much of the research in these settings is proprietary.

> ## BOX 7.1 What Is Health Services Research?
>
> The Institute of Medicine defines health services research as:
>
> a multidisciplinary field of inquiry, both basic and applied, that examines the use, costs, quality, accessibility, delivery, organization, financing, and outcomes of health care services to increase knowledge and understand the structure, processes, and effects of health services for individuals and populations.
>
> Several features of this definition are worth noting. First, health services research is a multidisciplinary field that draws from many academic and clinical disciplines such as economics, epidemiology, biostatistics, nursing, and medicine. Its boundaries are imprecise, particularly as they relate to policy and management studies and clinical research. A clinical trial, for example, could be categorized as health services research if the effectiveness of a health care technology or intervention was assessed in a "real-world" rather than in an ideal or highly controlled setting. Second, the reference to basic and applied research underscores the fact that health services research involves both questions about fundamental individual, organizational, and system behaviors and questions of direct practical interest to public and private decision makers. Third, by referring to both knowledge and understanding, the definition stretches the boundaries of the field to include work of a theoretical or conceptual nature. Finally, the definition includes research that can have either a group- or an individual-level focus.
>
> SOURCE: IOM, 1995.

Health services research can be defined broadly to include behavioral and psychological research (e.g., assessments of individuals' preferences in health care), evaluations of programs that may fall outside the purview of the traditional health care system (e.g., school-based health programs), and randomized controlled clinical trials (e.g., studies of the effectiveness of health care technologies in situations representative of community practice). The National Cancer Policy Board accepted a broad definition of health services research and for this review applied the rubric used by the National Library of Medicine to select projects for inclusion in its health services research database (i.e., HSRProj) (Box 7.2).

Status of Cancer-Related Health Services Research

Publications

Evaluating trends in research publications is one way to assess the level of activity within a discipline. A resource for tracking such studies is the National Library of Medicine (NLM) Medline bibliographic database, which stores information about individual citations including index terms used to characterize each article (articles are indexed according to a dictionary of medical subject headings called MESH terms).

   The volume of cancer-related health services research articles appears to have been relatively stable during the 1980s, but increased sharply in the 1990s according to Medline searches from 1980 to 1997. In 1997, there were more than 1,200 articles indexed that addressed health services research issues related to cancer (Figure 7.1). Although the number of health services research citations increased during this period, by 1997 they represented less than 3 percent of all cancer-related citations indexed in the medical literature (Figure 7.2). These trends reflect publications in English, but not necessarily articles written by U.S. investigators. Much of the literature reviewed in Chapter 5 was conducted in the United Kingdom and is represented here. Figures 7.1 and 7.2 therefore reflect trends in the general medical literature, not necessarily trends in the United States. These trends must be interpreted with caution because they may reflect changes in the way MESH headings are applied to index the literature rather than real increases in cancer-related health services research.

BOX 7.2 Topics in Health Services Research

Health services research may address, or be conducted for the purposes of understanding or improving, areas such as the following:

- need and demand for health care;
- availability and accessibility of health care;
- utilization of health care;
- patient preferences (e.g., for treatments, providers, settings);
- patient compliance with treatment;
- organization and delivery of health care (e.g., managed care versus fee for service);
- health care workforce;
- financing of health care (e.g., public and private third-party payment, capitation);
- costs, cost-effectiveness, cost–benefit, and other economic aspects of health care;
- patient and population health status or quality of life;
- outcomes of health care technologies and interventions;
- practice patterns and diffusion of technologies or interventions;
- quality assurance programs and techniques;
- guidelines, standards, and criteria for health care;
- health care administration and management;
- health education and patient instruction;
- health professions education;
- health planning and forecasting;
- legal and regulatory changes affecting the health care system (e.g., antitrust laws);
- data and information needed for health care decision making (e.g., report cards);

and
- clinical trials (including randomized controlled trials) of the effectiveness of health care technologies or interventions.

SOURCE: HSRProj, 1998.

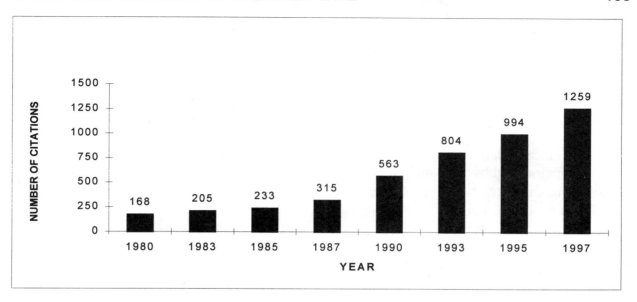

FIGURE 7.1 Medline citations for cancer-related health services research, 1980–1997. Research citations were identified in the NLM's Medline database using the MESH heading "neoplasms" (for cancer) and any one of the following major MESH headings "health services research," "quality of health care," and "quality assurance." The last terms encompass cancer citations addressing guideline adherence, outcomes and process assessment, accreditation, and health planning. Only articles published in English are counted.

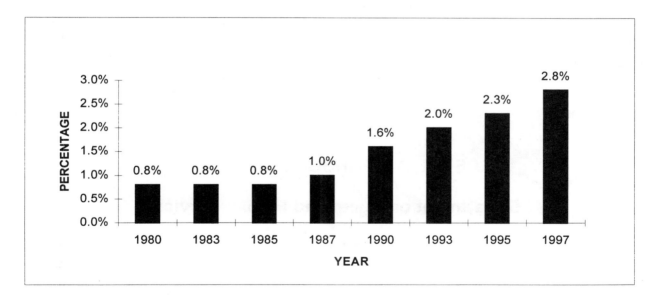

FIGURE 7.2 Medline citations for cancer-related health services research as a percentage of all cancer citations, 1980–1997. Percentages were calculated as the number of cancer-related health services research citations (as described in Figure 7.1) divided by the total number of citations identified using the "neoplasms" MESH term alone, for each given year. Only articles published in English are counted.

Research Support

A more direct way to assess the status of U.S.-based cancer-related health services research is to describe topics of investigation and levels of research spending. There is no one comprehensive source of information on health services research support, and as part of its review, the National Cancer Policy Board relied on the following sources:

- information catalogued in the HSRProj database (Health Services Research Project database) maintained by the National Library of Medicine—this database includes brief descriptions of ongoing extramural research sponsored by federal and state agencies, foundations, and other organizations;
- listings of research projects provided by some organizations (e.g., National Cancer Institute, Agency for Health Care Policy and Research, American Cancer Society);
- review of annual reports of research arms of certain agencies (e.g., the Department of Veterans Affairs);
- review of agency web sites (e.g., Department of Defense);
- informal contacts with agency representatives known to be involved in health services research (e.g., Health Care Financing Administration, Centers for Disease Control and Prevention); and
- meetings with senior agency representatives (i.e., Agency for Health Care Policy and Research, National Cancer Institute).

Despite the best efforts of the Board, the description of the nation's cancer-related health services research portfolio that follows may under- or over-estimate the actual level of research. Organizations varied in how they defined health services research and consequently, there is likely some inconsistency in what was included (or excluded) as a health services research activity. Furthermore, some health services research activities may have been missed because of limitations of research tracking systems. The review is limited to currently active research projects for most organizations.

FEDERALLY SPONSORED RESEARCH

Department of Health and Human Services

The Department of Health and Human Services (DHHS) includes the Public Health Service (PHS), which in turn oversees several sites that house cancer research: the National Institutes of Health (NIH), the Agency for Health Care Policy and Research (AHCPR), and the Centers for Disease Control and Prevention (CDC). Within DHHS, the Health Care Financing Administration (HCFA), which is organizationally parallel to the PHS, also supports applied cancer research. DHHS reports to Congress each year about the amount it spends on a number of health-related areas, including cancer (McGeary, 1999).

• The National Cancer Institute (NCI), one of the National Institutes of Health is the largest single provider of funds for cancer research ($2.4 billion in FY 1997).

• AHCPR estimated it spent $3.9 million for research on health costs, quality, and outcomes related to cancer (out of a research budget of $95 million).

• HCFA spends enormous amounts on cancer—$16.7 billion in FY 1997—mostly on medical services and care, but it has a small program of research (see below).

• CDC estimated that it spent $185 million on cancer-related programs in FY 1997. The categories included breast and cervical cancer ($139.7 million), cancer registries ($22.3 million), other chronic diseases ($8.1 million), infectious diseases ($450,000), environmental health ($1.7 million), and occupational safety and health ($12.7 million). All categories do not represent research programs. For example, the breast and cervical cancer program is an early detection program aimed at underserved populations. Deleting this program and assuming the rest of the activities are research would leave $45.3 million.

National Institutes of Health

National Cancer Institute. *Cancer Surveillance Research Program.* Many of NCI's health services research activities are housed in the Division of Cancer Control and Population Sciences, Cancer Surveillance Research Program (CSRP). CSRP develops information systems and methods needed to conduct cancer surveillance research and makes these resources available to investigators throughout the research community. The linked Medicare–SEER (Surveillance, Epidemiology, and End Results) database, for example, is now widely used to answer cancer-related health services research questions (www.dccps.ims.nci.nih.gov/ARB/SEERMedicare). CSRP-sponsored research evaluates trends in cancer related to risk factors, health behaviors, and health services and assesses the influence of these factors on cancer burden (e.g., cancer incidence, morbidity, mortality, survival). The division sponsors research related to patterns of care, diffusion of new technologies, cost of cancer care, and methodology and modeling.

Examples of health services research supported by the division include the following (Edwards, 1998a, b):

• *Patterns of Care studies*: SEER data are used to describe the dissemination of state-of-the-art cancer treatment and explanatory factors for variation in patterns of care. First conducted in 1987, samples of cases from SEER were obtained in 1988, 1989, 1990, 1991, 1995, and 1996. Currently, data are being collected on cases diagnosed in 1997 with cancer of the head and neck, cervix, childhood brain stem, and ductal carcinoma in situ of the breast. In previous years, cancer sites assessed have included: in situ and early-stage breast, colorectal, ovarian, urinary bladder, melanoma, non-small-cell lung, and childhood cancers. Annual budgets for the past three funding years ranged from $575,000 to $690,000 per year.

• *Prostate cancer outcomes study*: A longitudinal survey of 3,500 men with prostate cancer is underway regarding quality of life measured at 6 and 12 months and at 5 years following diagnosis (data collection to be completed in 1999). Practice patterns are also being assessed.

• *Breast Cancer Surveillance Consortium (a national mammography screening and outcomes database)*: The performance of mammography screenings (i.e., its sensitivity, specificity, predictive value) in a community setting is being evaluated in eight sites across the country as part of a congressionally mandated study under the Mammography Quality Standards Act of 1992. The major objectives of the consortium are to enhance understanding of the accuracy, cost, and quality of breast cancer screening; to foster collaborative research among consortium participants; to assess factors associated with variations in mammography practice, accuracy, and subsequent diagnostic evaluation; and to provide a foundation for the conduct of clinical and basic science research that can improve understanding of breast cancer etiology and prognosis. By the year 2000, the consortium will have data on nearly 3.2 million screening mammographic examinations and more than 24,000 breast cancer cases. Through 1999, total funding for the consortium is $17.2 million (NCI provides 85–90 percent of the total funding, with the remainder coming from CDC and the DoD). An additional $31 million for the period FY 2000 through FY 2004 will support the extramural research effort.

• *The SEER–Medicare database*: This is a collaborative effort of the NCI, the SEER registries, and HCFA to create a large population-based source of information for cancer-related epidemiologic and health services research. The database links cases in SEER cancer registries to claims records in Medicare's administrative database. The currently available linked file includes all Medicare data through 1994 for persons diagnosed with cancer through 1993. An update of the linkage, which will incorporate SEER cancer cases diagnosed in 1994–1996, will be completed in 1999.

The SEER–Medicare data offer an opportunity to examine patterns of care prior to the diagnosis of cancer, during the period of initial diagnosis, and during long-term follow-up. Topics that can be addressed with the linked database include patterns of care for specific cancers, the use of health services, and the costs of treatment. There is also the potential for longitudinal surveillance of the health care of persons with cancer. These data can be used to assess health care directed toward the prevention of disease or disability, as well as the restoration or maintenance of health (Edwards, 1997). Active projects using the linked SEER–Medicare database include analyses of

- trends in treatment of in situ breast cancer;
- total lifetime payments for elderly cancer patients;
- differences in patterns of care and cancer survival between health maintenance organizations (HMOs) and fee-for-service (FFS) providers;
- breast cancer treatment patterns and trends;
- prostate cancer detection practices; and
- trends and variations in initial treatment for early-stage prostate cancer.

HMO Cancer Research Network. The purpose of the Cancer Research Network (CRN) is to encourage the expansion of collaborative cancer research among health care provider organizations that are oriented to community care; have access to large, stable, and diverse patient populations; and are able to take advantage of existing integrated databases that can provide patient-level information relevant to research studies on cancer control and to cancer-related population studies. Beginning in 1999, NCI will fund the first CRN project—a consortium of 10 large, not-for-profit, research-oriented HMOs. The CRN will conduct four main projects (Martin Brown, Head, Health Services and Economics Section, Applied Research Branch, Cancer Surveillance Research Program, Division of Cancer Control and Population Sciences, NCI, personal communication, December 16, 1998):

1. The development of an administrative infrastructure to support research collaboration, data quality, and integrity and to develop methods and organizational approaches to increase the participation of managed care patients in NCI-approved clinical trials. The infrastructure will include a data-coordinating center and expert teams to provide organized scientific input in the areas of biostatistics, health economics, survey measures, pharmacoepidemiology, genetics, clinical trials management, and survivorship.

2. A study of the efficacy, reach, adherence to, and quality of delivery of smoking cessation programs in HMO practice settings.

3. A study of late-stage breast and invasive cervical cancer cases to elucidate the patient, provider, and system factors that contribute to preventing advanced disease.

4. A study of the effectiveness of the commonly used strategies of frequent mammography or prophylactic mastectomy, to prevent fatal breast cancer among women at increased risk for breast cancer.

Funding for this four-year extramural grant is approximately $4 million per year, with a total award of approximately $16 million.

The division has established an Outcomes Research Section to examine outcomes measures used in clinical trials and to monitor the national burden of cancer. The section will support research in the areas of measurement of quality of life, cost, and quality of care. Aspects of clinical trial organization and financing will also be addressed (e.g., integrating trials into routine care) (Martin Brown, Head, Health Services and Economics Section, Applied Research Branch, Cancer Surveillance Research Program, Division of Cancer Control and Population Sciences, NCI, personal communication, December 16, 1998).

Office of Cancer Survivorship. In 1996, NCI established the Office of Cancer Survivorship to develop and support a research agenda that explores the long- and short-term physical and psychological effects of cancer and its treatment. The office has provided $4 million to supplement existing cooperative agreements, grants, and contracts. An additional $700,000 was committed by the Susan Komen Foundation. Investigator-initiated research will be funded with an additional $3 million per year for five years. Most of the research funded to date has focused on treatment complications (e.g., effects of cancer treatment on gonadal function and reproductive health) and quality-of-life issues (e.g., quality of life for adult survivors of childhood leukemia), but a few awards have addressed health services research issues (e.g., medical care costs of cancer). Box 7.3 shows prioritized areas of research for the Office of Cancer Survivorship.

Health services research supported by the NCI is shown for breast cancer in Box 7.4, other cancer sites in Box 7.5, and other general research (i.e., not cancer-site specific) in Box 7.6.

Several other NIH institutes have supported extramural health services research (Table 7.1).

BOX 7.3 Prioritized Areas of Research for the
Office of Cancer Survivorship (OCS)

OCS has, to date, focused its research agenda on the issues of survivors who are at least two years post-treatment, because research data has been lacking for this group of individuals. Little information has been available about long-term cancer survivors (5-, 10-, and 15-year survivors) and the types of problems they face. OCS also aims to increase awareness of survivor issues among medical professionals and the general public. Prioritized areas of research include:

- prevalence of physiological and psychological long-term effects of cancer and its treatment,
- the risk of second cancers and the relationship between patients' risk levels and previous exposures, treatment received, and genetic predisposition,
- prevention and treatment of second cancers associated with treatment,
- issues related to reproductive and sexual functioning,
- the risk of cardiac disease in adults treated for childhood cancers and how to prevent this delayed treatment effect,
- the impact of cancer treatment on renal and cognitive function,
- effects of treatment on offspring of cancer survivors,
- treatment of premature menopause (e.g., with hormone replacement) and its effect on quality of life and the risk of recurrence,
- comparisons of cancer survivors with non-cancer patients to assess undesirable outcomes that could be prevented, either during the course of therapy or after therapy is completed,
- interventions to prevent long-term problems,
- behavior modification,
- patient education,
- surveillance and follow-up care for cancer survivors, and
- the economic impact of cancer.

A number of survivor groups have been overlooked in studies to date; these include patients with certain diagnoses, survivors representing various ethnic and socioeconomic groups, and the elderly. In addition, longitudinal survivorship studies have been lacking and instrumentation has been inadequate to measure quality of life over time.

SOURCE: Meadows A., presentation at the President's Cancer Panel, June 2, 1998.

BOX 7.4 Current Extramural Health Services Research Projects on Breast Cancer Supported by NCI

Prevention and Screening:
- Breast and cervical screening—older, low-income, rural women
- Increasing compliance with mammography guidelines
- Reducing barriers to the use of breast cancer screening
- Empowering physicians to improve breast cancer screening
- Increasing breast screening among rural minority women
- Improving breast and cervical cancer screening
- Maximizing mammography participation—a randomized trial
- Increasing breast screening among nonadherent women
- Promoting mammography screening in North Dakota
- Barriers to abnormal mammogram follow-up
- Mammography referral in primary care
- Breast cancer education through organized labor
- Mammographic practice and performance in the population
- Interventions for breast cancer screening behaviors
- Pilot for a community mammography and tumor registry
- Breast cancer surveillance (four projects)
- Cost-effectiveness analysis of breast cancer control for African Americans
- Case-control study of mammography
- Evaluating mammography claims data
- Public health study of mammogram interpretation
- Population-based approach to increase mammography use
- Follow-up evaluation of breast screening program project
- Breast and cervical cancer screening among Filipina women

Treatment:
- Data sources and patterns of care for breast cancer
- Multilevel compliance model of breast treatments
- Breast cancer patterns of care and morbidity
- Home-based moderate exercise for breast cancer patients
- Hierarchical modeling for assessing breast cancer care
- Breast cancer treatment protocols for Hawaii minorities
- Breast and Cervical Cancer Intervention Study
- Adjustment to breast cancer
- Patient barriers to breast cancer clinical trials
- Breast conserving surgery for the elderly
- Home care training for younger breast cancer patients
- Managing uncertainty—self-help in breast cancer
- Promoting self-help—underserved women with breast cancer
- Breast cancer in young women—population-based approach

SOURCES: Brenda Edwards, Associate Director, CSRP, DCCPS, National Cancer Institute, personal communication to Maria Hewitt, November 1998; http://www.nih.gov/grants/guide/pa; Martin Brown, Head, Health Services and Economics Section, Applied Research Branch, CSRP, DCCPS, NCI, personal communication to Maria Hewitt, December 1998; HSRProj, 1998.

BOX 7.5 Current Extramural Health Services Research Projects on Cancers Other than Breast Cancer Supported by NCI

Prevention and Screening:
- Prevention and control of skin cancer
- Cost-effectiveness of human papillomavirus screening for cervical cancer
- Abnormal Pap smears—what is cost-effective management?
- Single-visit cervical cancer prevention program
- Improving colorectal cancer screening
- Adding new fecal occult blood tests to sigmoidoscopy
- Enhancing diagnostic evaluation in colorectal cancer screening

Treatment:
- Prostate cancer in relation to vasectomy
- Cost-effectiveness of lung cancer chemotherapy
- Data resource for analyzing blood and marrow transplants
- Medical decision making in bone marrow transplantation
- Determinants of access to pediatric cancer care
- Minimally invasive surgery in children with cancer
- Staging and monitoring musculoskeletal sarcomas
- Pain relief in pancreatic cancer
- Minimal access surgery for pancreatic cancer
- Cancer and leukemia Group B—Minnesota Oncology Group
- Rehabilitation of patients with head and neck cancer
- CCSP in head and neck cancer rehabilitation
- Psychosocial factors in adjustment of bone marrow transplant survivors

SOURCES: Brenda K. Edwards, Division of Cancer Control and Population Sciences, National Cancer Institute, personal communication to Maria Hewitt, November 1998; http://www.nih.gov/grants/ guide/pa; Martin Brown, Head, Health Services and Economics Section, Applied Research Branch, CSRP, DCCPS, NCI, personal communication to Maria Hewitt, December 1998; HSRProj, 1998.

BOX 7.6 Current Extramural General Health Services Research Projects Supported by NCI

Prevention and Cancer Control (Including Early Detection):
- Community randomized trial of Hispanic cancer prevention
- Cancer control in North American Chinese women
- Community trial to increase cancer screening adherence
- Mujeres Protease/Women Protect Yourself—cancer screening
- Cancer control among Hispanic women—a research proposal
- Promoting cancer prevention among Vietnamese immigrants
- Increasing cancer screening in poor and minority women

Continued

BOX 7.6 *Continued*

- Detroit Cancer Control Intervention Project
- Los Angeles County Cancer Prevention Research Unit
- Data-based cancer control (several projects listed)
- New Hampshire interagency cancer control initiative
- Enhancing cancer control in a community health center
- Minority Cancer Control Research Program
- Florida cancer prevention and control project
- Cancer prevention and control
- Cancer Control Surveillance and Investigation System

Palliative Care:
- Pain education for elderly cancer patients at home
- Enhancing cancer pain control in American Indians
- Cancer pain relief skills for minority outpatients
- Pilot study of cancer pain
- Cancer pain management in community-based rural settings
- Development of a cancer pain interactive video disk
- Improving quality of life in advanced cancer
- Clinical management of cancer pain in U.S. nursing homes
- Patterns of care for cancer patients at end of life
- Aging—end-of-life care for hospitalized cancer patients
- Palliative training for caregivers of cancer patients

Rural Cancer Care:
- Rural partnership linkage for cancer care
- Clinical trials participation in a rural population
- Rural Cancer Care Project
- State-of-the-art cancer management in rural areas
- Role of telemedicine in rural cancer care

Special Populations—Racial or Ethnic Minority Groups:
- National Black Leadership Initiative on Cancer
- Spanish translation/validation—South West Oncology Group Quality of Life questionnaire

Cost Studies:
- Cost–quality trade-offs in cancer screening, diagnosis, and treatment
- Economic studies in cancer prevention, screening, and care
- Economics of cancer

Education:
- Por la Vida intervention model in cancer education
- Diana2 computer-based teaching of elder care

Clinical Trials:
- Impact of easy-to-read informed consent statements on clinical trials
- Barriers to Latino participation in clinical trials

Continued

BOX 7.6 *Continued*

Methodology:
- Claims data to assess cancer incidence, stage, and therapy
- Using claims data for cancer surveillance
- Cancer surveillance using health claims-based data system
- Statistical issues in the early detection of disease

Provider Issues:
- Survey of African-American physicians and patients
- Improving medical student communication with low-literacy adults

Other:
- Health care delivery systems and cancer outcomes
- Stress of cancer caregiving—analysis and intervention
- Utah center for alternative medicine research in cancer
- Supportive oncology—reducing the burden of cancer
- Patterns of Care study in radiation oncology

SOURCES: Brenda Edwards, DCCPS, National Cancer Institute, personal communication to Maria Hewitt, November 1998; http://www.nih.gov/grants/ guide/pa; Martin Brown, Head, Health Services and Economics Section, Applied Research Branch, CSRP, DCCPS, NCI, personal communication to Maria Hewitt, December 1998; HSRProj, 1998.

TABLE 7.1 Current Extramural Health Services Research Projects Supported Elsewhere at NIH and Listed on HSRProj

Institute	Project
National Institute on Aging	• Family and the health of African-American elderly: cancer prevention videos in a community setting • Health technologies' cost and outcomes in the elderly • Improving breast cancer care through patient activation • Caregiver responses to managing elderly patients at home • Breast and cervical cancer control in the elderly • Breast cancer prevention and control in older women
National Institute of Dental Research	• Patterns of care, outcomes, and cost of oral cavity pharyngeal cancer
National Eye Institute	• Collaborative Ocular Melanoma Study (2 grants) • Ocular melanoma (18 grants) • Quality of life—Collaborative Ocular Melanoma Study
National Library of Medicine	• New decision supports and databases for drug dosage • Using teledermatology to improve the ability of primary care physicians to recognize and treat skin cancers and other skin conditions in Oregon

SOURCE: HSRProj, 1998.

Agency for Health Care Policy and Research

AHCPR is the lead agency within DHHS charged with supporting research on health care quality, outcomes, cost, utilization, and access. The agency supports intramural research as well as an extramural grants program with a budget of $171 million (1999 appropriation) (www.ahcpr.gov). Support for intramural and extramural cancer-related health services research projects active since FY 1995 totals $20 million and represents an estimated 6 percent of the research budget during this period (Wendy Perry, AHCPR, personal communication to Maria Hewitt, December 1998).

Ongoing extramural research projects supported by AHCPR since FY 1995 are listed in Box 7.7.

BOX 7.7 Extramural Cancer-Related Health Services Research Projects Active Since FY 1995, AHCPR

Prevention, Screening, and Early Detection

1. General:
   - A physician insurer's impact on early cancer detection
   - Cancer prevention for minority women in a Medicaid HMO
   - Cancer screening of low-income and minority women
   - Genetic screening in primary care: ethics and policy
   - Efficacy of telemedicine colposcopy

2. Breast cancer:
   - Access to mammography for older women of color
   - Cost-effectiveness of MRI (magnetic resonance imaging) breast screening
   - Developing effective breast cancer risk information
   - Breast cancer screening policy and practice
   - Breast and colon screening evaluated by cancer mortality

3. Prostate cancer:
   - Couples' preferences for prostate cancer screening

4. Other cancers:
   - Screening for colorectal cancer
   - Evaluation of cervical cytology
   - Cost-effectiveness of preventing AIDS complications
   - Community physician diagnostic accuracy in colposcopy

Treatment

1. General:
   - Measuring quality by achievable benchmarks of care (ABC)
   - Risk factor for early unscheduled visits in cancer patients
   - A quality-of-life module for end-stage cancer patients
   - Adoption of cancer pain guidelines in managed care
   - Optimal policies for clinical lab quality control
   - Message and person effects on cancer treatment decisions

Continued

BOX 7.7 *Continued*

2. Breast cancer:
   - Care, costs, and outcomes of local breast cancer
   - Care, costs, and outcomes of breast cancer: elderly African Americans
   - Experiences of low-income women with breast cancer

3. Prostate cancer:
   - PORT-II for prostatic diseases
   - Enhanced accuracy of MI for staging prostate cancer
   - Comparison of treatment efficacy for prostate cancer
   - Treatment choices and outcomes in prostate cancer
   - Assessing therapies for BPH (benign prostatic hyperplasia) and localized prostate cancer

4. Other cancers:
   - Patterns of care and outcomes for colon cancer
   - Computerized decision support for posttransplant care
   - Quality outcomes in subacute and home care programs
   - Practice variations in pain control at the end of life
   - Using cancer registries to assess quality of cancer care
   - Internet multimedia cancer patient education system
   - Risk adjustment methods for hysterectomy complications

SOURCE: Wendy Perry, AHCPR, personal communication to Maria Hewitt, December 1998.

Evidence-Based Practice Program. The Evidence-Based Practice Program supports literature syntheses on clinical effectiveness, a resource for developing clinical practice guidelines or performance measures. Two cancer-related topics were among the first 12 topics assigned to the evidence-based practice centers: testosterone suppression treatment for advanced prostate cancer and evaluation of cervical cytology. In addition, two assessments will be completed in 1999: (1) an assessment of the management of cancer pain and (2) an analysis of the use of erythropoietin in hematology and oncology.

CONQUEST. CONQUEST (*C*omputerized *N*eeds-Oriented *QU*ality Measurement *E*valuation *Sys*tem) is a database of clinical performance measures, a resource for quality monitoring activities. Included are measures related to the management of several cancers (i.e., colorectal, lung, prostate, breast), the use of screening tests (i.e., mammography, Pap smear), and cigarette use.

Patient Outcomes Research Teams (PORTs). PORTs conduct research and disseminate findings related to common disorders. Two of the 14 conditions funded to date relate to cancer, prostate disease, and local breast cancer.

Clinical Trials. AHCPR's budget is insufficient to permit sole funding of major randomized clinical trials, although it has on a few occasions collaborated with other agencies (e.g., the Department of Veterans Affairs [VA] and several institutes within NIH) to take part in a larger comparative effectiveness study (U.S. Congress, 1994). AHCPR is, for example, supporting the Prostate Cancer Intervention Versus Observation Trial (PIVOT) in collaboration with NCI and VA. This randomized trial compares radical prostatectomy and palliative expectant management for the treatment of clinically localized prostate cancer. Information is being collected on patient outcomes such as functional status and quality of life. Costs and cost-effectiveness of alternative treatments are being assessed. Less than 5 percent of the total funding for this trial is from AHCPR.

Other Intraagency Agreements. In addition to the PIVOT trial, AHCPR sometimes transfers money to other agencies to support health services research. The Health Resources and Services Administration (HRSA), for example, received $100,000 to evaluate a multimedia education program on cervical cancer that was developed at NCI and the NLM for physicians, nurses, and other health care professionals. Funds were transferred to NCI to support an evaluation of minimal access surgery in cancer treatment (i.e., a comparative study of laparascopic versus open colectomy for the treatment of colon cancer). The assessment includes an analysis of cost-effectiveness. (AHCPR, personal communication to Maria Hewitt, December 1998).

Clinical Practice Guidelines. AHCPR no longer develops treatment guidelines, but it has recently issued guidelines on smoking cessation (1996) and the quality determinants of mammography (1994). In 1994, AHCPR published a practice guideline on cancer pain that will be updated with information forthcoming from an evidence practice center recently funded to review this topic. It has also recently issued a technical review of colorectal cancer screening (1998) (www.ahcpr.gov). AHCPR, in collaboration with the American Medical Association and the American Association of Health Plans, has developed a National Guideline Clearinghouse accessible by the Internet (www.guideline.gov). The website contains information on available guidelines, permits comparisons of guidelines recommendations, and facilitates communication among those involved in guideline development and dissemination (Stephenson, 1997). Of the first 414 guidelines accepted for inclusion, 45 relate to cancer (AHCPR, personal communication to Maria Hewitt, December 1998).

U.S. Preventive Services Task Force (USPSTF) and Put Prevention into Practice (PPIP). Since the 1980s, the USPSTF has evaluated scientific evidence for the effectiveness of clinical preventive services (e.g., screening tests, counseling, immunization, chemoprophylaxis) and produced age- and risk factor-specific recommendations for the services that should be included in a periodic health examination. PPIP is designed to help implement recommendations of the USPSTF. Roughly 20 percent of the services considered by USPSTF and PPIP relate to cancer detection or prevention.

Intramural Research Projects. Some of the research conducted by AHCPR staff concerns the quality of cancer care services (e.g., "Drive-through mastectomy: How common and who's driving?").

Basic Health Services Research. AHCPR supports research aimed at expanding the available array of quality measures. Some of these are not specific to cancer but could be relevant to cancer patients (e.g., quality measures for home and subacute care, health outcomes and quality-of-life measures for adolescents, aspects of clinician–patient interactions that improve patient satisfaction and outcomes) (Elaine Power, AHCPR, personal communication to Maria Hewitt, May 1998).

Research on Managed Care. To evaluate the effect of particular managed care policies on the quality of care provided to patients with chronic diseases (e.g., protocols governing the referral of patients to medical specialists, arrangements for paying physicians), AHCPR, in collaboration with HRSA (which is also part of DHHS) and the American Association of Health Plans Foundation, has recently funded a three-year research program. None of the conditions under study are cancers, but findings may be generalizable to cancer (www.ahcpr.gov/news/press/aahppr.htm).

Technology Assessment. AHCPR staff have evaluated the effectiveness of several cancer-related technologies including autologous peripheral stem cell transplantation, hematopoietic stem cell transplantation in multiple myeloma, and cryosurgery for recurrent prostate cancer following radiation therapy.

Health Care Financing Administration

Intramural Research—Office of Strategic Planning.   *Patterns and Outcomes of Cancer Care in the Medicare Population*. HCFA analysts are attempting to answer the following questions with the linked SEER–Medicare database:

- What are overall Medicare costs, by type and stage of cancer?
- What Medicare costs are specifically related to cancer care?
- What comorbidities are associated with cancer and how do they influence Medicare use and cost?
- What is the mix of care (on a per-person basis) among community hospitals, teaching hospitals, and cancer centers?
- What institutional factors influence the type of inpatient hospital care received by cancer patients?

Breast Cancer Treatment Patterns Among Medicare Enrollees in HMOs and FFS. The linked SEER–Medicare database has recently been analyzed to examine the use of breast conserving surgery (BCS) versus mastectomy for early-stage breast cancer cases in HMOs and FFS. The study also compared the distributions of stage at diagnosis between HMO and FFS enrollees and examined the use of adjuvant radiation therapy among BCS patients. The study included all early-stage breast cancer cases diagnosed in 1988–1993 among elderly women entitled to Medicare residing in SEER reporting areas. (USDHHS, 1998; Riley et al, 1999).

Mammography Utilization Initiative. Rates of mammography use have been published by age and race, at the state and county levels, for 1993. The mammography use data book will be updated with 1994 and 1995 Medicare data and disseminated to public health and cancer organizations to help target outreach activities to areas with particularly low utilization. The data will be placed on HCFA's Internet home page (USDHHS, 1998).

Hospice Use. The linked SEER–Medicare database will be analyzed to examine the sociodemographic (e.g., age, sex, race or ethnicity, income, education) and health care (e.g., HMO status) determinants of hospice use among beneficiaries with colorectal and lung cancer (diagnosed in 1992 and 1993). The hospice benefit was originally designed as an alternative to aggressive care for beneficiaries with terminal illnesses. Few studies, however, have examined the utilization and cost of health care services among hospice patients. This study will assess the level and type of services both prior to and during hospice care (R. Mentnech, Health Care Financing Administration, personal communication to Maria Hewitt, November 1998.).

Intramural Research—Center for Health Plans and Providers

Research Related to Payment Issues. Patterns of care and volume stability at the physician organization level will be studied using per capita measures of utilization for selected oncology services and for all Medicare services. The effect of the principal provider organization's characteristics, size, and case mix of oncology practice, as well as geographic location, on per capita costs will also be examined. These analyses will support the development of alternative service bundles and carve-out payments for the care of Medicare cancer patients. The linked SEER–Medicare database will be the principal source of data. The project is in the early development phase (USDHHS, 1998).

Research Training and Development. In an effort to promote research using its databases, HCFA has created the Research Data Assistance Center (ResDAC) to assist new researchers and promote familiarity with and use of its databases for research on Medicare and Medicaid issues. The initial ResDAC contract is with the University of Minnesota, which has formed a consortium with Boston University, Dartmouth College, and Georgetown University. ResDAC will facilitate and expedite the use of HCFA data for research on Medicare and Medicaid by providing education and training, improving researcher access to HCFA data, and providing expert consultation for researchers (USDHHS, 1998).

Extramural Research. According to the HSRProj database, HCFA has sponsored one extramural health services research project, "Estimating Mammography Utilization by Elderly Medicare Women."

Centers for Disease Control and Prevention

Most of the cancer-related health services research supported by CDC is funded through the National Center for Chronic Disease Prevention and Health, Division of Cancer Prevention and Control. The division plans and conducts epidemiologic studies and evaluations to identify the feasibility and effectiveness of cancer prevention and control strategies. Other activities include providing technical assistance to states, local public health agencies, and other health care provider organizations. Ongoing extramural research supported by the Division of Cancer Prevention and Control is shown in Box 7.8.

BOX 7.8 Current Extramural Health Services Research Projects Funded by CDC's National Center for Chronic Disease Prevention and Health, Division of Cancer Prevention and Control

General
- Validation of patient survey data on cancer screening
- Strategies for reaching Native American/Alaska Natives: case study
- Psychosocial issues in cancer prevention for Hispanics
- Research on psychosocial issues relating to intervention development for cancer prevention and control
- Media advocacy for cancer prevention and control
- Medicaid/Medicare claims data—diagnosis to treatment
- A symposium to facilitate the exchange of cancer data among HMOs and state and regional population-based registries
- Standardized staging classification of cancer
- Comprehensive cancer control

Breast and Cervical Cancer
- Case-control study of the efficacy of screening mammography: validation of self-reported mammography and analysis of screening and late-stage disease
- Behavioral research in urban/rural, minority, low-income communities: Breast and cervical cancer
- Intervention research project: Breast and cervical cancer
- Research on psychosocial issues related to breast and cervical cancer screening with older, uninsured or underinsured
- Mammography rescreening
- Rescreening among participants in the National Breast and Cervical Cancer Early Detection Program: Focus group data
- Mammography rescreening rates and risk factors
- Increasing rescreening in the Minnesota Breast and Cervical Cancer Early Detection Program

Prostate Cancer
- Socioeconomic correlates of prostate cancer among minority populations
- Content analysis of popular print media's portrayal of prostate cancer: Differences between newspapers and magazines targeted to the general public and African-American audiences
- Communication of prostate health information in primary care in predominantly African- American communities
- PSA effectiveness-case control study of prostate cancer screening and mortality
- PSA and colorectal cancer screening test utilization in the managed care environment
- Improving African-American men's knowledge of the prostate cancer screening dilemma
- Efficacy of balance sheets in prostate cancer screening decisions

Continued

BOX 7.8 *Continued*

- Informed decision making and prostate cancer screening
- Survey of knowledge, attitudes, and anticipated practices of physicians in training regarding prostate cancer screening
- Clarifying the treatment decision process and post-treatment quality of life factors among prostate cancer survivors
- Prostate cancer treatment and quality of life among minority populations with prostate cancer

Colorectal Cancer
- Increasing participation in colorectal cancer screening
- Barriers to participant's compliance in a flexible sigmoidoscopy screening program
- Compliance barriers to free-of-charge colorectal flexible sigmoidoscopy screening services in populations 60 to 64 years of age
- Proposal to develop and evaluate a colorectal cancer screening measure for Health Plan Employer Data and Information Set (HEDIS)
- Community assessments of the burden of colorectal cancer

SOURCE: Kevin Brady, Acting Deputy Director, Division of Cancer Prevention and Control, National Center for Chronic Disease Prevention and Health, CDC, personal communication to Maria Hewitt, March, 1999.

Other cancer-related health services research is conducted within other areas of CDC. Two projects were identified within the Epidemiology Program Office: Mammography utilization in an HMO, and treatment issues related to breast and cervical cancer. Within the National Center for Health Statistics, researchers are evaluating the role of social class and race/ethnicity on the incidence of cancer (HSRProj, 1998).

Department of Defense

Beginning in FY 1992, the U.S. Congress directed the Department of Defense (DoD) to manage several appropriations for an extramural grant program directed toward specific research initiatives. The United States Army Medical Research and Materiel Command (USAMRMC) constituted the office of the Congressionally Directed Medical Research Programs (CDMRP) to administer these funds. To date, between FY 1992 and 1999, $1.1 billion has been targeted by Congress for research on breast cancer, prostate cancer, ovarian cancer, neurofibromatosis, defense women's health, and osteoporosis. The CDMRP strives to identify gaps in funding and provide award opportunities that will enhance program research objectives without duplicating existing funding opportunities.

The three DoD programs targeted at cancer research include the following:

1. *Breast cancer:* Between FY 1992 and 1999, $883.8 million has been appropriated to the Breast Cancer Research Program (BCRP). Proposals are sought across all areas of laboratory, clinical, behavioral, and epidemiological research including all disciplines within the basic, clini-

cal, psychosocial, behavioral, sociocultural, and environmental sciences: nursing, occupational health, alternative therapies, public health and policy, and economics. In FY 1993–1994 the program applied the recommendations of the Institute of Medicine and focused on traditional research and infrastructure (IOM, 1997). In FY 1996, the program deemphasized traditional awards to fund innovative "idea awards" and clinical translational research. The BCRP also offers training support, such as predoctoral, postdoctoral, sabbatical, and career development awards.

2. *Prostate cancer:* Between FY 1997 and 1999, $135 million has been appropriated to the Prostate Cancer Research Program for basic and clinical research. The goals of the program are to pursue breakthrough ideas and approaches, prepare new scientists, encourage established investigators, and promote prostate cancer public awareness and education among the public. The program encourages innovative, multi-institutional, and multidisciplinary research and has funded new investigator awards, idea development awards, and minority population-focused training awards.

3. *Ovarian cancer:* Between FY 1997 and 1999, $27.5 million has been appropriated to the Ovarian Cancer Research Program. To date, comprehensive, multidisciplinary, preventive center grants have been funded to foster the development of a sustained national ovarian cancer research enterprise.

Extramural research identified in HSRProj is shown in Box 7.9.

BOX 7.9 Current Extramural Health Services Research Projects Funded by DoD

General
- Utilization of a national clinical trials infrastructure to evaluate breast cancer patient outcomes of importance in determining priorities for new care reform
- A randomized clinical trial to evaluate advanced nursing care for women with newly diagnosed breast cancer
- Decision modeling of psychosocial and clinical factors in assessing treatment alternatives for lobular carcinoma in situ
- Adding data accessibility and rule-based targeting data collection to the California cancer reporting system for breast cases
- Massachusetts cancer control evaluation project
- Development of a stochastic simulation model of the cost-effectiveness of promoting breast cancer screening
- Special sabbatical for training in health decision sciences with application to breast cancer treatment evaluation

Prostate Cancer
- Role of African-American churches in prostate cancer prevention
- Unbiased outcome estimates for conservative versus aggressive treatment of early-stage prostate cancer from retrospective data: an instrumental variables approach
- Assessing patient values toward prostate cancer genetic screening

Continued

BOX 7.9 *Continued*

- The effects of supportive and nonsupportive behaviors on the quality of life of prostate cancer patients and their spouses
  - Value-based decision making in prostate cancer early detection
  - Microsimulation model of the benefits and costs of prostate cancer screening and treatment

Breast Cancer

1. Prevention:
   - Psychoeducational group intervention for women at increased risk for breast cancer
   - Breast cancer information system designed to foster increased proactive prevention activities among minority populations

2. Screening:
   - Breast cancer screening by physical examination: a randomized clinical trial in the Philippines
   - Facility inreach strategy to promote annual mammography
   - Regional breast cancer screening network
   - Evaluation of multiple outcall intervention to increase screening mammography use among low-income and minority women

3. Treatment:
   - Surveillance after initial treatment for breast cancer: a population-based study of variation in outcomes of care
   - Follow-up care for older women with breast cancer
   - Cost-effectiveness of alternative treatments for local breast cancer in the elderly
   - Managing menopausal symptoms in breast cancer survivors
   - Psychoeducational group intervention for women at increased risk for breast cancer
   - Role of physician gender in variation in breast cancer care
   - Effects of meditation-based stress reduction in younger women with breast cancer
   - Psychological intervention for women with breast cancer

4. Other:
   - Emotional processing and expression in breast cancer patients: effects on health and psychological adjustment
   - Multigenerational breast cancer risk factors in African-American women
   - Knowledge and beliefs regarding breast cancer among elderly Puerto Rican women
   - Linkage of molecular and epidemiological breast cancer investigations with treatment data: a specialized registry
   - Establishment of the Fox Chase network breast cancer risk registry
   - Enhancing positive reactions to breast cancer risk appraisal
   - Methodology for case-control studies of breast cancer
   - Effects of a comprehensive coping strategy on clinical outcomes in breast cancer bone marrow transplant patients and primary caregiver

SOURCES: HSRProj 1998; S. Young-McCaughan, Deputy Director for Research Programs, CDMRP, personal communication to Maria Hewitt, December 1998.

Department of Veterans Affairs

The Department of Veterans Affairs (VA) Office of Research and Development supports intramural biomedical, rehabilitation, and health services research. Health services research focuses on conditions that are common among veterans, including cancer (especially prostate and lung). Recent initiatives have addressed factors affecting the delivery of health care such as managed care; the implementation of clinical practice guidelines; ethnic, cultural, and gender issues; continuity of care, and patient-centered care. VA support for cancer-related health services research totaled $9.5 million in fiscal years 1997 and 1998.

Eleven Centers of Excellence have been established to link health services research to patient and administrative needs and to provide technical expertise in certain areas, for example, the measurement of chronic disease outcomes, health economics, and tobacco use and cessation. Studies of cancer treatments, chronic pain, and end-of-life care are being conducted as part of the VA's quality improvement program, the Quality Enhancement Research Initiative (QUERI).

The VA is supporting two clinical trials with health services research components:

1. PIVOT, a randomized trial comparing radical prostatectomy versus palliative expectant management for the treatment of clinically localized prostate cancer (other sponsors include NCI and AHCPR); and

2. A VA cooperative trial to assess whether 18-F-Fluorideoxyglucose Positron Emission Tomography (PET) imaging can be used to accurately determine if solitary pulmonary nodules are malignant. The trial will assess the costs and benefits of this technology (e.g., avoidance of unnecessary procedures).

In 1998, the VA's Office of Research and Development began collaborating with the Department of Defense for studies on prostate diseases including prostate cancer.

Other VA intramural health services research is shown in Box 7.10.

BOX 7.10 Intramural Health Services Research Projects, Department of Veterans Affairs

General
- Assessing pain control in acute and chronically ill patients
- Implementation of clinical practice guidelines for smoking cessation
- The use of nurses to improve cancer patient pain outcomes

Prostate Cancer
- Impact of education on prostate cancer screening decisions
- Prospective study of patient preferences for prostatic cancer treatment
- Familial patterns in prostate cancer
- Effectiveness of screening for prostatic cancer
- Effects of age and race on prostate cancer outcomes
- Differences in patterns of care, risk factors, and health-related knowledge and beliefs among African-American and white men

Continued

BOX 7.10 *Continued*

- Prostate cancer-case controlled study of African-American versus white men, VA versus private sector
  - Quality of life and patient utility for veterans with prostate cancer

Breast Cancer
- Breast cancer among women veterans

Other Cancers
- VA marrow transplantation: potential demand, resource use, effectiveness
- Posttreatment management options for lung cancer patients
- Evaluation of compliance in colorectal tumor postoperative screening
- An evaluation of the risk factors for colon cancer and determination of follow-up intervals for screening
- Teledermatology: Diagnosing dermatologic lesions by digital imaging
- Comprehensive outcomes of nonmelanoma skin cancer

SOURCE: Department of Veterans Affairs, Office of Research and Development, Mary Jones, personal communication to Maria Hewitt, January 7, 1999.

PRIVATE ORGANIZATIONS FUNDING RESEARCH

American Cancer Society

The American Cancer Society (ACS) is the largest non-government funder of cancer research in the United States ($93.4 million in 1996) (McGeary, 1999).

Intramural Research Programs

Department of Epidemiology and Surveillance Research. *Assessment of the Quality of Treatment Data.* The ACS in collaboration with the American College of Surgeons and three state cancer registries (Illinois, Kentucky, Louisiana) is evaluating the completeness and quality of treatment data for patients with colon cancer. Different approaches to collecting data from both hospital and outpatient settings will be assessed with the aim of estimating the proportion of colon cancer patients who receive optimal treatment, given the stage of their disease at diagnosis. Data acquired in a more timely fashion could be used by clinicians, individual hospitals, and state health department officials as benchmarks to gauge the quality of care provided. Success in this feasibility study could lead to the study of other cancer sites in additional states. Funding for this feasibility study is less than $100,000 (P. Wingo, Department of Epidemiology and Surveillance Research, American Cancer Society, personal communication to Maria Hewitt, October 1998).

Patterns of Care Study. The ACS is analyzing the National Hospital Discharge Surveys from 1988 to 1995 to describe patterns of use of inpatient surgical procedures for treating cancers of the lung, colorectum, prostate, and female breast, by age, race, gender, and geographic region. This is an intramural research activity of the Department of Epidemiology and Surveillance Research (P. Wingo, Department of Epidemiology and Surveillance Research, American Cancer Society, personal communication to Maria Hewitt, October 1998).

Behavioral Research Center. Although not designed as health services research initiatives per se, several activities within ACS's Behavioral Research Center could have applications to health services research (ACS, 1998).

Population-Based Surveys of Cancer Survivors. The Behavioral Research Center is conducting two large population-based surveys of cancer survivors at a cost of $2 million for the pilot phases (Baker, VP Behavioral Research, ACS, personal communication to Maria Hewitt, October 1997). The first is the "Study of Cancer Survivors—Incidence." This survey of up to 100,000 cancer survivors is underway in a pilot phase and is designed as a 10-year prospective study of survivors enrolled within the first year after diagnosis of any one of the ten most common cancers (i.e., prostate, female breast, lung, colorectal, urinary bladder, non-Hodgkin's lymphoma, skin melanoma, uterine, kidney, ovarian). A population-based sample is being selected from area cancer registries in sufficient numbers to provide state-level estimates. The major aim of the survey is to examine the behavioral, psychosocial, treatment, and support factors that influence quality of life and survival of cancer patients. The survey is being fielded on a pilot basis in four states (Iowa, Minnesota, Wisconsin, Georgia), and plans are to extend the study to other states that have adequate cancer registration and an interest in participating. The survey includes a number of scales that have been validated (e.g., problems in daily living, physical and mental health functioning, problems with work) along with basic information about the cancer (type of cancer), treatment, health insurance, and site of health care. It should be possible, therefore, to examine quality-of-life issues by insurance or site of care, controlling for type of cancer (although it is unclear what information on comorbidity will be available).

The second survey is the "Study of Long-Term Cancer Survivors—Prevalence." This survey is a cross-sectional study of 6,000 long-term survivors (i.e., those who are 5, 10, and 15 years beyond diagnosis) of six cancers (prostate, breast, colorectal, bladder, melanoma, uterine). There will be 1,000 respondents for each type of cancer. Twenty-seven states have registries that were established in 1983 or earlier, and four SEER metro area registries also meet this requirement, which is necessary to identify 15-year survivors. Only 12 state registries and all four SEER registries have complete data (85 percent complete) for 1983, 1988, and 1993.

Complementary Therapies. Surveys of complementary therapies (e.g., acupuncture, visualization, yoga) have been conducted to determine the extent to which people with cancer are using these unconventional treatments and what their impact is on quality of life. In addition, surveys of oncology physicians, nurses, and social workers have been completed regarding the extent to which providers are aware of commonly used complementary therapies and whether they are supportive of cancer patients' use of these therapies.

Barriers to Care. Plans are underway to conduct research on factors that inhibit or are barriers to the participation of minorities and other special populations in prevention programs, screening, clinical trials, and effective treatment.

Extramural Research Program

Very little ACS extramural research is devoted to health services research, even when broadly defined to include behavioral, psychosocial, and quality-of-life research. Information from the ACS on institutional, research, and training grants in effect as of September 1, 1998, indicates that less than 5 percent of the total $171,336,000 grant program is allocated to health services research (Box 7.11). The brief descriptions of research projects included in the grant summary list do not always provide sufficient detail to allow one to distinguish between health services and other kinds of research. Consequently, this list may under- or overestimate the level of health services research support.

**BOX 7.11 ACS Extramural Grant Program Health Services
Research Support (as of September 1998)**

Breast Cancer

- Breast cancer recurrence: Promoting patient and family quality of life
- Community breast cancer screening
- Assessing and improving interval mammography screening
- Measuring quality of life utilities in BRCA1 and BRCA2 patients
- Psychological treatment of black women with breast cancer
- Telephone social support and education for adaptation to breast cancer

Colon Cancer

- Identification and targeting of counties deficient in colon cancer screening
- Colorectal cancer prevention in rural black churches

Prostate Cancer

- Development of the Cochrane Collaboration prostate cancer review
- Outcome studies of screening for prostate cancer
- Quality-of-life outcomes in men with localized prostate cancer
- Psychoeducational support groups for prostate cancer patients
- Patient utilities for health states in early-stage prostate cancer
- Quality of life and utilities for patients with prostate cancer

Continued

BOX 7.11 *Continued*

Prostate Cancer (*continued*)

- A physical activity quality-of-life intervention in androgen-ablated prostate cancer
- Effect of computer-based support on prostate cancer treatment decisions
- Nursing's impact on quality of life post-prostatectomy
- Facilitating participation in a prostate cancer family risk assessment program
- Life assessment for prostate cancer decision models
- Prostate-specific antigen screening and mortality from prostate cancer

Other Cancers

- Posttraumatic stress among mothers of children who survive cancer

Other

- Development of cost-effective models of cancer care
- Conversations about cancer: understanding how families talk through illness
- Comparing treatments using the Q-twist methodology
- Cancer-related health behaviors of Vietnamese youth: longitudinal study
- Legal reforms: effects of cancer diagnosis, treatment costs, outcomes
- Message framing, persuasion, and cancer prevention/detection
- Improving pain control: patient and family education
- Coaching patients with cancer to report sensory pain experience

SOURCE: ACS, 1998.

Several other private organizations support cancer-related health services research to a limited extent (Table 7.2).

TABLE 7.2 Current Extramural Health Services Research Projects Supported by Foundations or Private Organizations and Listed on HSRProj

Organization	Project
Robert Wood Johnson Foundation	Smoking and cancer screening: chronic disease prevention for older women
	Supporting quality improvement and Joint Commission on Accreditation of Healthcare Organizations standard setting for pain management in hospitals
	Research on cancer screening among Hispanic women
United Hospital Fund	Improving clinical care for early-stage breast cancer patients: changing physician practices
Aetna, Inc.	Preparing African-American men for decision making about prostate cancer and early detection
	Using performance measures to motivate process improvement: a randomized trial

SOURCE: HSRProj 1998.

The Cochrane Collaboration

Although not strictly health services research, the Cochrane Collaboration is a not-for-profit international organization that "aims to help people make well-informed decisions about healthcare by preparing, maintaining, and promoting the accessibility of systematic reviews of the effects of healthcare interventions" (Box 7.12). Evidence reviewed comes from a number of sources, with an emphasis on published and unpublished randomized clinical trials.

Since 1997, the Cochrane Cancer Network (http://www.canet.demon.co.uk) has coordinated the work of site-specific groups and plans to develop a database of all past and present controlled or randomized trials and systematic reviews in cancer. To date, the network has registered nearly 15,000 reports of controlled and randomized trials in cancer (www.canet.demon.co.uk). Cancer or cancer-related collaborative review groups that are registered or that are developing include:

- breast cancer,
- colorectal cancer,
- ear, nose, and throat disorders,
- eye cancer,
- gynecological cancer,
- head and neck cancer,
- hematological malignancies,
- liver cancer,
- lung cancer,
- oral cancer,
- pain, palliative, and supportive care,
- prostatic and urological cancers,
- skin cancer,
- stomach and pancreatic cancer, and
- tobacco addiction.

The Cochrane Cancer Network is developing a specialized database for cancer, called the Cancer Library in Europe, which will serve as a comprehensive source of information about cancer for consumer groups and other members of the cancer community (http://www.canet.demon.co.uk).

KEY FINDINGS

- Many public and private organizations are funding a diverse set of health services research topics, but with the information currently available, one cannot estimate total spending on cancer-related health services research. The best estimates suggest that it represents a very small share of total cancer research funding.

BOX 7.12 The Cochrane Collaboration

Health care professionals, consumers, researchers, and policy makers are overwhelmed with unmanageable amounts of information. In an influential book published in 1972, Archie Cochrane, a British epidemiologist, drew attention to our great collective ignorance about the effects of health care. He recognized that people who want to make more informed decisions about health care do not have ready access to reliable reviews of the available evidence.

In 1987, the year before Cochrane died, he referred to a systematic review of randomized controlled trials (RCTs) of care during pregnancy and childbirth as "a real milestone in the history of randomized trials and in the evaluation of care," and suggested that other specialties should copy the methods used. In the same year, the scientific quality of many published reviews was shown to leave much to be desired. As Cochrane had emphasized, reviews of research evidence must be prepared systematically and they must be kept up-to-date to take account of new evidence.

If this is not done, important effects of health care (good and bad) will not be identified promptly, and people using the health services will be ill-served as a result. In addition, without systematic, up-to-date reviews of previous research, plans for new research will not be well informed. As a result, researchers and funding bodies will miss promising leads and will embark on studies asking questions that have already been answered.

The Cochrane Collaboration Logo

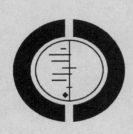

The Cochrane Collaboration logo illustrates a systematic review of data from seven randomized controlled trials, comparing one health care treatment with a placebo. Each horizontal line represents the results of one trial (the shorter the line, the more certain is the result); the diamond represents their combined results. The vertical line indicates the position around which the horizontal lines would cluster if the two treatments compared in the trials had similar effects; if a horizontal line touches the vertical line, it means that that particular trial found no clear difference between the treatments. The position of the diamond to the left of the vertical line indicates that the treatment studied is beneficial. Horizontal lines or a diamond to the right of the line would show that the treatment did more harm than good.

This diagram shows the results of a systematic review of RCTs of a short, inexpensive course of a corticosteroid given to women about to give birth prematurely. The first RCT was reported in 1972. The diagram summarizes the evidence that would have been revealed had the available RCTs been reviewed systematically a decade later: it indicates strongly that corticosteroids reduce the risk of babies' dying from the complications of immaturity. By 1991, seven more trials had been reported, and the picture had become still stronger. This treatment reduces by 30 to 50 percent the odds that the babies of these women will die from the complications of immaturity.

Because no systematic reviews of these trials were published until 1989, most obstetricians did not realize that the treatment was so effective. As a result, tens of thousands of premature babies probably suffered and died unnecessarily (and received more expensive treatment than was necessary). This is just one of many examples of the human costs resulting from failure to perform systematic, up-to-date reviews of RCTs of health care.

SOURCE: The Cochrane Collaboration, 1999.

• Currently funded health services research is addressing important issues related to the quality of cancer care, for example, the impact of managed care, patterns of care, outcomes studies, issues in cancer survivorship, cancer control in minority communities, barriers to access to cancer care, cancer surveillance, pain management, and end-of-life care.

• NCI appears to be the primary sponsor of cancer-related health services research. The health services research budget is not known, but quality-related research appears to represent a very small fraction of the overall NCI research budget ($2.4 billion in FY 1997).

• AHCPR has a small budget ($171 million in 1999) and a limited but balanced (by cancer site) portfolio of extramurally funded cancer health services research. An estimated 6 percent of the research budget is spent on cancer-related health services research. AHCPR is developing an infrastructure for evidence synthesis and is disseminating information about clinical practice guidelines, both or which have relevance to cancer care.

• Analysts at NCI and HCFA are conducting important cancer-related health services research with the linked SEER–Medicare claims file. NCI and HCFA are attempting to assist new researchers and to promote familiarity with, and use of, this database.

• DoD is supporting breast, prostate, and ovarian cancer research through its Congressionally Directed Medical Research Programs, but very few of the awards are for health services research.

• Very few private organizations (e.g., foundations) appear to be funding cancer-related health services research. The American Cancer Society has an extramural research budget of $171 million of which 5 percent of support is devoted to health services research. The ACS is internally funding the development of two very large surveys of cancer survivors, which will provide valuable information about the experience of cancer, especially quality-of-life issues.

• The Cochrane Collaboration, an international organization devoted to synthesizing the results of clinical trials, has begun to organize groups based on cancer site.

REFERENCES

American Cancer Society. 1998a. *American Cancer Society Extramural Grants Programs in Effect September 1, 1998.* Atlanta, GA: American Cancer Society.

American Cancer Society. 1998b. *Behavioral Research Center: Program Description and Progress Report.* Atlanta, GA: American Cancer Society.

Brown M. 1998. Head, Health Services and Economics Section, Applied Research Branch, Cancer Surveillance Research Program, personal communication to Maria Hewitt, December 16, 1998.

The Cochrane Collaboration. 1999. http://hiru.mcmaster.ca/cochrane/default.htm.

Edwards BK. 1997a. Associate Director, Cancer Surveillance Research Program, Division of Cancer Control and Population Sciences, National Cancer Institute. Presentation to National Cancer Policy Board. Washington, D.C.

Edwards BK. 1997b Briefing Book prepared for National Cancer Policy Board. Updated by personal communication.

Edwards, BK. 1998. Associate Director, Cancer Surveillance Research Program, Division of Cancer Control and Population Sciences, National Cancer Institute, personal communication to Maria Hewitt, November 2, 1998

Eisenberg JM. 1998. AHCPR focuses on information for health care decision makers. *Health Services Research* 33(4):767–785.

HSRProj Database (Health Services Research Project Database). 1998. http:// www.ahsr.org.

IOM (Institute of Medicine). 1995. *Health Services Research: Work Force and Educational Issues.* Field MJ, Tranquada RE, Feasley JC, eds. Washington, D.C.: National Academy Press.

IOM. 1997. A Review of the Department of Defense's Program for Breast Cancer Research. Committee to Review the Department of Defense's Breast Cancer Research Program. Washington, D.C.: National Academy Press.

McGeary, M. 1999. *Cancer Research Funding in the United States.* Draft presented to National Cancer Policy Board, Washington, D.C.

Riley GF, Potosky AL, Klabunde CN, et al. 1999. Stage at diagnosis and treatment patterns among older women with breast cancer: An HMO and fee-for-service comparison. *Journal of the American Medical Association* 281(8):720–726.

Stephenson J. 1997. Revitalized AHCPR pursues research on quality. *Journal of the American Medical Association* 278(19):1557.

U.S. Congress, Office of Technology Assessment. 1994. *Identifying Health Technologies That Work: Searching for Evidence.* OTA-H-608. Washington, D.C.: U.S. Government Printing Office.

U.S. Department of Defense. 1998. *Congressionally Directed Medical Research Programs: Prostate Cancer Research Program.* http://cdmrp.army.mil/prostate.

U.S. Department of Health and Human Services, Health Care Financing Administration. 1998. *Active Projects Report: Research and Demonstration in Health Care Financ*ing. Washington, D.C.

U.S. Department of Veteran Affairs, Office of Research and Development. 1997. *Refining Research Priorities: New Initiatives Meeting Veteran Needs.* Washington, D.C.

8

Findings and Recommendations

The findings and recommendations listed in Box 1.1 are based on the evidence reviewed in previous chapters, which includes literature reviews, compilations of data, and summaries of key findings. Detailed discussions and references can be found in those chapters and are merely summarized here.

**BOX 8.1 Findings and Recommendations of the
National Cancer Policy Board Cancer Care System**

What Is the State of the Cancer Care "System"?

The National Cancer Policy Board has concluded that for many Americans with cancer, there is a wide gulf between what could be construed as the ideal and the reality of their experience with cancer care.

What Is Quality Cancer Care and How Is It Measured?

Health care can be judged as good to the extent that it increases the likelihood of desired health outcomes and is consistent with current professional knowledge. The first step in assessing quality of care is establishing which attributes of care are linked to optimal outcomes (e.g., survival, enhanced quality of life). Large, carefully designed clinical trials are usually necessary to establish which specific processes of care or treatments are effective.

Continued

BOX 8.1 *Continued*

Next, observations of current medical practice—for example, through reviews of a sample of medical records—reveal the extent to which effective care is being applied. Measures of quality may assess structural aspects of the health care delivery system (e.g., hospital case volume), processes of care (e.g., use of screening), or outcomes of care (e.g., survival, quality of life).

What Problems Are Evident in the Quality of Cancer Care and What Steps Can Be Taken to Improve Care?

Based on the best available evidence, some individuals with cancer do not receive care known to be effective for their condition. The magnitude of the problem is not known, but the National Cancer Policy Board believes it is substantial.

The National Cancer Policy Board has identified some specific ways to improve cancer care, which require systemic changes in the health care system and in the components that deal directly with cancer. Implementation of these recommendations may vary by locality and by system of care with, for example, different mechanisms needed in rural versus urban areas, or for particularly high-risk or underserved populations.

Cancer care is optimally delivered in systems of care that:

Recommendation 1: Ensure that patients undergoing procedures that are technically difficult to perform and have been associated with higher mortality in lower-volume settings receive care at facilities with extensive experience (i.e., high-volume facilities). Examples of such procedures include removal of all or part of the esophagus, surgery for pancreatic cancer, removal of pelvic organs, and complex chemotherapy regimens.

Recommendation 2: Use systematically developed guidelines based on the best available evidence for prevention, diagnosis, treatment, and palliative care.

Recommendation 3: Measure and monitor the quality of care using a core set of quality measures. Cancer care quality measures should

- span the continuum of cancer care and be developed through a coordinated public–private effort;
- be used to hold providers, including health care systems, health plans, and physicians, accountable for demonstrating that they provide and improve quality of care;
- be applied to care provided through the Medicare and Medicaid programs as a requirement of participation in these programs; and
- be disseminated widely and communicated to purchasers, providers, consumer organizations, individuals with cancer, policy makers, and health services researchers, in a form that is relevant and useful for health care decision-making.

Recommendation 4: Ensure the following elements of quality care for each individual with cancer:

- that recommendations about initial cancer management, which are critical in determining long-term outcome, are made by experienced professionals;

Continued

BOX 8.1 *Continued*

- an agreed-upon care plan that outlines goals of care;
- access to the full complement of resources necessary to implement the care plan;
- access to high-quality clinical trials;
- policies to ensure full disclosure of information about appropriate treatment options;
- a mechanism to coordinate services; and
- psychosocial support services and compassionate care.

Recommendation 5: Ensure quality of care at the end of life, in particular, the management of cancer-related pain and timely referral to palliative and hospice care.

How Can We Improve What We Know About the Quality of Cancer Care?

The following recommendations relate to information needs:

Recommendation 6: Federal and private research sponsors such as the National Cancer Institute, the Agency for Health Care Policy and Research, and various health plans should invest in clinical trials to address questions about cancer care management.

Recommendation 7: A cancer data system is needed that can provide quality benchmarks for use by systems of care (such as hospitals, provider groups, and managed care systems).

Toward that end, in 1999, the National Cancer Policy Board will hold workshops to:

- identify how best to meet the data needs for cancer in light of quality monitoring goals;
- identify financial and other resources needed to improve the cancer data system to achieve quality-related goals; and
- develop strategies to improve data available on the quality of cancer care.

Recommendation 8: Public and private sponsors of cancer care research should support national studies of recently diagnosed individuals with cancer, using information sources with sufficient detail to assess patterns of cancer care and factors associated with the receipt of good care. Research sponsors should also support training for cancer care providers interested in health services research.

What Steps Can Be Taken to Overcome Barriers of Access to Quality Cancer Care?

The following recommendations are concerned with access to quality care:

Recommendation 9: Services for the un- and underinsured need to be enhanced to assure entry to, and equitable treatment within, the cancer care system.

Recommendation 10: Studies are needed to find out why specific segments of the population (e.g., members of certain racial or ethnic groups, older patients) do not receive appropriate cancer care. These studies should measure provider and individual knowledge, attitudes, and beliefs, as well as other potential barriers to access to care.

The remainder of this chapter is organized around the following five questions:

1. What is the state of the cancer care "system"?
2. What is quality cancer care and how is it measured?
3. What cancer care quality problems are evident and what steps can be taken to improve care?
4. How can we improve what we know about the quality of cancer care?
5. What steps can be taken to overcome barriers to access to quality cancer care?

WHAT IS THE STATE OF THE CANCER CARE "SYSTEM"?

Health care in the United States is superb at its best, but there is a growing recognition that for many people in many situations, it is not at its best (Chassin et al., 1998). Observers have noted serious and extensive problems in health care quality and have called for urgent action. Although a few health plans, hospitals, and integrated delivery systems have made impressive efforts to improve their quality of care, and some success has been achieved, there are in general no clear models of exemplary delivery systems in this country (Chassin et al., 1998). The IOM National Roundtable on Health Care Quality concluded that current attempts to improve quality will not succeed unless major, systemic efforts are undertaken to overhaul the way in which health care services are delivered, physicians are educated and trained, and quality is assessed (Chassin et al., 1998).

The National Cancer Policy Board began its deliberations on quality by trying to describe what an ideal cancer care system would look and feel like from the vantage point of an individual receiving cancer care. The NCPB suggested that, for many, excellence in cancer care would be achieved if individuals had:

- access to comprehensive and coordinated services;
- confidence in the experience and training of their providers;
- a feeling that providers respected them, listened to them, and advocated on their behalf;
- an ability to ask questions and voice opinions comfortably, to be full participants in all decisions regarding care;
- a clear understanding of their diagnosis and access to information to aid this understanding;
- awareness of all treatment options and of the risks and benefits associated with each;
- confidence that recommended treatments are appropriate, offering the best chance of a good outcome consistent with personal preferences;
- a prospective plan for treatment and palliation;
- a health care professional responsible (and accountable) for organizing this plan in partnership with each individual; and
- assurances that agreed-upon national standards of quality care are met at their site of care.

The NCPB then described at least some aspects of a cancer care *system* that would support such an ideal state of care. A system of ideal cancer care would

- articulate goals consistent with this vision of quality cancer care;
- implement policies to achieve these goals;
- identify barriers to the practice and receipt of quality care and target interventions to overcome these barriers;
- further efforts to coordinate the currently diverse systems of care;
- ensure appropriate training for cancer care providers;
- have mechanisms in place to facilitate the translation of research to clinical practice;
- monitor and ensure the quality of care; and
- conduct research necessary to further the understanding of effective cancer care.

The NCPB has concluded that for many Americans with cancer, there is a wide gulf between what could be construed as the ideal and the reality of their experience with cancer care.

There is no national cancer care program or system of care in the United States. Like other chronic illnesses, efforts to diagnose and treat cancer are centered on individual physicians, health plans, and cancer care centers. The ad hoc and fragmented cancer care system does not ensure access to care, lacks coordination, and is inefficient in its use of resources. The authority to organize, coordinate, and improve cancer care services rests largely with service providers and insurers. At numerous sites in the federal government, programs and research directly relate to the quality of cancer care, but in no one place are these disparate efforts coordinated or even described. Efforts to improve cancer care in many cases will therefore be local or regional and could feasibly originate in a physician's practice, a hospital, or a managed care plan. Because cancer disproportionately affects the elderly, the Medicare program could be an important vehicle for change. Certainly, issues related to quality cancer care have to be addressed at the national and state levels, in coordination with other quality-of-care efforts. Of note is the creation of organizations to implement recommendations of the President's Advisory Commission on Consumer Protection and Quality in the Health Care Industry. The commission recommended that broad national aims for quality improvement be set with specific measurable objectives and that, within each national aim, standardized sets of indicators be developed for use in all sectors of the health care system (President's Advisory Commission, 1998).

WHAT IS QUALITY CANCER CARE AND HOW IS IT MEASURED?

Health care can be judged as good to the extent that it increases the likelihood of desired health outcomes and is consistent with current professional knowledge (IOM, 1990). In practical terms, poor quality can mean

- overuse (e.g., unnecessary tests, medication, and procedures, with associated risks and side effects);
- underuse (e.g., not receiving a lifesaving surgical procedure); or
- misuse (e.g., medicines that should not be given together, poor surgical technique).

Quality care means providing patients with appropriate services in a technically competent manner, with good communication, shared decision making, and cultural sensitivity.

The first step in assessing quality of care is establishing which attributes of care are linked to optimal outcomes (e.g., survival, enhanced quality of life). Large, carefully designed clinical trials are usually necessary to establish which specific processes of care or treatments are effective. Early detection of breast cancer through screening mammography, for example, has been shown to reduce mortality significantly for women age 50 and older. Other types of research, notably health services research, also have a role to play in defining high-quality care. Next, observations of current medical practice—for example, through reviews of a sample of medical records—reveal the extent to which effective care is being applied. Measures of quality may assess structural aspects of the health care delivery system (e.g., hospital case volume), processes of care (e.g., use of screening), or outcomes of care (e.g., survival, quality of life). Each of these dimensions of quality could be assessed to provide complementary information.

WHAT PROBLEMS ARE EVIDENT IN THE QUALITY OF CANCER CARE AND WHAT STEPS CAN BE TAKEN TO IMPROVE CARE?

More is known about the quality of care for breast cancer than for any other kind of cancer. Treatment of early breast cancer saves lives, and early detection through screening contributes to early diagnosis, when treatment is most effective. When established quality measures have been used to assess the care women receive, the following quality problems have been identified:

- underuse of mammography to detect cancer early;
- lack of adherence to standards for diagnosis (e.g., inadequate biopsies, poor reporting of pathology studies);
- inadequate patient counseling regarding treatment options; and
- underuse of radiation therapy and adjuvant chemotherapy after surgery.

The consequences of these lapses in care are, in some cases, reduced survival and, in others, compromised quality of life.

Based on the best available evidence, some individuals with cancer do not receive care known to be effective for their condition. The magnitude of the problem is not known, but the National Cancer Policy Board believes it is substantial. The reasons for failure to deliver high-quality care have not been studied adequately, nor has there been much investigation of how appropriate standards vary from patient to patient.

The means for improving the quality of cancer care, which involve changes in the health care system, are the first five of a total of ten recommendations of the National Cancer Policy Board. Implementation of these recommendations may vary by locality and by system of care with, for example, different mechanisms needed in rural versus urban areas, or for particularly high-risk or underserved populations.

Cancer care is optimally delivered in systems of care that:

RECOMMENDATION 1: Ensure that patients undergoing procedures that are technically difficult to perform and have been associated with higher mortality in lower-volume settings receive care at facilities with extensive experience (i.e., high-volume facilities). Examples of such procedures include removal of all or part of the esophagus, surgery for pancreatic cancer, removal of pelvic organs, and complex chemotherapy regimens.

Many aspects of the delivery of health care can potentially affect its quality. There is convincing evidence of a relationship between treatment in higher-volume hospitals and better short-term survival for individuals with several types of cancer for which high-risk surgery is indicated (e.g., pancreatic cancer, non-small-cell lung cancer). Several studies show very large effects, with lower-volume hospitals having postsurgical mortality rates two to three times higher than hospitals that do more such procedures. A dose–response effect is also evident to support the finding that as volume increases, so do good outcomes. The findings cut across cancer types and systems of care, sharing the common element of complicated medical or surgical intervention. Although estimates are imprecise, a relatively large share of high-risk surgery is taking place in lower-volume settings (e.g., from one-quarter to one-half of surgical procedures for pancreatic cancer).

More limited data show a relationship between surgery performed at higher-volume hospitals and better outcomes for men with prostate cancer who undergo radical prostatectomy and for women who undergo breast cancer surgery. A few studies of the management of other types of cancer (i.e., testicular cancer, leukemia) also show a relationship between higher volume and better outcome. This volume–outcome relationship appears to be strong, and consistent with findings from other areas of complex care (e.g., coronary revascularization procedures).

Even in the absence of extensive data for each particular cancer type and stage, evidence strongly indicates that health outcomes are better in high-volume settings for highly technical cancer management.

RECOMMENDATION 2: Use systematically developed guidelines based on the best available evidence for prevention, diagnosis, treatment, and palliative care.

Total quality improvement initiatives, disease management programs, and implementation of clinical practice guidelines all have the potential to improve care within health systems. Information about clinical practice can serve as a powerful tool to change physician and patient behavior and to improve the use of effective treatments. The experience with oncology practice guidelines has been mixed, however, with some examples of success, but other examples of failure to change provider behavior or outcomes. Many guideline efforts have failed because of flaws in the way the guidelines were developed or implemented. Evidence suggests that care can be improved when providers themselves are involved in shaping guidelines and when systems of accountability are in place. Such efforts must be intensified.

RECOMMENDATION 3: Measure and monitor the quality of care using a core set of quality measures.

Once effective care has been identified through the research system, mechanisms to develop and implement measurement systems are needed. Translating research results into quality monitoring measures is a complex process that will require significant research investments. There is now a broad consensus about how to assess some aspects of quality of care for many common cancers (e.g., cancers of the breast, colon, lung, prostate, and cervix), but specific measures of the quality of care for these cancers are still being developed and tested within health delivery systems.

Systematic improvements in health care quality will likely only occur through collaborative efforts of the public and private sectors. As large health care purchasers, both sectors have a stake in improving the quality of care, and both sectors have knowledge and experience concerning quality measurement and reporting. Each sector has unique strengths (President's Advisory Commission, 1998):

- Private-sector organizations have the capacity to act quickly in response to rapid changes in the health care system.
- Public-sector organizations can provide safeguards to ensure public accountability (e.g., adequate representation of stakeholders, open proceedings).

A public–private collaborative approach has recently been recommended by the President's Advisory Commission on Consumer Protection and Quality in the Health Care Industry, and some initial implementation steps are being taken.

Cancer care quality measures should span the continuum of cancer care and be developed through a coordinated public–private effort.

To ensure the rapid translation of research into practice, a mechanism is needed to quickly identify the results of research with quality-of-care implications and ensure that it is applied in monitoring quality. In a few areas, evidence suggests that care does not meet national standards for interventions known to improve care. After primary prevention, cancer screening is the most effective method to reduce the burden of cancer, yet screening is underused. It is often health care providers who can be held accountable for the underuse of cancer screening tests. One of the strongest predictors of whether a person will be screened for cancer is whether the physician recommends it, and evidence suggests that physicians order fewer cancer screening tests than they should. Even when screening is accomplished, many individuals fail to receive timely, or any, follow-up of an abnormal screening test. Both screening and follow-up rates can be improved with interventions aimed both at those eligible for screening and at health care providers (e.g., reminder systems). Implementation of accountability systems can greatly increase participation in cancer screening.

Cancer care quality measures should be used to hold providers, including health care systems, health plans, and physicians, accountable for demonstrating that they provide and improve quality of care.

There are many opportunities to exert leverage on the health care system to improve quality. Quality assurance systems are often not apparent to consumers, but have the potential to greatly affect their care:

- large employer groups are holding managed care plans accountable for quality performance goals;
- the Health Care Financing Administration (HCFA, which funds Medicare and the federal component of Medicaid) requires Medicare and Medicaid health plans to produce standard quality reports; and
- state Medicaid programs are beginning to include quality provisions in their contracts with plans and providers.

Six of ten new cancer cases occur among people age 65 and older and, consequently, Medicare is the principal payer for cancer care. There is generally a lack of quality-related data from fee-for-service providers from whom most Medicare beneficiaries receive their care. Information systems are, however, in place that allow the reporting on a regional basis of some quality indicators (e.g., cancer screening rates) relevant to those in fee-for-service systems. For Medicare beneficiaries in managed care plans, accountability systems should incorporate core measures of quality cancer care.

Cancer care quality measures should be applied to care provided through the Medicare and Medicaid programs as a requirement for participation in these programs.

The collection, reporting, and analysis of information about the quality of cancer care will be expensive. Many segments of the health care industry will invest in information systems to maximize efficiency and to stay competitive, however, some may require incentives to provide patient-level data.

Information about quality cancer care is becoming more available to individuals with cancer (or at risk for cancer), but it is not yet easily accessible or understandable to consumers. A number of potential quality indicators can be listed, but most have not been evaluated to assess their ultimate value for consumers. It is unclear, for example, how the following indicators affect an individual's experience of care or health care outcomes:

- a physician's board certification,
- a hospital's approval status, for example, as determined by the American College of Surgeons' Commission on Cancer, and
- a health plan's accreditation status and quality scores from the National Committee for Quality Assurance.

By the time a diagnosis of cancer is made and individuals have a clear reason to seek quality care, it is often too late to switch health plans. Also, even if they wanted to, most people do not have access to alternative plans. Individuals may use available quality indicators to choose doctors and hospitals within their plans, and perhaps to choose alternative courses of treatment, but evidence suggests that individual consumers can exert only a modest "market" pressure for quality improvement through access to better information about the quality of cancer care. Large purchasers such as employers, are likely to exert more leverage, and to have designated staff to assess alternative plans.

Cancer care quality measures should be disseminated widely and communicated to purchasers, providers, consumer organizations, individuals with cancer, policy makers, and health services researchers, in a form that is relevant and useful for health care decision-making.

Quality measures enable consumers and purchasers to judge the quality of a system of care by its performance relative to evidence-based standards.

> **RECOMMENDATION 4: Ensure the following elements of quality care for each individual with cancer:**
>
> • **that recommendations about initial cancer management, which are critical in determining long-term outcome, are made by experienced professionals;**
> • **an agreed-upon care plan that outlines goals of care;**
> • **access to the full complement of resources necessary to implement the care plan;**
> • **access to high-quality clinical trials;**
> • **policies to ensure full disclosure of information about appropriate treatment options;**
> • **a mechanism to coordinate services; and**
> • **psychosocial support services and compassionate care.**

Some elements of care simply make sense—that is, they have strong face validity and can reasonably be assumed to improve care unless and until evidence accumulates to the contrary. This recommendation amounts to a statement of the ideal, based on principles of cancer care articulated by cancer survivors. Details of how to interpret and apply the principles will vary according to health plan, cancer type, stage of disease, and preferences of the individual needing care.

> **RECOMMENDATION 5: Ensure quality of care at the end of life, in particular, the management of cancer-related pain and timely referral to palliative and hospice care.**

Cancer is the second leading cause of death in the United States. A strong body of evidence suggests that the experience of dying for many with cancer can be greatly improved with better palliative care (IOM, 1997).[*] Many individuals with cancer suffer pain needlessly and have their treatment preferences ignored. Practice guidelines are available to assist health care providers in this area, but they have not been adopted widely. Financial barriers limit effective care for people at the end of life. Additional studies are needed to identify nonfinancial barriers to appropriate end-of-life care.

---

[*]The NCPB paper "Issues in End-of-Life Care for People with Cancer: Interviews with Selected Providers and Researchers" supplements the 1997 IOM report, *Approaching Death: Improving Care at the End of Life*.

HOW CAN WE IMPROVE WHAT WE KNOW ABOUT THE QUALITY OF CANCER CARE?

For many aspects of cancer care, it is not yet possible to assess quality because the first step in quality assessment has not been taken—the conduct of clinical trials. Consequently, for many types of cancer, answers to the following basic questions are not yet available:

- How frequently should patients be evaluated following their primary cancer therapy, what tests should be included in the follow-up regimen, and who should provide follow-up care?
- What is the most effective way to manage recurrent cancers, or cancers first identified at late stages?

> **RECOMMENDATION 6: Federal and private research sponsors such as the National Cancer Institute, the Agency for Health Care Policy and Research, and various health plans should invest in clinical trials to address questions about cancer care management.**

For some questions regarding cancer management, a health services research component could possibly be integrated into a clinical trial designed to assess the efficacy of a new treatment. For other questions, innovative units of randomization could be used, for example, randomizing providers (instead of patients) to test different clinical management strategies. Such trials have been used to assess educational and service delivery topics (e.g., colorectal screening performed by nurse clinicians, counseling patients to quit smoking) (U.S. Congress, OTA, 1994).

> **RECOMMENDATION 7: A cancer data system is needed that can provide quality benchmarks for use by systems of care (such as hospitals, provider groups, and managed care systems).**

Toward that end, in 1999, the National Cancer Policy Board will hold workshops to:

- identify how best to meet the data needs for cancer in light of quality monitoring goals;
- identify financial and other resources needed to improve the cancer data system to achieve quality-related goals; and
- develop strategies to improve data available on the quality of cancer care.

The second step of quality assessment involves surveillance—making sure that evidence regarding what works is applied in practice. Ideally, quality assessment studies would include recently diagnosed individuals with cancer in care settings representative of contemporary practice across the country, using information sources with sufficient detail to allow appropriate comparisons.

The available evidence on the quality of cancer care is far from this ideal. In fact, it is difficult to judge the quality of current practice from the published literature because

- many studies were conducted in the 1980s and do not reflect current practice;

- many studies are difficult to interpret because dissimilar groups of patients were compared (e.g., there are insufficient controls for important clinical characteristics such as the presence of diseases other than cancer);
- studies are confined to a small group of patients, in one or a few institutions, states, or health plans, making it difficult to generalize to all patients with cancer; and
- studies are often based on data from cancer registries, which do not capture important aspects of care (e.g., outpatient treatment may not be included).

Two national databases are available with which to assess the quality of cancer care, but each has limitations.

1. The Surveillance, Epidemiology, and End Results (SEER) cancer registry, maintained by the National Cancer Institute (NCI), when linked to Medicare and other insurance administrative files, has been valuable in assessing the quality of care for the elderly and other insured populations. It is also useful in identifying a sample of cases for in-depth studies of quality-related issues. The SEER registry, however, covers only 14 percent of the U.S. population in certain geographic locations, so it may not adequately represent the diversity of systems of care. Finding ways to capture measures of process of care, treatment information, and intermediate outcomes— and to improving the timeliness of reporting—would enhance the registry's use in quality assessment.

2. The National Cancer Data Base (NCDB), a joint project of the American College of Surgeon's Commission on Cancer and the American Cancer Society, now holds information on more than half of all newly diagnosed cases of cancer nationwide and includes many of the demographic, clinical, and health system data elements necessary to assess quality of care. A limitation of the NCDB is the absence of complete information on outpatient care. The NCDB has not yet been widely used to assess quality of care, but has great potential for doing so.

Existing data systems must be enhanced so that questions about quality of care can be answered comprehensively, on a national scale, without delays of many years between data collection and analysis. An effective system would capture information about

- individuals with cancer (e.g., age, race and ethnicity, socioeconomic status, insurance or health plan coverage);
- their condition (e.g., stage, grade, histological pattern, comorbid conditions);
- their treatment, including significant outpatient treatments (e.g., adjuvant therapy, radiation therapy);
- their providers (e.g., specialty training);
- site of care delivery (e.g., community hospital, cancer center);
- type of care delivery system (e.g., managed care, fee-for-service); and
- outcomes (e.g., satisfaction, relapse, complications, quality of life, survival time, death).

It may be costly and difficult to obtain all of the desired data elements for all individuals with available sources, so sampling techniques could be used to make the task manageable for targeted studies. Alternatively, it may be feasible to link some databases (e.g., those describing structural aspects of care such as hospital characteristics) to other existing databases. It is unlikely that one single database can meet all of the various objectives of such systems, for example, cancer surveillance, research, and quality monitoring. Data systems need to be monitored to assure accuracy, and should be automated to improve the timeliness of quality data. Data gathered into national databases, in particular, should be made available quickly for analysis by investigators and evaluators.

> **RECOMMENDATION 8: Public and private sponsors of cancer care research should support national studies of recently diagnosed individuals with cancer, using information sources with sufficient detail to assess patterns of cancer care and factors associated with the receipt of good care. Research sponsors should also support training for cancer care providers interested in health services research.**

Grants to support the analysis of data that focus on pressing health policy questions, especially about how the organization and financing of cancer care affect the processes and outcomes of care, should be a high priority. Methodologic research is also needed to improve the quality of cancer-related health services research, for example, to develop tools for "case-mix" adjustments to reduce the potential for bias inherent in observational cancer research.

An annual report that provides a description of the status of cancer-related quality-of-care research, and summarizes relevant published literature in the area would serve as a valuable resource for health services researchers and those involved in quality assessment. Such a report would also help organizations set priorities for research, ensure that their research portfolios address important quality-of-care questions, and ensure that their research programs are complementary and coordinated.

WHAT STEPS CAN BE TAKEN TO OVERCOME BARRIERS OF ACCESS TO QUALITY CANCER CARE?

> **RECOMMENDATION 9: Services for the un- and underinsured should be enhanced to ensure entry to, and equitable treatment within, the cancer care system.**

Cancer is among the most expensive conditions to treat, and individuals with cancer and their families invariably bear some of the financial burden. Most individuals diagnosed with cancer are elderly and have Medicare coverage, but an estimated 7 percent of individuals facing a new diagnosis of cancer lack any health insurance at all. For these individuals, cancer can be catastrophic to their finances as well as their health. The problem that affects far more individuals, however, is underinsurance—health plans and insurance coverage offer some, but often incomplete, protection against the high costs of cancer care. High deductibles, copayments or coinsurance, and coverage caps can all contribute to high out-of-pocket expenditures. Medicare, for example, was estimated to cover only 83 percent of typical total charges for lung cancer and 65 percent of charges for breast cancer in 1986. Some individuals have additional protection through other insurers (e.g., Medigap policies or Medicaid), but despite this, the financial burden of cancer can be substantial even among those covered by a health plan. Limits on prescription drug coverage, an expensive and widely used benefit (e.g., outpatient pain medications), are a particular problem for many with cancer because the drugs are often expensive. A limited number of free services or financial assistance programs are available to people with cancer, but they do not substitute for adequate insurance coverage for cancer treatment.

> **RECOMMENDATION 10: Studies are needed to find out why specific segments of the population (e.g., members of certain racial or ethnic groups, older patients) do not receive appropriate cancer care. These studies should measure provider and individual knowledge, attitudes, and beliefs, as well as other potential barriers to access to care.**

While access problems persist throughout cancer care, overcoming barriers to screening and early detection is a priority because after primary prevention, the greatest improvements in outcomes will be realized by identifying cancers early, when treatments are most effective. Moreover, initial planning is extremely important for many types of cancer, because failure on the first treatment severely limits subsequent treatment options due to the nature of cancer progression. Evidence suggests that much of the disparity in mortality by race could be reduced by improving access to primary care and cancer screening.

A number of public and private programs have enhanced access to care. The Centers for Disease Control and Prevention's National Breast and Cervical Cancer Early Detection Program provides screening for women unable to afford care. A few states have launched special programs to pay for cancer care for the poor and uninsured (e.g., the Maryland program for women with breast cancer). Many pharmaceutical companies have patient assistance programs to help defray the costs of expensive chemotherapy drugs. These programs and services cannot substitute for adequate insurance coverage for cancer treatment, but they can ease the financial burden for those eligible to receive them.

Although having health insurance coverage improves access, it does not guarantee good care. Several factors other than insurance status and cost can prevent people from "getting to the door" of a health care provider. These include fear of a diagnosis of cancer, distrust of health care providers, language, geography, and difficulties in getting through appointment systems. Incomplete understanding of cancer risk or certain beliefs, such as the belief that one is not at risk or that nothing can be done to change one's fate may also prevent people from seeking care. Once "in the door," other barriers to access may surface when attempting to navigate the system: for example, getting from a primary care provider to a specialist. Within the system, providers may have difficulty communicating with patients or have insufficient staff to coordinate care and provide all the services patients need. The cancer care system is complex, and different barriers may impede access to care at different phases.

Individuals who have low educational attainment or are members of certain racial or ethnic minority groups face higher barriers to receiving cancer care and tend to have less favorable outcomes than other groups.[*] Limited access to primary care and cancer screening contributes to having cancer diagnosed at later stages when prognosis is worse. Differences in treatment by race have been well documented; however, it appears that the effect may actually be more closely related to social class than to race.

---

[*]Research in this area sponsored by the National Institutes of Health is addressed in the 1999 IOM report *The Unequal Burden of Cancer: An Assessment of NIH Research and Programs for Ethnic Minorities and the Medically Underserved* (IOM, 1999).

Those of advanced age also appear to be vulnerable in the cancer care system. Older people are less likely than younger people to receive effective cancer treatments, despite evidence that the elderly can tolerate and benefit from them. Some undertreatment is explained by provider attitudes toward treating the elderly, who are perceived as less willing or able to tolerate aggressive treatment. Some undertreatment may also be due to patient preferences and unwillingness to experience the side effects of certain treatments.

REFERENCES

Chassin MR, Gavin RW. 1998. The urgent need to improve health care quality. Institute of Medicine National Roundtable on Health Care Quality. *Journal of the American Medical Association* 280(11):1000–1005.

IOM (Institute of Medicine). 1990. *Medicare: A Strategy for Quality Assurance*, KN Lohr, ed. Washington, D.C.: National Academy Press.

IOM. 1997. *Approaching Death: Improving Care at the End of Life*. MJ Field, CK Cassel, eds. Washington, D.C.: National Academy Press.

IOM. 1999. *The Unequal Burden of Cancer: An Assessment of NIH Research and Programs for Ethnic Minorities and the Medically Underserved.* MA Haynes, BD Smedley, eds. Washington, D.C.: National Academy Press.

National Cancer Advisory Board. 1994. *Cancer at a Crossroads: A Report to Congress for the Nation.*

National Cancer Policy Board. 1998. *Taking Action to Reduce Tobacco Use.* RM Cook-Deegan, ed., Washington, D.C.: National Academy Press.

National Center for Health Statistics. 1997. *Healthy People 2000 Review.* Hyattsville, MD: Public Health Service.

President's Advisory Commission on Consumer Protection and Quality in the Health Care Industry. 1998. *Quality First: Better Health Care for All Americans*. Washington, D.C.

SUPPORT Principal Investigators. 1995. A controlled trial to improve care for seriously ill hospitalized patients. The study to understand prognoses and preferences for outcomes and risks of treatments (SUPPORT). *Journal of the American Medical Association* 274(20):1591–1598.

U.S. Congress. Office of Technology Assessment. 1994. *Identifying Health Technologies That Work: Searching for Evidence.* Washington D.C.: U.S. Government Printing Office.

Glossary

activities of daily living: self-care abilities related to personal care, such as bathing, dressing, eating, and continence.

adenocarcinoma: cancer that starts in glandular tissue (e.g., breast, lung, thyroid, colon, pancreas).

alkylating agents: a family of anticancer drugs that combine with a cancer cell's DNA to prevent normal cell division.

allogeneic transplantation: bone marrow transplant in which the donor marrow is obtained from a person who is not an identical twin and then given to the patient.

ambulatory care: the use of outpatient facilities—doctors' offices, home care, outpatient hospital clinics and day-care facilities—to provide medical care without the need for hospitalization. Often refers to any care outside a hospital.

androgen ablation: elimination of adrenal and testicular sources of male hormones, such as testosterone, from the prostate; used to treat end-stage prostate cancer.

aneurysm: circumscribed dilation (ballooning out) of an artery or a heart chamber, often due to an acquired or congenital weakness of the wall of the artery or chamber.

anthracycline: antitumor antibiotic that has shown activity in a wide range of hematological malignancies and solid tumors; believed to exert antitumor effects through direct binding to DNA.

antiandrogen therapy: treatment that entails blocking the production of or binding to male hormone receptors on cell surfaces, for example, to reduce stimulation of testosterone-induced growth of prostate cancer.

arthroplasty: creation of an artificial joint to correct the stiffening or fixation of a joint; an operation to restore as far as possible the integrity and functional power of a joint.

autologous bone marrow transplant: bone marrow transplant in which the donor marrow is obtained from the patient, stored, and then given back to the patient following the anticancer treatments.

axillary node-negative: lymph nodes in the armpit (axillary nodes) that do not show evidence of cancer.

benign prostatic hyperplasia (BPH): a noncancerous enlargement of the prostate gland that produces bothersome lower urinary tract symptoms in aging men.

biologic response modifiers: naturally occurring substance produced by cells that stimulate or modulate the growth and function of multiple cells, including immune cells, bone marrow cells, and tumor cells; examples include interferon, interleukin, colony-stimulating factors, and monoclonal antibodies.

bone marrow: the inner, spongy core of bone that produces blood cells.

bone scan: picture of the bones using a radioactive dye that shows injury, disease, or healing; may be used to determine if cancer has spread to the bone, if anticancer therapy is successful, and if affected areas are healing.

brachytherapy: radiotherapy in which the source of irraditaion is placed close to the surface of the body or within a body cavity; e.g., application of radium to the cervix.

BRCA 1: gene located on the short arm of chromosome 17; when damaged (mutated), a woman is at greater risk of developing breast and/or ovarian cancer compared to women who do not have the mutation.

BRCA 2: mutation of this gene, located on chromosome 13, is associated with increased risk of breast cancer.

breast-conserving surgery: surgery to remove a breast cancer and a small amount of tissue around the cancer, but without removing the entire breast or surrounding tissues.

case mix: the characteristics of a health care facility's patient population for a given period of time, classified by such factors as individual sociodemographic characteristics, disease, diagnostic or therapeutic procedures performed, method of payment, duration of hospitalization, and intensity and type of services provided.

census tract level: geographic unit used by the census bureau to designate areas within a county.

cisplatin: a chemotherapy agent containing platinum with antitumor activity; binds DNA and interferes with DNA synthesis.

colposcopy: examination of the vagina and cervix by means of an endoscope; generally takes place after an abnormal Pap smear.

conformal radiation therapy: this technique uses conventional linear accelerators equipped with computer-controlled collimators to produce a high-dose radiation volume that conforms to the tumor with great precision.

craniotomy: an operation on the cranium; incision into the cranium.

cryosurgery: the use of a special cold probe as a surgical instrument; it is used to destroy cancer tissues by freezing it.

cystitis: inflammation of the urinary bladder.

debulking: procedure to remove as much of the cancer as possible; reducing the "bulk" of the cancer.

ductal carcinoma: a very early form of breast cancer confined to cells lining the breast ducts, as opposed to the glandular tissue of the breast.

echography: the location, measurement, or delineation of deep structures by measuring the reflection or transmission of high frequency or ultrasonic waves.

endarterectomy: excision of diseased tissues surrounding the lumen of an artery.

endoscopy: a procedure in which the doctor looks inside the body through a lighted tube called an endoscope.

etiology: the science and study of the causes of disease and their mode of operation.

exenteration: removal of internal organs and tissues, usually radical removal of the contents of a body cavity, such as all the pelvic organs.

extracapsular extension: invasion of a tumor beyond the capsule surrounding its organ of origin, for example if prostate cancer invades beyond the capsule surrounding the prostate or tumor near a joint extends beyond the joint capsule.

febrile neutropenia: fever associated with a low neutrophil count.

germ cell: reproductive cells produced by the ovaries (eggs) or the testis (sperm).

Gleason score: grade of tumor of the prostate; based on glandular differentiation.

hematopoietic stem cells: cells in the bone marrow from which all cells in the circulating blood are derived.

hospice: a discrete site of care in the form of an inpatient hospital or nursing home unit or a freestanding facility; an organization or program that provides, arranges, and advises on a wide range of medical and supportive services for dying patients and their families and friends; an approach to care for dying patients based on clinical, social, and metaphysical or spiritual principles.

kappa coefficient: used to measure the strength of agreement between two data gatherers for interval, ordinal, or nominal-level variables.

Karnofsky performance status: a scale of objective criteria for the quality of life, which is used for patients with incapacitating diseases; the scale was developed for patients with cancer and of use in AIDS.

laparascopic colectomy: excision of part or all of the colon using a laparoscope passed through the abdominal wall.

lesion: abnormal area, may be benign or malignant.

leukemia: any cancer of the blood-forming tissues characterized by production of leukocytes: white blood cells.

lobular carcinoma in situ: a very early type of breast cancer that develops within the milk-producing glands (lobules) of the breast and does not penetrate through the wall of the lobules.

local recurrence: recurrence of a tumor at its original location.

lumpectomy: complete surgical removal of a cancerous breast lump with little adjacent breast tissue.

luteinizing hormone-releasing hormone (LHRH): a hormone released from the hypothalamus that triggers the secretion of luteinizing hormone from the anterior pituitary.

lymphadenectomy: excision of the lymph nodes.

lymphoma: cancer that begins in the lymphatic system, such as in the lymph nodes, spleen, and thymus.

magnetic resonance imaging (MRI): a technique that employs a magnetic field to provide images of the internal structure of the body; computer-generated images from the magnetic frequencies correspond to particular structures in the body.

managed care: an entity that assumes both the clinical and financial responsibility for the provision of health care for a defined population.

margin: border between a tumor and normal tissue.

mastectomy: excision of all or part of the breast.

medical oncologist: physician who specializes in the diagnosis and treatment of cancer, especially in the use of chemotherapy to treat cancer.

metastasis: the spread of cancer from its original site to one or more additional body sites.

modified radical mastectomy: removal of the breast, skin, nipple, areola, and most of the axillary lymph nodes on the same side, leaving the chest muscles intact.

neoadjuvant therapy: use of anticancer drugs before initial surgery or radiation treatment.

neutropenia: low neturophil (a type of white blood cell) count; this is associated with high risk of infection.

nonseminomatous: subtype of testicular cancer.

open colectomy: removal of part or all of the colon through abdominal surgery.

orchiectomy: removal of one or both testes.

palliation: the act of relieving or soothing a symptom, such as pain, without actually curing the cause.

palliative care: treatment of symptoms associated with the effects of cancer and its treatment.

pancreatico-duodenectomy: excision of all or part of the pancreas together with the duodenum.

perioperative: around the time of operation.

peripheral stem cell: a cell collected from blood that is capable of producing diverse cell types.

pneumonectomy: surgery to remove part or all of the lung.

proctitis: inflammation of the mucous membrane of the rectum.

prostate specific antigen: a protein found in the blood that may be elevated in patients with prostate cancer.

Q-twist (Quality-Adjusted Time Without Symptoms or Toxicity): a statistical technique that brings quality of life factors into the analysis of treatment regimens.

quadrantectomy: a partial mastectomy in which the quarter of the breast that contains tumor is removed.

radiation oncologist: physician who specializes in the diagnosis and treatment of cancer, especially in the use of x-rays (radiation) to treat cancer.

radical prostatectomy: the removal of the prostate and the surrounding tissue as a treatment for prostate cancer.

randomized (clinical) trial: an experiment designed to test the safety and efficacy of a medical technology in which people are randomly allocated to experimental or control groups, and outcomes are compared.

seed implants: technique in which the radioactive source is placed in close proximity to the malignancy and provides a predictable dose of radiation to a confined area.

segmental resection: removal of the lump and a small amount of surrounding breast tissue.

spiculated mass: tumor with highly irregular, spiked appearance—usually associated with invasive ductal and lobular carcinoma.

staging: the determination of the anatomic extent of a cancer.

stress incontinence: involuntary discharge of urine due to anatomic displacement which exerts an opening pull on the bladder orifice, as in straining or coughing.

thoracotomy: incision into the chest wall.

tumor necrosis factor: a substance produced by certain white blood cells that kills cancer cells.

tumor–node–metastasis (TNM): standard nomenclature for the staging of tumors according to three basic components: the size of the primary tumor (T), involvement of regional lymph nodes (N), and metastastis (M). Numbers are used to denote size and degree of involvement; for example, 0 indicates undetectable and 1, 2, 3, and 4, a progressive increase in size or involvement.

Acronyms

AAHC/URAC:	American Accreditation Health Care Commission, Inc./URAC
AARP:	American Association of Retired Persons
ABC:	achievable benchmarks of care
ACCC:	Association of Community Cancer Centers
ACoS:	American College of Surgeons
ACoS-COC:	American College of Surgeons, Commission on Cancer
ACR:	American College of Radiology
ACS:	American Cancer Society
AHCPR:	Agency for Health Care Policy and Research
AIDS:	acquired immunodeficiency syndrome
AJCC:	American Joint Committee on Cancer
AMA:	American Medical Association
ASCO:	American Society of Clinical Oncology
BC/BS:	Blue Cross/Blue Shield
BCQ:	Breast Cancer Chemotherapy Questionnaire
BCRP:	Breast Cancer Research Program
BCS:	breast-conserving surgery
BCT:	breast-conserving therapy
BPH:	benign prostatic hyperplasia
CABG:	coronary artery bypass graft
CARES:	Cancer Rehabilitation Evaluation System
CCOP:	Community Clinical Oncology Program
CDC:	Centers for Disease Control and Prevention
CDMRP:	Congressionally Directed Medical Research Programs
CHOP:	Community Hospital Oncology Program

C.I.:   confidence interval
CML: chronic myelocytic leukemia
CONQUEST: Computerized Needs-Oriented Quality Measurement Evaluation System
CRN: Cancer Research Network
CSRP: Cancer Surveillance Research Program
CT: computerized tomography

DHHS: Department of Health and Human Services
DOCS: Documented Outcomes Collection System
DoD: Department of Defense
DRE: digital rectal exam

ERISA: Employee Retirement Income Security Act

FACCT: Foundation for Accountability
FDA: Food and Drug Administration
FFS: fee-for-service
FLIC: Functional Living Index—Cancer
FOBT: fecal occult blood test

GAO: General Accounting Office

HCFA: Health Care Financing Administration
HD: Hodgkin's disease
HEDIS: Health Plan Employer Data and Information Set
HIV: human immunodeficiency virus
HLA: human leukocyte antigen
HMO: health maintenance organization
HRSA: Health Resources and Services Administration

ICD-9:   *International Classification of Diseases,* 9th edition
IMS: Indicator Measurement System
IOM: Institute of Medicine
IPA: independent practice association

JCAHO: Joint Commission on Accreditation of Heathcare Organizations

LHRH: luteinizing hormone-releasing hormone

MCO: managed care organizations
MESH: medical subject headings

NCAB: National Cancer Advisory Board
NCCN: National Comprehensive Cancer Network

NCCS:	National Coalition of Cancer Survivors
NCDB:	National Cancer Data Base
NCI:	National Cancer Institute
NCPB:	National Cancer Policy Board
NCQA:	National Committee for Quality Assurance
NHL:	non-Hodgkin's lymphoma
NIH:	National Institutes of Health
NLM:	National Library of Medicine
NSCLC:	non-small-cell lung cancer
NSGCT:	nonseminomatous germ cell tumors
OASIS:	Outcomes and Assessment Information Set
OR:	odds ratio
PBGH:	Pacific Business Group on Health
PCE:	Patient Care Evaluation
PDQ:	Physician Data Query
PHS:	Public Health Service
PIVOT:	Prostate Cancer Intervention Versus Observation Trial
PLCO:	prostate, lung, colorectal, and ovarian
PORT:	Patient Outcomes Research Teams
PPIP:	Put Prevention into Practice
PPO:	preferred provider organizations
PRO:	peer review organizations
PSA:	prostate-specific antigen
PTCA:	percutaneous transluminal coronary angioplasty
RCT:	randomized controlled trials
ResDAC:	Research Data Assistance Center
RP:	radical prostatectomy
RR:	relative risk
SEER:	Surveillance, Epidemiology, and End Results Program
SSA:	Social Security Administration
SSI:	Supplemental Security Income
TNM:	tumor–node–metastasis
TQM:	total quality management
TRUS:	transrectal ultrasound
USAMRMC:	United States Army Medical Research and Materiel Command
USPSTF:	United States Preventive Services Task Force
VA:	Department of Veterans Affairs

Index

T